7TH EDITION

D1236108

Nutrition Counseling and Education Skills: A Guide for Professionals

Betsy B. Holli, EdD, RDN, LDN
Professor Emeritus
Department of Nutrition Sciences
Dominican University
River Forest, Illinois

Judith A. Beto, PhD, RDN, LDN, FAND
Professor Emeritus
Department of Nutrition Sciences
Dominican University
River Forest, Illinois

Research Associate, Nephrology and
Hypertension
Loyola University Chicago, Health
Sciences
Maywood, Illinois

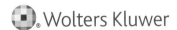
. Wolters Kluwer

Philadelphia • Baltimore • New York • London
Buenos Aires • Hong Kong • Sydney • Tokyo

Acquisitions Editor: Jonathan Joyce
Product Development Editor: John Larkin
Marketing Manager: Leah Thomson
Production Project Manager: Kim Cox
Design Coordinator: Holly McLaughlin
Manufacturing Coordinator: Margie Orzech
Prepress Vendor: S4Carlisle Publishing Services

Seventh edition

Library of Congress Cataloging-in-Publication Data

Names: Holli, Betsy B., author. | Beto, Judith A., author.
Title: Nutrition counseling and education skills : a guide for professionals / Betsy B. Holli, Judith A. Beto.
Description: 7th edition. | Philadelphia : Wolters Kluwer Health, [2018] | Includes bibliographical references and index.
Identifiers: LCCN 2016047763 | ISBN 9781496339140
Subjects: | MESH: Diet Therapy | Nutrition Therapy | Patient Education as Topic—methods | Health Communication—methods | Counseling—methods
Classification: LCC RM214.3 | NLM WB 18 | DDC 615.8/54—dc23 LC record available at https://lccn.loc.gov/2016047763

CCS1216

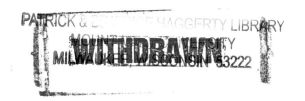
To our extended families, professional
colleagues, and dedicated students who have
contributed to our nutrition communication
and education skills over the years.

BBH and JAB

Preface

Effective communication skills are essential for all nutrition professionals, whether working in clinical, community, management, research, or food service settings. A major challenge is to learn, develop, and apply the necessary knowledge and skills while practicing them in one's professional and personal life.

The scope of practice of nutrition professionals is rapidly expanding to wider and more diverse audiences. The Accreditation Council for Education in Nutrition and Dietetics (ACEND) standards remain grounded in the core communication, counseling, and education skills essential for professional practice, which are the focus of the book. These competencies are mirrored in international practice as well.

The Nutrition Care Process (NCP) is the basis for the Standards of Practice and Standards of Professional Performance. The Nutrition Care Process Terminology (eNCPT) provides a means to connect practice intervention with outcomes in the age of the electronic medical record.

Here are a few of the changes in the 7th edition:

- The Table of Contents is divided into three sections: Communication Skills, Counseling for Health Behavior Change, and Education Skills. Some chapters are reordered and renumbered.
- Case studies are reformatted as a Case Challenge found at the beginning of each chapter with Case Analysis questions interwoven throughout.
- Chapter 1 reflects the expanding scope of nutrition practice in the United States as well as globally.
- References are found at the back of the book grouped by chapter.
- Instructor and student support materials are expanded and available on thePoint, the publisher's website.
- The standardized Nutrition Care Process Terminology (eNCPT) is no longer available in print, but electronically from the Academy of Nutrition and Dietetics (AND).

Effective nutrition interventions are based on evidence-based theories, models, and strategies; clinical nutrition principles; and the knowledge of a variety of behavioral science and educational approaches. There is evidence that interventions based on theories are more effective than those without a theoretical basis and that health professionals need to customize (or individualize) the choice of theory or model to the client's specific situations. Interventions that are based on theories or models, such as the Health Belief Model, behavioral theory, social-cognitive theory, motivational interviewing, or the transtheoretical model of behavior change, are found in the chapters.

The dramatic increase in overweight and obesity among adults and children worldwide is a major threat to overall health. The purpose of our interventions is active behavior change in diet and physical activity to improve health and to prevent and/or control a chronic disease.

Acknowledgments

We thank Hope T. Bilyk, MS, RD, LDN, Assistant Professor, Department of Nutrition, College of Health Professions, Rosalind Franklin University of Medicine and Science, North Chicago, Illinois, for her review of the chapter on Communication and Cultural Competence. Diane Rigassio Radler, PhD, RD, Associate Professor, Department of Nutritional Sciences and Director, Institute of Nutrition Interventions, Rutgers University, New Jersey, continues as a chapter contributor on Counseling for Behavior Modification.

We thank John Larkin, Project Manager of Wolters Kluwer Health, Health Professions, for his assistance throughout the preparation of the manuscript and ancillaries. Some photographs were obtained from the US Department of Agriculture and the CDCP Public Health Image Library.

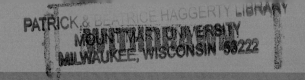
Contents

Communication Skills

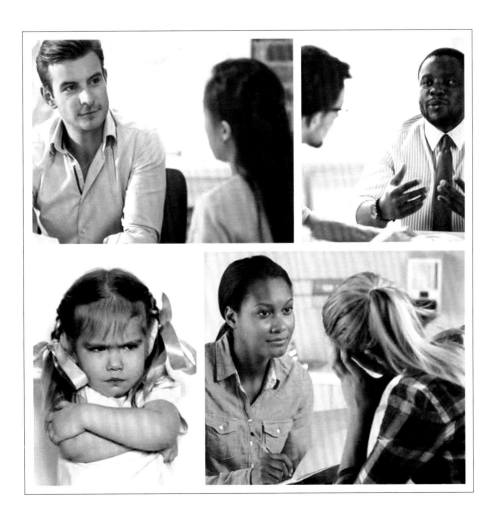

Expanding Scope of Nutrition Practice

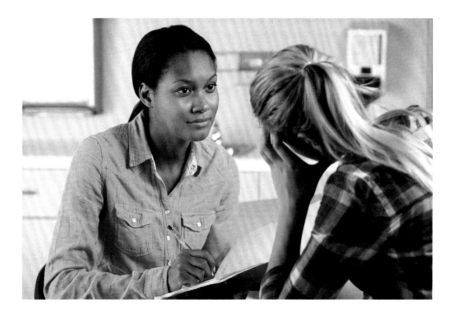

Objectives

- Discuss the origin of people's food habits or behaviors.
- Describe the use of the Scope of Practice Framework.
- Describe the four parts of the Nutrition Care Process.
- Explore evolving areas of practice in nutrition

Karen, a 35-year-old married woman, made an appointment with a Registered Dietitian Nutritionist (RDN) in private practice to get counseling for weight loss and maintenance. Karen works full-time as a secretary at a bank, often going out to lunch with coworkers. Her husband is in computer sales. They have three children ranging in age from 6 to 10 years, and all are in school. Karen's mother comes to watch the children after school until she arrives home. Karen is 5'5" tall and weighs 170 lb. She weighed 135 lb when she was married 12 years ago.

Karen described her daily schedule. She gets up early to make breakfast and to help the children get ready for school. After work, she is tired and the children are hungry and clamoring for dinner, so she describes dinner as a "rush job" or something brought in. After cleaning up, she helps the children with homework, does laundry or other housework, attends evening activities at the school, runs errands, gets the children to bed, and then goes to bed herself. She describes herself as "exhausted."

Never doubt that a small group of thoughtful, committed citizens can change the world. Indeed, it is the only thing that ever has.

—Margaret Meade

Introduction

Counseling, and education knowledge and skills have been recognized since the beginning of the nutrition profession as essential for successful clinical and management practice. These basic communication techniques are still required today in the United States by the Academy of Nutrition and Dietetics for the credential of Registered Dietitian Nutritionist (RDN) and Nutrition and Dietetic Technician, Registered (NDTR). Similar communication and counseling skills are required by the global community of nutrition professionals as well.[1–4]

The International Confederation of Dietetic Associations (ICDA) represents more than 41 international dietetics organizations comprising more than 160,000 members worldwide. The ICDA's definition of "a dietitian is a person with a qualification in nutrition and dietetics, recognized by national authority(s). The dietitian applies the science of nutrition to the feeding and education of individuals or groups in health and disease."[5]

Specific educational competencies vary between member groups, but counseling and education knowledge and skills are required universally. Practitioners may be called dietitians or nutritionists and may have country/area-specific licensure requirements.[6] Some of the dietetic associations that are members of the ICDA include The Academy of Nutrition and Dietetics, Dietitians Association of Australia, Dietitians of Canada, and the European Federation of the Association of Dietitians.[5]

Nutrition professionals have expanded their practice settings, particularly over the last decade to include hospitals, academic health science centers, long-term care facilities, corporate wellness programs, interdisciplinary practice in areas such as sports nutrition or weight loss, public health agencies, private practice, or corporate management. Most practitioners are responsible for assessing nutritional status, selecting diagnoses, intervening through counseling, and evaluating what clients and patients are doing successfully and what they may need to change. The goal is to help people change their eating behaviors for improving their health and reducing the risk of chronic diseases. Health behavior change holds the promise of reducing the risk of preventable diseases and improving the health of those with medical problems.

This chapter discusses the expanding scope of practice in nutrition. Government initiatives are reviewed that direct population-based public health knowledge and programs for health behavior change. The Academy of Nutrition and Dietetics' Scope of Practice framework forms the parameters of competent practice. The Nutrition Care Process (NCP) model uses the Nutrition Care Process Terminology (eNCPT) to drive the cycle of nutrition care. Finally, new areas of evolving practice are explored.

Origin of Food Habits or Behaviors

People's food habits, often described as food behaviors, originate beginning in childhood and evolve over time. Why do people eat the way they do? In physiologic response to hunger, of course, but food choices and eating are far more complex. Cultural, social, economic, environmental, and other factors are involved in food selection in addition to individual choice, patterns, and personal taste.[7] There are many cues to eating in our daily lives. The consumption of food eaten away from home at commercial food service establishments continues to increase.

Nutrition practitioners counsel people who need to make changes in their food habits, using intervention strategies to motivate and improve people's success at change. Food selection is a part of a complex behavioral system that is shaped by a vast array of variables. Food is essential to life, but the dietary patterns and choices people make can directly affect health. Food and lifestyle choices often change an individual's risk for many chronic diseases including heart disease, stroke, diabetes, and some cancers.[8] Successful nutrition counseling and education require an understanding of why clients eat the way they do and then using this knowledge to develop appropriate interventions.

CASE ANALYSIS 1

What lifestyle factors may help or hinder Karen in adhering to different food choices?

Having positive rather than negative cognitions or thoughts helps a person to make changes. Cognitions may be influenced by attitudes, perceptions, and feelings. There is a big difference between "Nutrition is important and this is worth the effort for my health" and "It's too much trouble and I feel OK anyway." Attitudes are thought to influence peoples' decisions and actions. People may eat not only for physiologic reasons such as hunger but also for psychological reasons, such as anxiety, depression, loneliness, stress, and boredom, as well as due to positive emotional states, such as happiness and celebrations. Food may assuage guilt as well as lead to guilt feelings.[7]

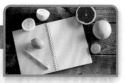

SELF-ASSESSMENT 1

List three things that influence your choices of foods.

Knowledge of what to eat is certainly a first step in influencing healthful food choices, but it is probably overrated. There are individuals who know what to eat and yet do not do it. When people do not eat healthfully, some counselors redouble their efforts in educating as if the problem is lack of knowledge. The relationship between what people know about food and nutrition and what they eat is a very weak one. Other factors may be taking precedence and need to be explored. Knowledge helps only when people are ready and motivated to change. Thus, there are many influences on food choices, including cognitive, sociocultural, physical, and geographical factors. The nutrition counselor needs to explore all of them to understand the client, the client's motivation for change, and the appropriate intervention to use. Figure 1-1 summarizes some of the variables motivating changes in people's food choices and health behaviors. In subsequent chapters of this book, specific counseling strategies are provided to address areas such as cognitive and behavioral change along with an entire chapter discussing cultural components.

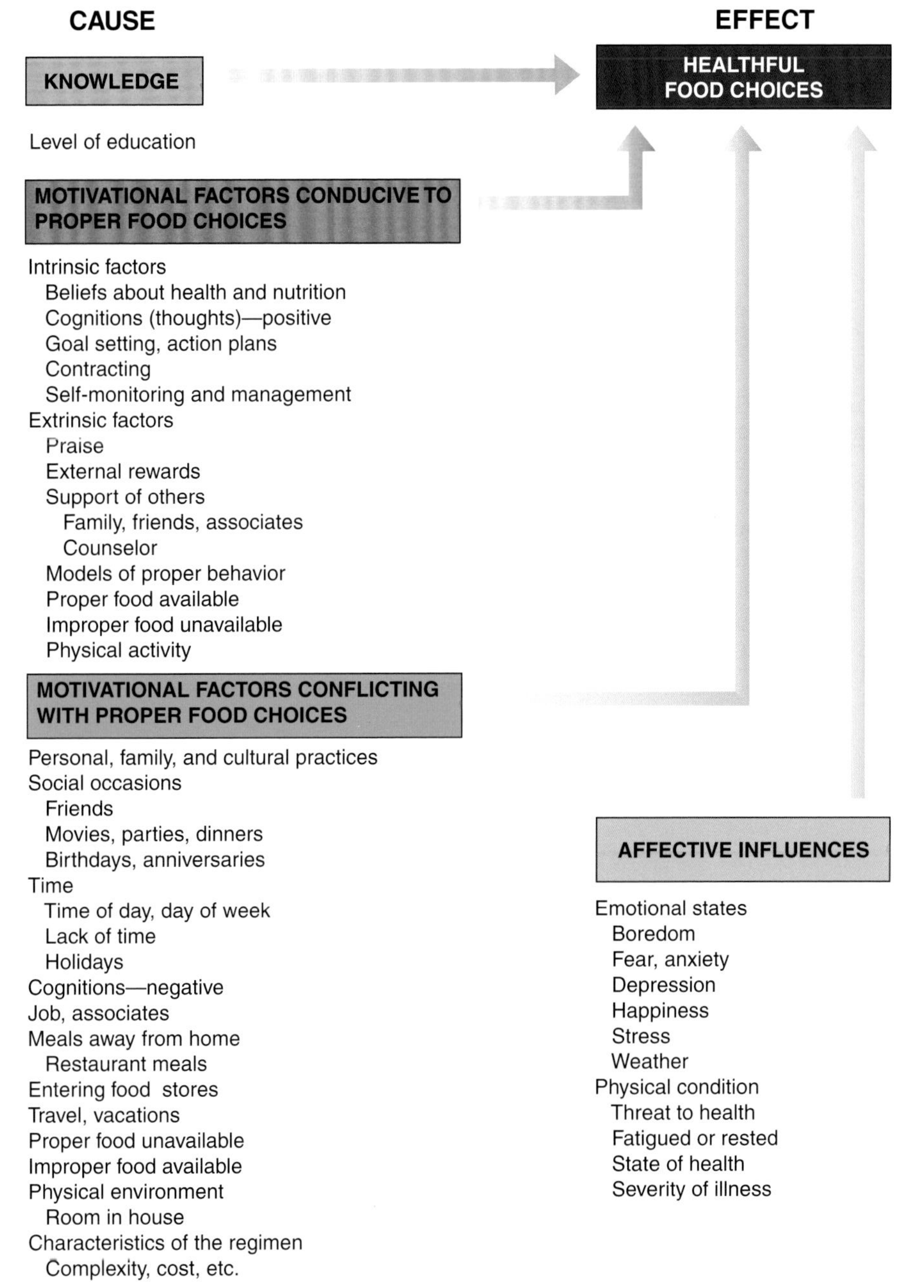

CAUSE   **EFFECT**

| KNOWLEDGE | | HEALTHFUL FOOD CHOICES |

Level of education

| MOTIVATIONAL FACTORS CONDUCIVE TO PROPER FOOD CHOICES |

Intrinsic factors
  Beliefs about health and nutrition
  Cognitions (thoughts)—positive
  Goal setting, action plans
  Contracting
  Self-monitoring and management
Extrinsic factors
  Praise
  External rewards
  Support of others
    Family, friends, associates
    Counselor
  Models of proper behavior
  Proper food available
  Improper food unavailable
  Physical activity

| MOTIVATIONAL FACTORS CONFLICTING WITH PROPER FOOD CHOICES |

Personal, family, and cultural practices
Social occasions
  Friends
  Movies, parties, dinners
  Birthdays, anniversaries
Time
  Time of day, day of week
  Lack of time
  Holidays
Cognitions—negative
Job, associates
Meals away from home
  Restaurant meals
Entering food stores
Travel, vacations
Proper food unavailable
Improper food available
Physical environment
  Room in house
Characteristics of the regimen
  Complexity, cost, etc.

| AFFECTIVE INFLUENCES |

Emotional states
  Boredom
  Fear, anxiety
  Depression
  Happiness
  Stress
  Weather
Physical condition
  Threat to health
  Fatigued or rested
  State of health
  Severity of illness

Figure 1-1 ■ Variables motivating change in food choices and health behavior.

Government Public Health Initiatives

Many government agencies have developed public health education initiatives to improve the health outcomes of populations. The United States Department of Agriculture, for example, has ongoing programs to evaluate the status of the American public and provide guidelines for improving health. The National Health and Nutrition Evaluation Survey (NHANES) is an ongoing, federally funded longitudinal program that provides data on a randomized set of children and adults of varying ages by collecting data on dietary intake and anthropometrics.[9] This dataset is often used by investigators to conduct research on health trends over time correlated to behavior changes.

ChooseMyPlate

The United States Department of Agriculture "ChooseMyPlate" gives a positive and visual message of how to select foods for each meal.[10] On the plate, fruits and vegetables should make up half of the diet, with more vegetables than fruits. The other half should include grains and protein, such as meat, poultry, and fish, with more grains than proteins. Dairy is shown on the side. Adaptations to the ChooseMyPlate program include application in school environments and in group settings, and electronic support with a website and accompanying interactive online resources (Figure 1-2).[11,12]

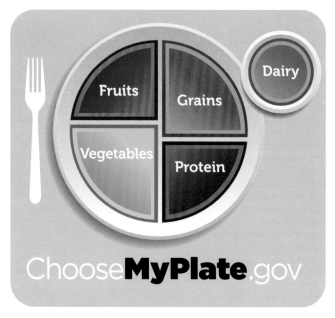

Figure 1-2 ■ http://ChooseMyPlate.gov.
Source: US Department of Agriculture.

Dietary Guidelines for Americans

The United States Department of Health and Human Services (HHS) sponsors updates to the Dietary Guidelines for Americans at regular intervals. The most current edition (2015–2020) summarizes a consensus of scientific, evidence-based nutrition recommendations for a healthy diet, which are revised every 5 years. The chairperson of the Dietary Guidelines Advisory Committee was Barbara Millen, DrPH, RDN from Boston.[13] The guidelines are the basis for nutrition counseling and education programs and federal food assistance programs. They are intended for healthy people and those at high risk for chronic diseases. Poor diet and physical inactivity are important factors contributing to the epidemic of overweight and obesity and are associated with major causes of morbidity and mortality in the United States. More than one-third of children and more than two-thirds of US adults are overweight or obese.[8]

Healthy People 2020

Healthy People 2020 is a set of national goals and objectives designed to guide health promotion and disease prevention efforts to improve people's health over a 10-year period. It is released by the US HHS each decade. More than forty health topics are found on the website. The challenge is to avoid preventable and chronic diseases from occurring. Heart disease, cancer, and diabetes mellitus are responsible for 7 out of 10 deaths among Americans annually. A healthy diet helps reduce the risk of overweight and obesity, heart disease, high blood pressure, type 2 diabetes, dyslipidemias (poor lipid profile), some cancers, and other conditions.[8,13]

CASE ANALYSIS 2

What suggestions or alternatives can you give Karen to overcome any problems using any of the public health initiatives described above? How could she use the ChooseMyPlate program in her family unit?

International Health Guidelines

Table 1-1 provides selected examples of international health guidelines that are applicable to country-specific or general world populations including the United States. The World Health Organization (WHO) maintains a global focus as well as an individualized focus by countries and regional areas of health and nutrition interest. The Food and Agriculture Organization (FAO) of the United Nations also monitors food-focused guidelines. The majority of health guidelines are updated regularly and are individualized to their intended audiences.[13-15]

Country	Health Guideline	Organization
Australia	Australia Guide to Health Eating www.eatforhealth.gov.au	Australian Government, National Health and Medical Research Council, Department of Health and Ageing
Canada	Canada's Food Guide www.hc-sc-gc.ca	Health Canada, Office of Nutrition Policy and Promotion
International	Global Targets/Country-specific guidelines who.int/nutrition/en fao.org/nutrition	World Health Organization, Food and Agriculture Organization of the United Nations
Philippines	Philippines Dietary Reference Intake (PDRI) 2015 fnri.dost.gov.ph	Food and Nutrition Research Institute, Department of Science and Technology
United States	ChooseMyPlate ChooseMyPlate.gov	United States Department of Agriculture, Food and Nutrition Services
United States	2015–2020 Dietary Guidelines health.gov/dietaryguidelines	United States Department of Health and Human Services, United States Department of Agriculture

Table 1-1 ■ List of Selected Government Population-Focused Health Guidelines

Food and Health Survey Results

How much do people already know about nutrition and health and how are food choices affected? In 2015, the International Food Information Council Foundation conducted the tenth Food & Health Survey about consumer attitudes toward food safety, nutrition, and health.

The survey found the following[16]:

- More than three-quarters (78%) say they would rather hear information about *what to eat* versus *what not to eat*. This was up 7% from 2014 for the strongly agree response category.
- About 84% (up from 76% in 2011) are trying to lose or maintain their weight. The two highest barriers were lack of willpower (37%) and lack of time (31%).
- About 76% are trying to cut calories by consuming more water and low- or no-calorie beverages.

- About 57% rate their health as very good to excellent, yet 55% of survey group was overweight or obese.
- Consumers are trying to eat more fruits and vegetables (82%).
- About 70% are trying to eat more foods with whole grains.
- About 69% are cutting back on foods that are higher in added sugar.
- About 68% are consuming smaller portions.
- More than half of Americans (51%) admit our food supply would be higher in cost if processed foods were eliminated and 45% state food would become less convenient.
- Lower income survey respondents are concerned about rising food costs and are more likely to spend extra money, if available, on food.
- Taste (83%), price (68%), and healthfulness (60%) continue to be top three drivers of food purchases.
- About 60% (compared to 70% in 2013) have confidence in the safety of the US food supply.
- Consumers use the food label to determine before they buy the product for expiration date (51%), nutrition facts panel (49%), ingredients (40%), serving sizes and amount per container (36%), and brand name (27%). Only 11% report not using the food label.
- The time reported to prepare dinner: 19% less than 15 minutes, 52% between 15 and 44 minutes, and 29% more than 45 minutes.

Access to technology continues to change healthcare for both professionals and their clients. In 1995, only 1 in 10 Americans had Internet access compared with about 80% of adults in 2015. The number of individuals with a smartphone only increased to 13% (up from 8% in 2013). The greatest increase in replacing home phone, cable, and internet service with only smartphone technology occurred in African-American and rural populations. Clients with access may arrive at appointments with medical and nutrition information.[17]

Scope of Practice Framework

The Scope of Practice Framework from the Academy of Nutrition and Dietetics provides guidance on what is within the practitioner's skill set or scope of practice. For RDNs and NDTRs, it delineates core responsibilities at the entry level of practice based on formal education, knowledge, skills, and training or foundation knowledge set by the Accreditation Council of Education in Nutrition and Dietetics (ACEND).[1,18,19] The first level of the Scope of Practice Framework uses the NCP as a framework for decision-making in nutrition care.[20] NCP is a required knowledge area in accredited education programs, in the credential examinations for RDN and NDTR conducted by the Commission on Dietetic Registration

(CDR), and has been incorporated into the Standards of Practice and of Professional Performance.[1,18–21]

The second level provides evaluation resources, such as Standards of Practice (SOPs) and Standards of Professional Performance (SOPPs), at the entry level and advanced levels of practice and includes the Academy Code of Ethics (Figure 1-3). Finally, there are decision aids or tools for those considering new roles or activities. As dietetics professionals refer to these materials, they guide practice, and the decision tree assists in personal assessment of competence. It is important to note that these standards are for scope of theoretical credential practice, but actual application of practice may be further defined by licensure. Licensure occurs typically on a state level, whereas credentials occur on a national level. For example, an RDN credential is attained by passing a national competency examination administered by the CDR. However, individual licensure must be obtained for practice within each state resulting in a licensed dietitian nutritionist (LDN) status which requires the RDN credential but also payment of an annual fee at the state level.

As part of the Scope of Practice, the Academy develops standards for evaluating the quality of practice and performance of RDNs and NDTRs. SOPs and SOPPs are tools for professionals to use in self-evaluation and to determine the education and skills necessary to advance from a generalist to specialty and advanced levels of dietetics practice. The SOPs are based

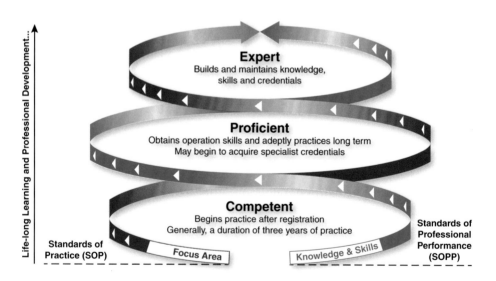

Figure 1-3 ■ Standards of practice and standards of professional performance for registered dietitian nutritionists (competent, proficient, and expert).

Source: ©Academy of Nutrition and Dietetics. Reprinted with permission.

on the four steps in the NCP of nutrition assessment, nutrition diagnosis, nutrition intervention, and nutrition monitoring and evaluation and are related to patient care.[20] The SOPPs contain six dimensions of professional performance, including the following: provision of services, application of research, communication and application of knowledge, utilization and management of resources, quality in practice, and competency and accountability.

Practice-specific SOPs and SOPPs have also been developed in areas such as disordered eating and eating disorders, integrative and functional medicine, extended care settings, diabetes care, oncology nutrition care, sports dietetics, and management of food and nutrition systems to name a few.[22] Many of these practice-specific SOPs and SOPPs form the basis of specialty credentials. For example, the Certified Specialist in Renal (CSR) documents competence in the defined standard of practice in nephrology care at the expert level.[23]

Nutrition Care Process

The NCP is a tool created to advance the profession of dietetics and to achieve "strategic goals of promoting the demand for nutrition professionals and to help them be more competitive in the marketplace."[20] An initial workgroup created the stepwise process to describing how nutrition professionals provide care to patients/clients. It was evident that a standardized taxonomy would assist in communicating the results of nutrition care and a standardized nutrition language would evolve. The NCP provides a method to address practice-related problems and make decisions about nutrition interventions. The nutrition professional obtains and interprets data about a possible nutrition-related problem and its causes. The framework aids thinking and decision making that RDNs use to guide professional practice.

The NCP uses the official international dietetics and nutrition terminology (eNCPT), a standardized set of terms which is only available electronically. These terms are also used for documentation in the medical record. Use in an electronic medical record, but not a paper record, requires permission from the Academy of Nutrition and Dietetics since the language is protected by copyright.[24] Adoption of a standardized eNCPT language will enable electronic medical records to be searched for NCP and outcomes. This, in turn, will provide evidence for health outcomes that can be attributed to nutrition intervention—and link to evidence-based reimbursement for RDN counseling and education.

NCP is used by nutrition professionals when delivering quality nutrition care to patients, clients, and other groups. There are four interrelated, sequential steps in a standardized process: (1) nutrition assessment, (2)

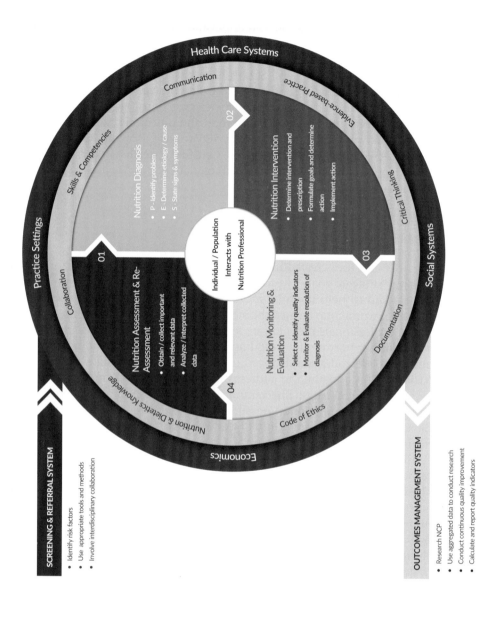

Figure 1-4 ■ The nutrition care process model.

Source: ©Academy of Nutrition and Dietetics. Reprinted with permission.

nutrition diagnosis, (3) nutrition intervention, and (4) nutrition monitoring and evaluation. Each step provides information for the following step. However, if new information is obtained and a reassessment is needed, previous steps may be revisited. NCP begins after the patient is referred by a health professional or identified at possible nutritional risk (Figure 1-4).[20]

Step 1: Nutrition Assessment

The purpose of nutrition assessment is "to obtain, verify, and interpret data needed to identify nutrition-related problems, their causes, and significance."[18] Nutrition-related data are obtained from patients/clients, the medical record, and other family members and health professionals. There are five categories of data to collect: (1) a food/nutrition-related history is often obtained by interviews; (2) anthropometric measurements, such as height, weight, and body mass index (BMI); (3) results of biochemical data, medical tests, and procedures in the medical record; (4) nutrition-focused physical findings, such as appetite and physical appearance; and (5) a client personal history, some of which is in the medical record. Data are compared with standards and interpreted.[20]

In the assessment step, the nutrition professional gathers in advance data or information about the patient or client that may have an impact on treatment. Information that is unavailable from the medical record may be obtained during an interview, such as a food and nutrition history. Factors that may have an impact on food and nutrient intake include the role in family, occupation, socioeconomic status, educational level, cultural and religious beliefs, physical activity, functional status, cognitive abilities, and housing situation. For example, the counselor may discover that the individual has been on a previously prescribed diet (eNCPT terminology code FH 2.1 representing Food/Nutrition-Related History main category, 2.1 Diet History assessment term).[20,24]

The counselor may collect data on current eating patterns or habits; on physical, social, and cognitive environments; and on previous attempts to make dietary changes. The physical environment includes where meals are eaten (at home or in restaurants and in which rooms of the home) and events that occur while eating (socializing, watching television, or reading). The social environment, which may or may not be supportive, includes family members, friends, social norms, and trends involved with eating behaviors (e.g., meeting friends for dinner, popular food items, and beverages when tailgating). The cognitive or mental environment involves the client's thoughts and feelings about food and his or her self-image and self-confidence. It concerns what clients say to themselves about their food habits and life, since personal thoughts may or may not promote successful change. Positive thoughts, such as "I love a steak and baked potato" or "My favorite snacks are potato chips and beer," may support continued eating.

There may be negative and self-defeating thoughts or thoughts of failure, boredom, stress, and hunger. Examples include "It's too difficult," "It's not worth it," "I can't do it," "I've been on diets before, always failed, and regained all of the weight I lost," or "I'm happy the way I am and don't want to change." These may also support continued eating.

Since behavior is influenced by beliefs and attitudes, the counselor may need to explore these in relation to the medical condition, nutrition, food choices, and health. The client's literacy level and any language barriers should also be noted.

If a problem is identified, the assessment of nutritional status provides baseline information from which to determine the nutrition diagnosis and establish interventions that are realistic. Once all of the data for the assessment are collected, the counselor must integrate and assimilate what she or he has read, heard, and observed to distinguish relevant from irrelevant data, identify discrepancies and gaps in the data, and finally organize the data in a meaningful way and document the assessment.[20]

CASE ANALYSIS 3

What would be a potential nutrition assessment for Karen? How would you express the potential nutrition assessment using the eNCPT?

Step 2: Nutrition Diagnosis

The purpose of the nutrition diagnosis is "to identify and describe a specific nutrition problem that can be resolved or improved through treatment/nutrition intervention by a nutrition professional."[20] The nutrition diagnosis is what the RDN is treating independently and differs from the medical diagnosis identified by the physician.

The data from the nutrition assessment are used to label the nutrition diagnosis. The nutrition diagnosis is organized into three categories: (1) intake (NI), such as amount of food or nutrients consumed compared with needs; (2) clinical (NC), such as problems related to medical or physical conditions; and (3) behavioral–environmental (NB), such as attitudes, beliefs, and the person's physical environment. For example, the medical diagnosis for a dialysis patient may be "kidney failure" but the nutrition diagnosis terminology using the eNCPT may be "NI-5.10.2 excessive potassium intake" or "NB-1.1 food- and nutrition-related knowledge deficit."[20,24]

The nutrition diagnosis, selected from the list of diagnoses from the eNCPT terminology, is written in a PES statement describing the problem (P), its etiology (E) or cause, and signs and symptoms (S) or evidence data.[20] The format of the PES statement is "nutrition problem label related

Problem (P)	Etiology (E)	Signs and Symptoms (S)
Specific nutrition diagnosis	Related to etiology	As evidenced by signs and symptoms
Overweight (NC-3.3)	Related to excessive energy intake (NI-1.5)	As evidenced by significant fast-food consumption and weight gain up to 10 lb in 3 mo (FH-1.2.2.3)

Table 1-2 ■ Example of the PES System Integrating Nutrition Care Process Terminology Codes

Nutrition Diagnostic: NC, Clinical; NI, Nutrition Intake; Nutrition Assessment and Monitoring and Evaluation: FH, Food/Nutrition-Related History.

to ____ as evidenced by ____." The problem (P) *related to* etiology (E) *as evidenced by* signs/symptoms (S). The problem (P) or nutrition diagnosis label describes alterations in the person's nutritional status. It is followed by etiology (E), the potential cause or contributing factors, and is linked to the diagnosis by the words "related to." The signs/symptoms (S) are the data used by the nutrition practitioner to determine that the person has the specified nutrition diagnosis and is linked to the etiology by the words "as evidenced by."[20] Table 1-2 is an example of the PES.

Documentation is essential throughout the NCP and is a process that supports all four steps.[20] After selecting the most essential diagnoses to work on, the system of charting may be reoriented to capture, in one to two sentences, the diagnosis based on the assessment. The recommendation is to document the diagnosis in the three-step PES. The PES could be entered into the notes section of an electronic medical record or remain as a written chart note in other documentation systems.

CASE ANALYSIS 4

What would be a potential nutrition diagnosis for Karen? How would you express the potential nutrition assessment using the eNCPT? Write a PES statement for Karen.

Step 3: Nutrition Intervention

Nutrition intervention is defined as "purposefully planned actions intended to positively change a nutrition-related behavior, environmental condition, or aspect of health status for an individual (and his or her family or caregiver), target group, or the community at large."[18] The purpose is "to resolve or improve the identified nutrition problem by planning and implementing appropriate nutrition interventions that are tailored to the patient/client's needs."[18] The intervention is directed by the etiology or causes of the nutrition problem described in the PES statement.

There are four general categories of eNCPT interventions: (1) food and/or nutrient delivery (ND), such as meals, supplements, or alternative feeding methods; (2) nutrition education (E), such as providing information and skills to modify eating behaviors to improve health; (3) nutrition counseling (C) to create individualized nutrition plans to improve health; and (4) coordinated nutrition care (RC), such as coordination with or referral to other healthcare providers. There are two interrelated components: a planning stage and the implementation stage. For example, the intervention strategy might be motivational interviewing, C-2.1 followed by E-2.2 skill development.[20,24]

The nutrition intervention incorporates the client's goals. The goals suggest the information, knowledge, and skills the client needs to make dietary changes. The counselor judges what information to provide, how much information can be absorbed at each session, at what educational or literacy level, and what handouts and media to use as supplements. The amount of information to provide and the best method of doing so must be individualized and matched to the client's cultural influences.

The intervention may include nutrition education or counseling, for example, about the following topics and activities: reading food labels, adapting recipes, menu planning, restaurant or carry-out meals, principles of healthful eating, food safety, nutrients in selected foods, nutritional supplements, nutrition misinformation, fat, carbohydrate, sodium, or calorie counting, nutrient–drug interactions, managing appetite, and the relationship of nutrition to the health problem. In addition, the client needs to know about physical activity, self-monitoring of diet and activity, and self-management. Problem-solving interventions for meal planning, food preparation, and food purchasing may be needed. Culturally sensitive interventions are important in meeting the needs, desires, and lifestyles of ethnic clients.

The counselor may suggest others with whom the client can discuss the goals, since a public commitment may make it more likely for goals to be accomplished. Self-monitoring records of food intakes and environments should be brought to the next appointment as a way for clients and the counselor to learn about factors affecting eating behaviors and as

CASE ANALYSIS 5

What would be a potential nutrition intervention for Karen? How would you express the potential nutrition assessment using the eNCPT?

a demonstration of the commitment to change. Clients' personal records, observations, and analyses of their environment contribute to the personal awareness and understanding.

Step 4: Nutrition Monitoring and Evaluation

The purpose of nutrition monitoring and evaluation is to "determine the amount of progress made and whether goals/expected outcomes are met."[18] The nutrition professional identifies patient/client outcomes relevant to the nutrition diagnosis, intervention plans, and goals. To determine progress, the practitioner identifies changes in behaviors, goals, or standards of care that are desired as the result of the nutrition care. This involves monitoring, measuring, and evaluating any changes in nutrition care indicators, the patient/client's previous status, reference standards, and the differences between assessment and reassessment.[18]

Monitoring is the follow-up step while evaluation is the comparison step, whether it is comparison to the last visit or comparison to a standard. After ascertaining progress, one may need to modify recommendations to promote progress to the goals. The determination of what the intervention should be as well as the evaluation mechanisms are individualized, but the Academy Evidence Analysis Library provides the framework for basing the NCP on available evidence of best practices.[25] An outcome, for example, is the measured result of the client's changes due to the counseling and education process. There are four categories of outcomes organized in nutrition monitoring and evaluation: (1) food/nutrition-related history outcomes, such as changes in dietary intake, physical activity, or knowledge and behaviors; (2) anthropometric measurement outcomes, such as weight, height, and BMI; (3) biochemical data, medical tests, and procedure outcomes including lab data and tests; (4) nutrition-focused physical finding outcomes, such as physical appearance and appetite.[20,24]

Outcome data identify the benefits of medical nutrition therapy in patient and client care. In using these systems of quality control, nutrition counselors may wish to evaluate several things: (1) the success of the client in following the goals set and in implementing new eating behaviors; (2) the degree of success of the nutrition intervention, including its strengths and weaknesses; and (3) their own personal skills as counselors.

CASE ANALYSIS **6**

What would be a potential nutrition monitoring and evaluation plan for Karen? How would you express this using the eNCPT?

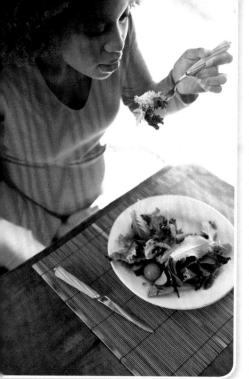

Having the right food available is helpful.

Nutrition Care Process Chains

It has been challenging to track the effect of nutrition intervention on changes in health patterns. With the NCP, the concept of "chains" has been formulated as a method to document RDNs are using evidence-based guidelines in their counseling content by linking health outcome data with RDN intervention and client change through electronic medical record searches. By tracking these changes over time, data can be collected that provides evidence that reimbursement for RDN services will result in cost-effective improvements in health outcomes. RDN reimbursement has already been approved by the Center for Medicare Services (CMS) for selected clients with diabetes and chronic kidney disease. RDNs must obtain a CMS provider number to bill and receive reimbursement directly. Internationally, reimbursement policies for nutrition services vary.[26]

The counselor should document using electronic records of the client's issues and goals, the factors influencing them, and the intervention for future measurement of client change. Examples of outcomes are changes in weight, glycemic control, blood pressure, lipid and other laboratory values; patient acceptance; progress at self-management; and improvement in knowledge, skills, dietary changes, and lifestyle changes. These indicate the impact of the intervention and can be used to evaluate the effectiveness of the treatment. The counselor and client should engage in evaluation jointly

Enthusiasm for change may decline during the first week and even more during the second week as obstacles develop. Therefore, frequent follow-up

CASE ANALYSIS 7

Write a potential nutrition care process "chain" plan for your work with Karen? How would you evaluate your effectiveness of treatment and document the cost-effectiveness of your professional time for future reimbursement?

appointments should be scheduled if possible. Acute care settings may not provide the opportunity for follow-up. Referrals to nutrition professionals in outpatient settings or in private practice may be necessary, since one session with a client is insufficient to promote long-term change in health practices. Communication is fundamental to each step in the process. Based on the nutrition assessment, clear documentation of the nutrition problem (diagnosis) and the treatment intervention will link measured outcomes to nutrition practice.

Evolving Scope of Practice in Nutrition

New areas of practice are continually evolving in the field of nutrition. A few will be highlighted here, but these examples only illustrate a small portion of the new and exciting areas of practice that are yet to be defined. The Subjective Global Assessment tool and nutrition physical examination examines patients for changes in oral mucosa, skin integrity, and nutrient deficiencies to formulate nutrition diagnoses and corresponding nutrition interventions.[27,28] Some practitioners are exploring advanced clinical skills examination principles that may one day be tested using standardized patients such as is currently done in medicine, osteopathic medicine, and podiatry.[29] An advanced practice audit conducted in 2013 funded by the CDR provided initial practice patterns that could eventually be used to develop an advanced practice credential examination.[30]

The concept of nutrition assessment using narrative medicine is also being explored. This technique builds upon motivational interviewing skills. It provides the ability to include subjective and detailed narrative prose in addition to the NCP. An example of narrative medicine documentation:

> The patient sat in the room with a lifeless expression, not wanting to make eye contact. He had just learned that his kidneys were failing and dialysis would soon be required. What to eat or not to eat was the last thing on his mind. Mr. Smith was instead focused on how he could continue to work and support his family.[31]

Finally, new practice settings are being explored. The area of emerging nutrition practice within integrated healthcare teams is evolving in patient-centered "whole-person" philosophy medical "homes" and accountable care organizations. These systems are shifting from a traditional fee-for-service model to a more comprehensive "total" care viewpoint. These integrated systems are rewarded for financially for improving health and wellness outcomes. The RDN has an integral basis in determining

Support sustainable farming practices and ecologic agriculture innovation
Encourage international food security and public policy collaboration
Promote farm-to-fork and fork-to-table global education initiatives
Advocate for safe and nutrition-conscious food processing
Partner with retailers to market healthy food options and programs
Educate consumers on evidence-based food preparation and storage methods
Raise awareness for comprehensive reduction of food waste/wasted food

Table 1-3 ■ Professional Initiatives to Link Agriculture, Nutrition, and Health

Adapted from Volgiano C, Steiber A, Brown K. Linking agriculture, nutrition, and health: The role of the Registered Dietitian Nutritionist. J Acad Nutr Diet. 2015;115:1710–1714; and Volgiano C, Brown K, Miller AM, et al. Plentiful, nutrient-dense food for the world: A guide for Registered Dietitian Nutritionists. J Acad Nutr Diet. 2015;115:2014–2018.

nutrition diagnosis, delivering appropriate nutrition interventions, and taking credit for client change in health risk reduction.[32]

Globally, groups have met to consider health economics of medical nutrition therapy in disease-related malnutrition and food insecurity.[15] Evidence-based nutrition guidelines have begun to evolve to advance research and practice. Ongoing monitoring and evaluation will be needed to direct public health policy and standards. An area of rising interest is the direct linking of agriculture, nutrition, and health (Table 1-3). Internationally, more than 30% of the food grown for human use is wasted or never available for use. Some nutrition professionals have already begun to move their area of influence to the role of farmer and direct food producer.[33,34] Future areas of practice are evolving rapidly in new and exciting directions.

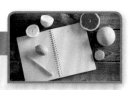

SELF-ASSESSMENT 2

What is an area of nutrition practice that you would like to explore or envision as developing in the future?

Summary

The current and expanding scope of the nutrition professional roles rely on communication, counseling, and education skills. Translating the science of nutrition and government health initiatives into practical application is fundamental to nutrition whether applied to communities, groups, families, or individuals in diverse areas such a food preparation, purchase, or intake. The art of communication is also essential in manager and leadership roles. All practitioners need the ability to communicate and work effectively with their employees, with coworkers and team members on their same level, with superiors who are in authority, and with customers, patients, and clients. The Scope of Practice Framework assists us in considering present and future boundaries of practice and providing quality, safe care to those we serve. The use of the NCP standardized language and eNCP terminology improves our communication in providing effective and quality nutrition care linked to positive health outcomes.

Review and Discussion Questions

1. List five influences on people's food habits or behaviors.
2. What are the major three components of the Standards of Practice Framework?
3. What are the four steps in the Nutrition Care Process (NCP)?
4. What does the nutrition professional do at each of the four steps in the NCP?

Suggested Activities

1. With someone trying to make changes in food choices, discuss the changes and the factors influencing the changes, including any opportunities, challenges, or barriers. What are the factors influencing the person?
2. Select a dietary regimen, such as increased fiber, restricted sodium, reduced calorie, or reduced fat and cholesterol, and follow it yourself for 7 days. Keep a daily record of all foods eaten. How easy or difficult was it to comply with the dietary change for a week? What factors helped or hindered your adherence?
3. Watch 2 hours of television or examine two current magazines. What food products are advertised? What are the messages? How do these ads influence food choices? Compare with peers.

CHAPTER 2

Communication

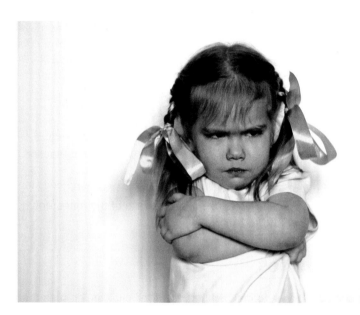

Objectives

- List the components of the communication model.
- Discuss ways to make verbal communication supportive and effective.
- Explain the use of paraphrasing.
- Explain examples of nonverbal behaviors.
- Discuss the impact of diversity on communication.
- Relate ways to improve listening skills.
- Identify common communication barriers and how to overcome them.

Joan Stivers, Nutritionist, noted on the medical record that her patient, John Jones, age 63, was 5'11" tall and weighed 250 lb. A retiree, he was just diagnosed with type 2 diabetes mellitus. Joan stopped by his hospital room, introduced herself, and told him that the purpose of her visit was to discuss his current food intake. During the conversation, Mr. Jones and his roommate were watching a baseball game on television, and periodically commented briefly on the plays and players. Finally, Mr. Jones said, "You need to talk with my wife, not me. She does the cooking." Just then, the physician entered the room.

You only have one chance to make a good first impression.

—Gary Dessler

Introduction

Today's technology makes communicating easier. We are connected by texting, email, smart phones, instant messaging, Twitter, and Facebook. But for health professionals, relating to others in person is necessary. Face-to-face skills need to be developed for communicating with individuals, groups, and the public. The Academy of Nutrition and Dietetics recognizes "expertise in verbal communication," as core competencies for communicating effectively with patients, clients, customers, and other professionals.[1,2] Providing "accurate and truthful information in communicating with the public" is required by the Code of Ethics.[3]

Communication skills are the foundation for interviewing, counseling, and educating patients, clients, and the public, as well as for efforts to assist people in changing their dietary and health behaviors. Nutrition counselors and health professionals deliver nutrition care and education in a collaborative partnership with patients, clients, and caregivers. Patient- and client-centered counseling as part of an intervention, for example, requires competent communication, counseling, and education skills.[1]

Well-developed communication skills increase the likelihood of the professional's success with clients and staff. Communication with other members of the healthcare team is important in identifying those in need of nutrition care and then in communicating with patients and clients about nutrition-related issues. Those in food service management and positions coordinating human resources communicate with staff and others regularly. As professionals advance to higher levels of authority in management, communication skills are essential in working effectively with people.

This chapter introduces the interpersonal communication process, including verbal and nonverbal communication, and listening skills. A model of the communication process is presented and discussed, followed by an explanation of the implications of the process for verbal, nonverbal, and listening behaviors. The impact of diversity on communication is addressed.

Communication Defined

A simple definition is that communication is "the process of acting on information" and about transmitting verbal and nonverbal messages in which "meaning is co-created simultaneously among people."[4] A professional needs the ability to use language that is appropriate to the client's or staff's level of understanding, the ability to develop a relationship with clients or staff, the ability to talk in a way that relieves anxiety, the ability to communicate in a way that ensures being able to recall information, and the ability to provide people with feedback.

Effective communication requires that the message is understood clearly as intended by the speaker; it achieves the intended effect; and it is ethical and truthful.[4] Differences in culture, gender, age, education, background, and other factors can be sources of misunderstanding. Effective and ethical communication requires listening carefully, understanding the person's story, and maintaining confidentiality.[5]

Among the focus areas in the government's Healthy People 2020 initiative is to bring better health to all citizens. Communication contributes to health promotion as well as disease prevention efforts. The plan is to use health communication and health information technology (IT) to improve population health outcomes and healthcare quality in order to achieve health equity.[6] Among the objectives are new opportunities to reach the culturally diverse and those with limited literacy skills who may face disparities in access to health information.[6,7]

Health literacy has been defined as "a constellation of skills that contribute to the ability to perform basic reading and numerical tasks for functioning in the health care environment and acting on health care information."[8] Low literacy is associated with poor understanding of written or spoken medical advice affecting health and is prevalent in certain groups, such as the less educated, those of lower cognitive ability, persons of certain social and ethnic groups, and the elderly.[7]

Communication skills are learned. One's speaking, listening, and the ability to understand verbal and nonverbal messages need to continue developing. Putting the principles into practice requires conscious efforts, repeated attempts, and many trials. With practice, in a relatively short time, you will notice a difference in the way others respond to you. Honing the skills, however, is an ongoing process and begins with an understanding of the many elements included in the interpersonal communication exchange.

Interpersonal Communication Model

Complicated processes are easier to grasp when they can be visualized in a model. The model is a graphic illustration to aid one's understanding. Studying the communication model to understand the role of each component is essential for professionals who are intent on expanding and improving their own communication repertoire.

Components of the Communication Model

The elements included in the communication model are the following: sender, receiver, the message itself, both verbal and nonverbal, feedback, and barriers. They are depicted graphically in Figure 2-1.

Sender

Senders of the message originate the thought or emotion, encode it into words, and speak first.

Receiver

Receivers or listeners attempt to decode or make sense of the message and usually interpret and transmit simultaneously. They may be listening to what is being said, filtering the message through their past experiences,

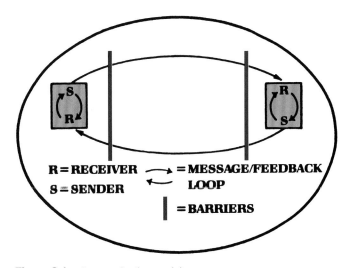

Figure 2-1 ■ Communication model.

values, or biases, while thinking about what they are going to say when the sender stops talking. Even when silent, it is impossible for receivers in a two-way communication transaction not to communicate. They may be reacting nonverbally with a flushed face or bored look, for example, depending on their inferences from the message. Senders interpret the receivers' appearance and demeanor and adjust subsequent communication accordingly. Thus, the two parties are sending and receiving simultaneously.

Message

The message is the information that is communicated to another. The receiver interprets two messages, the actual verbal message and the nonverbal message inferred from the sender and the environment. Nonverbal inferences arise from the perceived emotional tone of the sender's voice, facial expression, dress, gestures, tone of voice, choice of words, diction, and pronunciation, as well as from the communication environment.

Feedback

Since the communication process can be fraught with error, misunderstanding, or misinterpreted by the recipient, feedback is helpful. The term "feedback" refers to both verbal and nonverbal responses to messages. It insures that the message is understood and that the communication is successful. In face-to-face communication, the sender is talking while looking at the other person. The other person's verbal and nonverbal reactions to the sender's message, whether agreement, surprise, boredom, or hostility, are examples of feedback.

After the first few seconds, face-to-face communication becomes a simultaneous two-way sending-and-receiving process. While senders are talking, they are receiving nonverbal reactions from receivers. Based on these reactions, they may change their tone, speak louder, use simpler language, or in some other way adjust their communication. One can expect that feedback will vary with a person's experience, education, gender, and cultural group.[4] In many non-Western cultures, it can be subtle and circuitous, while the sender may prefer a more direct acknowledgment.

In written communication, writers cannot clarify the content for readers because they do not see them. Even when writers carefully select words for the benefit of their intended readers, written communication is generally less effective than one-on-one verbal communication because of the inability to adjust written language in response to the feedback from readers.

Barriers

Barriers, sometimes called noise or interference, can distort communication, and interfere with the understanding of the message. These factors include the unique attributes inherent in senders and receivers, such as the physiologic state of each communicator at the moment. Other factors include the room size, shape, color, temperature, and furniture arrangement. Interference can result from a ringing telephone or a television set.

No two people are exactly alike. Feelings of anxiety, fear, or apprehension may distort the message.[9] Because no one has shared in the exact life experiences of another, no two people understand language in precisely the same way. The sophisticated communicator needs to understand these dynamics and compensate or safeguard accordingly, so that the intended message is the one received.

Bear in mind that individuals have a limited capacity for processing information. When it exceeds our ability, the result is information overload. People may select, ignore, or forget, resulting in less effective communication.[9] Words mean different things to different people, and misinterpretation of the message may result. Meanings are in people, not in words.

Today's clients and employees, more than ever, originate from a wide variety of cultural and ethnic backgrounds. People from a different group increase the likelihood of a miscommunication in a verbal exchange. Words imply different things in different languages and people have different values, experiences, perceptions, and frames of reference.[9] Distortions can stem from psychological interference as well, including bias, prejudice, and closed-mindedness.

Psychological interference in healthcare patients may be due to fear of illness and its consequences. The job of senders is to generate in receivers those meanings for language that are closest to the sender's own. Because meanings are not universal, they can be affected by both external and internal influences. The communication environment, cultural differences, the distance between speakers, lighting, temperature, and colors are a few of the variables that can affect meanings ascribed to a message. These variables can be barriers and account for the difficulty in generating in others the meanings a person intends.

Interpersonal Communication

When focused on relationship-centered care, effective interpersonal communication should lead to better health outcomes for patients and clients. Improving patient knowledge and understanding, responding to emotions, and encouraging patient self-management are helpful. Communication outcomes may be affected by many factors, such as health literacy, provider communication, personal preferences, level of education, income, employment, occupation, neighborhood, culture, and urban or rural location. These shape interpersonal communication and health. How a person deals with illness influences health behavior change.[10]

While behavior change theories focus on actual behavioral change, interpersonal communication theories are based on the relationship between patient and provider. This may include family members and friends who can influence a person's health and illness may be included.[10] Relationships can affect goals and tasks associated with health behavior change. A relationship with trust and rapport promotes disclosure and openness in communication and affects how health behavior change is negotiated by the parties.

The patient or client is an expert on his or her own life, health, experiences, and relationships. Shared decision-making, negotiated dialog with the patient, development of empathy, and respect and removal of judgments allow for trust and openness.[10]

Relationship-centered care assumes that the provider and patient have a relationship characterized by respect, mutual trust, and engagement.[10] After the patient's feelings are understood and satisfied, one commits to goals and plans for treatment.

Patient–provider communication is important in affecting health outcomes. Interpersonal communication develops in a relationship between the provider and the patient or client in influencing health behavior change. Healing relationships respond to the person as well as the task of exchanging health information and providing patient self-management information. Helping and supporting people in managing their own health promotes self-management.

CASE ANALYSIS   1

What are the barriers to communication in the case challenge?

Verbal and Nonverbal Communication

We use two languages daily, our verbal language and our nonverbal or body language. Although both verbal and nonverbal communication occur simultaneously during interactions, they are discussed separately here in the context of their influence on the communication process.

Verbal Communication

To keep the communication channel open between the client or employee and the professional, one needs to know how to create a supportive climate. A supportive climate is one in which as one person speaks, the other listens, attending to the message rather than to his or her own internal thoughts and feelings. This creates a climate of trust, caring, and acceptance. A defensive climate, which occurs when the other person is feeling threatened or upset, creates the opposite effect, with the listener "shutting down." When this happens, there is little point in continuing the interaction because the message is no longer penetrating. Maintaining a supportive climate becomes especially crucial when the professional is attempting either to discuss a topic viewed differently, or to resolve conflict and defuse anger.

The verbal guidelines for creating a supportive communication climate are (1) to be aware of one's choice of words and discuss problems descriptively rather than evaluatively;

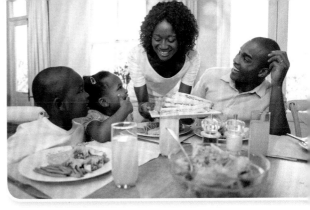

Families communicate at meal time.

Source: Pillitteri A. Maternal & Child Health Nursing, *4th ed.* Philadelphia, PA: Lippincott Williams & Wilkins; 2003.

(2) describe situations with a problem orientation in interpreting messages rather than in a manipulative way; (3) offer alternatives provisionally rather than dogmatically; (4) treat people as equals listening thoughtfully; and (5) be empathic rather than neutral or self-centered responding sensitively.[4]

Descriptive Rather Than Evaluative

Ordinarily, when approaching topics that tend to provoke defensiveness in clients, such as weight gain, professionals should think through the discussion before engaging the client, so that the problem area is exposed descriptively rather than evaluatively. Whenever people feel as if others are judging their attitudes, behavior, or the quality of their work, they show an increased tendency to become defensive. Such comments as "You don't seem to be trying," or "You don't care about cooperating," are based on inferences rather than facts. So when the other's response is "I do care," or "I am too trying," the framework for an argument is set, with no way of proving who is right or wrong.

Instead of making judgments regarding another's behavior or attitudes, the safest and least offensive way of dealing with a touchy issue is to describe the facts as objectively as possible. For example, when the professional tells a client that his or her continuing to eat ice cream and potato chips several times each day is discouraging to her as the client's counselor, she is confronting the problem without being evaluative. The client can then address the topic rather than argue about the professional's evaluation of poor adherence.

In a work-related situation, accusing an employee who has arrived late several mornings of being "irresponsible" and "uncaring" is likely to provoke a hostile response or cold silence. The employee may believe that being late does not warrant a reprimand. There may, in fact, be a reasonable explanation about which the manager should inquire. Describing how being late is causing problems for coworkers and causing work to back up is honest and descriptive and allows for nondefensive dialogue.

Problem-Oriented Rather Than Manipulative

Orienting people to a problem rather than manipulating them promotes a supportive communication climate. Frequently, when people want others to appreciate their point of view, they lead them through a series of questions until the other reaches the "appropriate" insight. This is a form of manipulation and provokes defensiveness as soon as respondents realize they are being channeled to share the other's vision.

> **EXAMPLE**   "Several weeks ago, you agreed that you were going to stop eating ice cream and potato chips; however, each week you acknowledge eating them. About a month ago, you agreed to switch to fresh fruit as a snack, but that has not occurred."

A discussion with the client would be more productive if the counselor took a direct problem-oriented approach.

> **EXAMPLE**   "In the past 6 weeks, you have gained 3 lb. With the dietary changes we planned, we anticipated a 4-to-5-lb weight loss. There seems to be a discrepancy here. Let's discuss what might explain the weight gain."

Employees and clients respect the professional when they believe the individual is being straightforward.

After the professional plans opening remarks descriptively rather than evaluatively, one should allow for collaborative problem solving without preplanned solutions. Creative, superior, and long-lasting solutions are more likely to occur when each person hears out the other fully, is heard in return, and when the client initiates the solution.

In the previous examples, the counselor's subsequent remarks depend on how the person responds to the directive to explain the problem. The professional needs to give the person time to think; this often means waiting for an answer. The practitioner needs to learn the discipline of sitting through the tension of silence supportively until the client or employee responds.

Frequently, the first explanations are those that people believe will not upset or shock the counselor. The "real" reasons, however, may not be revealed until the client or staff member feels secure enough to risk shocking the professional without fear of being humiliated or embarrassed. In other words, after the first explanations are offered, professionals would do best simply to repeat in their own words or paraphrase what they have understood. Only when the clients or employees are comfortable enough will they be able to express their authentic reactions, questions, or answers.

Provisional Rather Than Dogmatic

When offering advice to clients or helping them to solve problems, counselors should give advice provisionally rather than dogmatically. "Provisionally" implies the possibility of the practitioner changing the options, provided that additional facts emerge. It keeps the door open for clients to add information. A dogmatic prescription might be, "I know this is the way to solve your problem." A provisional prescription might be, "Here are several alternatives you might consider," or "There may be other ways of handling this problem; perhaps you have some ideas too, but here are things you might consider."

Equal Rather Than Superior

In discussing issues, the two parties should regard each other as equals and work collaboratively. Whenever the possibility of defensiveness exists, even between persons of equal rank, any verbal or nonverbal behavior that the other interprets as superiority generates a defensive response.

In the relationship between professionals and clients, or managers and employees, the professional's tendencies to emphasize status or rank may arise unconsciously from a desire to convince the other to accept his or her recommendations. Comments such as the following may cause the other to feel inferior or angry: "As a consumer, you may find this difficult to understand. Just do what I recommend; I've been doing this for 10 years." Certainly, there is nothing wrong with professionals letting clients know that they are educated and competent. However, the manner in which it is done is crucial. A more effective and subtle way is to make it clear that you don't have all the answers and to say, "I have studied this problem and dealt with other clients who have similar situations. I am interested, however, in incorporating your own thoughts and plans into the solution. You must be satisfied and willing to try new eating habits."

An employee making a recommendation to a manager that the manager had tried unsuccessfully in the past might be told, "If I were in your shoes, I would think the same thing. Someday when you are more experienced, you'll know why it won't work." The subtle underscoring of the inferior relative status of the subordinate could be enough to cause a defensive battle. The professional could have succeeded with a comment, such as "I can understand why you say that. I have thought the same myself, but when I tried, it was not successful." Showing respect for the client's and employee's intelligence and life experiences and recognizing their human dignity facilitates cooperation.

In conflict resolution, problem solving, and the discussion of any issues that may be threatening to the other person, collaboration is far more effective than trying to persuade the person to act according to the professional's recommendations. Collaboration has other virtues as well. People feel more of an obligation to uphold solutions that they themselves have participated in designing. If clients are trying the professional's solution, they may feel little satisfaction in proving that he or she was right; however, if the solution is one that was arrived at through collaboration, there is genuine satisfaction in proving its validity. Two people sharing insights, knowledge, experience, and feelings can generate creative thought processes in each other, which in turn generates other ideas that otherwise would not have emerged.

Empathic Rather Than "Neutral"

Empathy is "an emotional reaction that is similar to the reaction being experienced by another person."[4] We feel what the other person feels. Ask yourself: "Am I able to understand the other person's experiences as if I were experiencing them?" The skill of empathy is especially important when there is bias in healthcare, such as may occur with obese people.

Empathy is mentioned frequently in the skill of listening and is discussed later in the chapter. Empathy conveys that the professional is fully present and actively engaged in the interaction. Lacking empathy may leave patients, clients, and staff feeling misunderstood.[9]

To be effective in working with clients and employees, professionals must be able to demonstrate in some way their desire to understand the other's feelings. This "demonstration" might be an empathic response to comments, where the listener tells the other that he or she is attempting to understand both the speaker's content and feelings. For example, a client might say, "For my entire life I have eaten salty foods; they are a part of my culture. I don't know what my life will be like without them." The professional might then respond, "You seem to be worried that the quality of your life will change because of the dietary recommendations."

If the professional is accurate in the empathic remarks, the client will acknowledge it and probably go on talking, assured that the person listens. If the professional is wrong, however, the client will clarify the judgment and continue to talk. Thus, the counselor need not be accurate in inferring the other's feelings as long as he or she is trying to understand them. In addition, empathic responses allow the professional to respond without giving advice, focusing instead on the individual's need to talk and to express concerns. Before clients or staff can listen to the professional, they must express their concerns; otherwise, while the practitioner is talking, the clients or staff are thinking about what they will say when the individual stops talking.

An employee who has asked to be released from work on a busy weekend to attend a family gathering might receive the following neutral response: "No offense, but a rule is a rule. If I make an exception for you, others will expect it too." The employee would still feel sad about working, but would feel less antagonistic toward the supervisor, with the following empathic response: "I realize how badly you feel about not being able to attend the family party. I feel sorry myself having to refuse your request, but I can't afford to let you have the day off." The supervisor, by letting the subordinate know that he or she understands the subordinate's underlying feelings and is sympathetic, uses the most effective means of defusing the person's disappointment.

How should the professional respond to Mr. Jones? What should be the next steps?

Paraphrasing, a Critical Skill

Paraphrasing is restating in your own words what the other person has said and it is often done with empathy.[4] Most people have not incorporated the skill of paraphrasing into their communication repertoire. Even after people realize how vital this step is and begin to practice it in interactions, they may feel uncomfortable, self-conscious, or fear others may think they are "showing off." A hint for the professional feeling awkward about asking clients and staff to paraphrase would be to ask for the paraphrase by acknowledging one's own need to verify that what was heard is what the other intended. For example: "To be sure I understand your concern, you seem to be saying . . ."

> **EXAMPLE**   "I know that I don't always explain as well as I should, and that frequently, people have questions. Just to be sure I clearly covered the information, would you mind explaining in your own words how you will plan your meals?

Of course, it takes less time to ask, "Do you understand?" However, asking this question is less effective. Because of the perceived status distinction between the helper and the person being helped, the latter may be ashamed to admit that he or she does not understand. When persons of perceived higher status ask others if they "understand," almost always the answer is, "yes." This phenomenon is likely when working with some ethnic clients.

Another possibility is that the client or staff member honestly believes that he or she understands, and for that reason answered, "yes." The understanding, however, may include some alteration of the original message, in the form of substitution, distortion, or addition. The skill of paraphrasing needs to become second nature and automatic for professionals to verify important instructions, feelings, and significant client or staff disclosures.

Because of the anxiety attached to being in the presence of another of perceived higher status, the client or staff member may be less articulate than usual when describing symptoms or explaining a problem. The professional should paraphrase to verify that he or she understands the message as the "sender" intends. One should try to avoid sounding too clinical with such comments as "What I hear you saying is. . ." Instead, keep the language clear, simple, and natural. A comment such as "I want to make sure I understand this; let me repeat what you are saying in my own words" is more natural.

Two points need to be emphasized regarding paraphrasing: (1) Not everything the other person says needs paraphrasing. It would become a distraction. Paraphrasing is essential only when the discussion is centered on critical information that must be understood. (2) Paraphrasing often leads to additional disclosure and therefore provides further information.

People are so accustomed to being with others who do not really listen that when they are with someone who proves that he or she has been paying attention by repeating the content of what has been said, they usually want to talk more. For the professional, this additional information can be valuable. Another benefit is that after the client or staff member has expressed all questions and concerns and has cleared his or her mental agenda, he or she is psychologically ready to sit back and listen or to solve problems.

By talking too much or too soon, the professional may not be able to convey all of the message to the other, who may be using the difference in time between how fast the professional speaks and how fast the client's own mind processes information to rehearse what he is going to say next.[4] The human mind operates 4 to 10 times faster than human speech.

CASE ANALYSIS 3

What did Mr. Jones' verbal statements tell you about his attitudes toward his health problem?

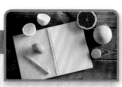

SELF-ASSESSMENT 1

Directions: Paraphrase the following:

1. Client: "I've been overweight most of my life. I've tried many different diets: I lose a few pounds, and gain it all back."
2. Employee: "I don't know why you want to keep changing things around here. Our old manager was satisfied with our procedures."

Nonverbal Communication and Image Management

Communication that creates meaning for people, but is not verbal or written, is called "nonverbal."[4] Of the two messages received simultaneously by receivers,

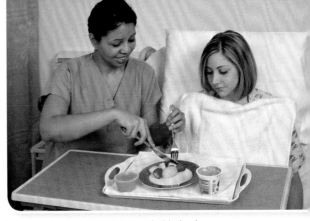

Be aware of the person's nonverbal behaviors.

Source: Springhouse. Lippincott's Visual Encyclopedia of Clinical Skills. Philadelphia, PA: Wolters Kluwer Health; 2009.

verbal and nonverbal, the nonverbal is the larger component and more influential and believable. As receivers of messages, people learn to trust their interpretations of nonverbal behaviors more than the word choices consciously selected by the sender. Intuitively, they know that control of nonverbal behavior is generally unconscious, whereas control of verbal messages is usually planned and deliberate.

Nonverbal messages communicate our feelings toward others and are critical to relationships. However, it is important to develop awareness in using nonverbals in interactions as well as to recognize them in others.[4] Our nonverbal messages are more believable than our verbal ones.

"A picture is worth a thousand words." What is your picture like? Even before we speak, we may be judged by our clothing and appearance.[11,12] Dress and appearance are consciously selected and are nonverbal communication vehicles. Makeup, hairstyle, clothing, and accessories represent who you are and your self-image. Professional image is difficult to define, but it is an impression one creates at the first meeting and most people recognize it. Personal appearance, including clothing, hairstyle, and accessories, are among the most important elements of the image.

Simple well-tailored clothes in neutral colors, such as a skirt or slacks with a blouse or sweater are examples for women. A shirt, tie, slacks, and dress shoes are examples for men as the goal is to look professional and conservative.[4] One should avoid clothes that are too tight, short, or trendy, piercings, flip flops, sweats, excessive jewelry, chipped nail polish, and uncovered body art. Clients who are unable to relate to your appearance may have trouble relating to your message and question your competence.[4,11]

In meeting new people, we begin making judgments immediately, based on nonverbals, such as noticing eye contact, appearance, and whether or not the handshake is strong or limp.[4] Chief nonverbal vehicles inherent in speakers are facial expression, tone of voice, eye contact, gestures, posture, and touch, with meanings varying among cultures.[4] The receivers of communication notice nonverbal behavior in clusters.

If the professional is listening to a client, for example, but shifting papers and looking at a computer screen with a bored look, the client will not believe the person is interested. Ordinarily, people do not notice posture, eye contact, or facial expression isolated from the other nonverbal channels. For this reason, professionals need to monitor all nonverbal communication vehicles so that together the clusters are congruent with one another as well as with the verbal messages.

Nonverbal behaviors vary widely among different groups with each having its own body language. Although similarities exist, the meanings of behaviors differ among groups, as the way people behave is learned early in life. Our own history influences our ideas of what a person "is" or "should be." These variations may require professionals to adapt their nonverbal behaviors. If the client shows any sign of resisting or objecting to the professional's eye contact or touch, for example, the professional should cease immediately. Communication competence requires "the ability to adapt one's behavior towards another person in ways that are appropriate to the other person's culture or ethnic group."[4]

CASE ANALYSIS 4

What do you notice about Mr. Jones's nonverbal behaviors?

Facial expression is usually the first nonverbal trait noticed. "Smile and the world smiles with you." What do you look like when you are happy? Or when you are bored or worried? A relaxed face with pleasant smile indicates a friendly, approachable climate and makes a good first impression.[12] A supportive tone of voice is one that is calm, controlled, energetic, and enthusiastic.

Eye contact includes gazing in a way that allows the communicator to encounter the other visually—to the extent of being able to notice the other's facial and bodily messages. Besides being an excellent vehicle for feedback, eye contact makes the person feel visible and ensures the other person of the professional's interest and desire to communicate. Posture is best when leaning somewhat toward, rather than away from, the person. Large expansive gestures may be interpreted as a show of power and generally should be avoided.

Touch is a vehicle for feedback that can work positively. Through a gentle touch, a pat, or a squeeze of the hand, one can communicate instantly a desire to solve a problem without offending. Touch can communicate affection, concern, and interest faster than these messages can be generated verbally. Although an individual may look calm, controlled, and totally at ease, a touch may reveal nervousness and insecurity.

Professionals Must Be Alert to Nonverbal Signals from Others

Besides the professional's concerns with the environment and his or her own verbal and nonverbal behavior in creating a trusting climate, one must also be sensitive to nonverbal cues in others. Even though the practitioner is being open, caring, and attending to his or her own behavior, the internal anxiety, confusion, nervousness, or fear in people may be causing them to misunderstand. Two requirements for effective interpersonal communication are to observe the nonverbal cues in others and then respond to them in an affirming way.[11]

If the client or employee is nodding the head to suggest understanding, for example, but looks puzzled, the professional needs to verify understanding by having the person paraphrase or summarize important instructions or dietary recommendations. If the client is flushed, has trembling hands, or tears rolling down the cheeks, the professional may need to deal directly with relieving anxiety. Until the individual is relaxed enough to concentrate, optimal two-way communication is unlikely.

After talking with one another for only a few minutes, both the professional and the client can sense the "warmness" or "coldness" of the other, as well as the degree of the other's concern. If the speaker has a pleasant expression, and looks directly into the eyes of the listener while talking, he or she might be generating inferences in the listener of being a caring person. After the initial positive impression has been created, the impression tends to spread into other areas not directly related to the behavior originally observed.

The process can work in reverse as well. If the professional does not look at the client while talking or touches the client too firmly and has an unpleasant facial expression, the inferences being created may be negative—arrogance, lack of concern, indifference, and "coldness." Even though these initial reactions, both positive and negative, may be inaccurate, faulty first impressions are common. The professional might not be given a second chance to win the client's trust and cooperation.

Positive Affect Must Be Consistent

Seeing clients or employees regularly gives practitioners and managers an opportunity to reinforce or alter the perceptions the other person has of them. A person who is cold, aloof, and uncaring on a daily basis, and suddenly, because it is time to conduct a meeting, acts differently, the individual will not be believed. Practitioners need to be consistent in adding positive inferences to the impressions of their staff and clients.

Not only is it important to generate concern through your own nonverbal behavior and disposition, it is also essential to control, whenever possible, the communication environment so that it, too, leads to positive inferences while eliminating barriers. Attractive offices, pastel-colored rooms, soft lighting, comfortable and private space for counseling, and comfortable furniture all can add to the client's or staff member's collective perception. Piles of papers on a desk, a ringing mobile phone, and constant interruptions must be replaced with privacy and quiet.[11] Because so much counseling takes place in a clinical setting, more attention must be given to creating an inviting atmosphere.

Among the requirements for effective and successful interpersonal communication is the need for the professional to send verbal and nonverbal messages that are congruent with one another. A client may hear a practitioner say, "I want to help you; I'm concerned about your health and the possible recurrence of your heart problem as a result of your food choices." But if the client sees the practitioner taking notes and checking a watch rather than looking at the client, the contradictory second message of impatience will be more intense than the stated message of concern. The professional may have said all the "right" words, but is judged as insincere. Helping professionals and managers who do not genuinely like working with people are ultimately destined to fail.

Diversity

In recent years, the US population has become more racially and ethnically diverse.[13,14] With the increasing diversity, professionals need knowledge and skills related to cultural competence in communication. The United States is becoming a multi-racial country due to shifts in demographic makeup resulting from immigration and fertility rates with the number of babies born here increasing. In 2011, more minority babies were born than White babies.[13] More children are members of minorities, that is, Black, Hispanic, Asian, and other non-White races.

As the baby boomers grow older and there is a lack of White immigration, the White population is expected to decline. Population projections based on the 2010 census show that White people will become a minority in the 2040s. It is predicted that there will be no racial majority in the United States after 2046.[13]

Communicating health and nutrition education is affected by cultural influences. People from other cultures have their own communication style, languages, practices, beliefs, values, customs, and foods. Cultural understanding and competence are needed to communicate effectively with racial, ethnic, cultural, and linguistically diverse groups.[14] Developing these abilities takes time.

Cultural practices, health beliefs, dealing with illness, and literacy may be influential. Interactions with people who are culturally and linguistically different from oneself should be based on mutual respect, trust, empathy, tolerance, genuine interest, and nonjudgmental responses. Responding to the person as well as exchanging information with simple words about dietary practices in a supportive environment enhances the communication relationship.

One needs to be aware of one's own cultural values, assumptions, and beliefs, but have the ability to function with people from diverse ethnic and cultural backgrounds.[15] Printed materials in the person's culture and other resources are available on the Internet.

Blacks were the largest minority until 2000. Currently, Hispanics are the largest minority group followed by Asians. Overall, Hispanics are less educated than the total population and rank lower on English language usage.[13] As the country becomes more racially diverse, this is affecting educational, medical, and other institutions.

Because there is a risk in self-disclosure, ethnic groups vary in how much they disclose and to whom. Women tend to disclose more than men. Americans may disclose a wider range of information including personal information than Japanese, Chinese, and Asians. People in collectivist cultures, such as China and Japan, follow cultural norms, disclose less, and work for the good of the group. Self-disclosure is affected by competence, involvement, and perceived similarity to oneself. In collectivist cultures, sentences are rarely begun with "I" and people avoid calling attention to themselves, while Americans are more direct.[13]

Nonverbal behaviors should reflect openness, respect, concern, and interest by listening actively and moderating cultural variables, such as touch, eye contact, facial expression, physical space, and use of gestures. Do you make eye contact as you meet someone? Levels of personal space are determined by one's cultural background. Preferences for spatial distance vary, for example, and some stand closer when talking. Vocal qualities, such as pitch, volume, rate, tone, and resonance will differ. Our verbal behaviors should indicate respect, empathy, and nonjudgmental concern, invite questions, and integrate the person's ethnic values and beliefs.

A patient-centered approach to communication competency may consist of assessing cross-cultural issues; exploring the meaning of the illness; inquiring about the social context of living; and engaging in collaborative negotiation. In the healthcare industry, as many as 20 different languages may be encountered among patients and staff. It is impossible to learn all of them, but we should learn those used most often.

Listening Skills

Listening to someone is probably the most ancient of healthcare skills. Listening is "the process of receiving, constructing meaning from, and responding to verbal and nonverbal messages."[4] Most of us are egocentric or focused on ourselves and may have difficulty focusing on communication from others that does not relate directly to us. Well-developed listening skills are a foundation for effective interpersonal relationships and quality care of healthcare providers. Whether working with individuals or groups, more than anything else, people want to be listened to and lack of listening leads to dissatisfaction.[4]

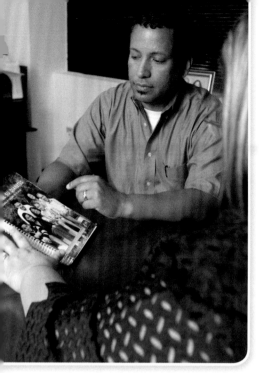

Listening is an essential skill.
Source: CDC/Amanda Mills.

An individual with average intelligence can process information mentally at speeds that are faster than human speech. Most people speak 125 words per minute, while some people can listen up to 600 to 800 words per minute.[4] As a result, people have time to be thinking about other things simultaneously. Two days later, most of us remember only 25% to 50% of what we heard. This is true of both clients and employees. Thus, while nutrition practitioners are listening to their clients or staff members talk, they have time to be thinking about other things. Clients, patients, and staff must believe that they are heard and understood and that the listener is genuinely interested in the message. A person-centered attitude based on empathy, congruence, and unconditional positive regard is helpful.

Everyone has had the experience of listening to a speaker and letting the mind wander to other topics. From the speaker's clothes, shoes, jewelry, diction, and speech patterns, people may tend to fill in details and develop an elaborate scenario while listening. The process of good listening involves learning to harness your attention so that you are able to concentrate totally on the speaker's message, both verbal and nonverbal. Development of these skills is not difficult, but it does require a conscious effort and perseverance.

Listening ability can be enriched only when the person desires such enrichment and is willing to follow the training with practice. The following is a list of five of the most common issues and barriers related to poor listening[4]:

1. Most people have a limited and undeveloped attention span.
2. People tend to stop listening when they have decided that the material is uninteresting and tend to pay attention only to material they "like" or see an immediate benefit in knowing.
3. Listeners tend to trust their intuition regarding the speaker's credibility, basing their judgments more on the speaker's nonverbal behavior than on the content of the message.
4. Listeners tend to attach too much credibility to messages heard on electronic media, such as the internet, television, movies, and so forth.
5. Communication is inhibited by judging, bias, prejudice, giving advice, providing solutions, and ignoring the concerns of the person.

What would you say about Mr. Jones's listening skills?

Active listening is a learned skill and requires focusing on what another is saying. Listening can be improved with practice. It is not a new skill, but an effort to eliminate the things that interfere with listening. The most important step in such improvement is resolving to listen more actively and efficiently.[4] The following are specific suggestions for improving listening:

- *Remember to listen carefully while remaining silent.* Give your undivided attention and remind yourself of the intent to listen carefully. Summarize the major facts, take notes, or make an outline of major points. Note when your mind drifts off to your own concerns and avoid distractions.[4]

- *Be objective.* The communication situation should be approached with the attitude of objectivity, with an open mind, and with a spirit of inquiry. Try repeating the message mentally as it is said. Do not formulate your response.

- *Watch for clues from the speaker.* Just as one uses bold type and italics in writing, speakers use physical arrangement, program outlines, voice inflection, rate, emphasis, voice quality, and bodily actions as aids to help the listener determine the meaning of what is being said and its importance.

- *Take your time.* Listeners need to make use of the thinking–speaking time difference and to remind themselves to concentrate on the speaker's message. They must use the extra time to think critically about the message, search for meaning and understanding, to relate it to what they already know, to consider the logic of the arguments, and to notice the accompanying nonverbal behavior—all simultaneously.

- *Find the real meaning.* Listeners need to look beyond the actual words to determine what the speaker means, and to determine whether the clusters of accompanying nonverbal behavior are congruent with the verbal message. Paraphrase the information.

- *Respond to confirm your understanding.* Listeners need to provide feedback to the speaker, either indirectly through nonverbal reactions or directly through paraphrasing, reflecting, restating, or summarizing, to verify that what is being understood by the listener is what the speaker intends. A nod of the head or "un huh" indicates you are listening.

Giving accurate feedback is the best way to prove that another person's message has been heard and understood.[4] It creates an atmosphere of trust in which people feel free to communicate openly without fear. Ultimately, the most valuable way to improve listening skills is ongoing practice, putting oneself in difficult listening situations, and concentrating.

2 CHAPTER

Summary

The chapter introduces verbal and nonverbal communication skills, listening skills, a model of the communication process, diversity, and cultural communication. Suggestions are presented for improving the nutrition and health professional's communication competence with clients and staff. To develop these skills, readers must begin to attempt new behaviors and put into practice what has been read. When people have the opportunity to try out new communication behaviors, forces within them tend to pull them toward their past behavior. Even when the old strategies are unsuccessful, they generally tend to be repeated. Competent professionals must communicate effectively with patients, clients, staff, customers, and other professionals.[1,2]

Review and Discussion Questions

1. In the helping professions, what conveys the professional's effectiveness with clients and staff?
2. Explain the components of the communication model.
3. How are verbal and nonverbal communications linked?
4. What can you do to identify and resolve barriers to communication?
5. What are the verbal guidelines for creating a supportive COMMUNICATION climate?
6. Describe an EMPATHIC response.
7. Of the two MESSAGES received simultaneously by receivers, which is more influential, the verbal or nonverbal? Give an example of making a verbal message unbelievable using a nonverbal message.
8. What are the most common barriers to listening?
9. What are some SPECIFIC suggestions for improving listening?

Suggested Activities

1. After filling out the questions below, join with classmates in groups of three to share and discuss your responses with one another.
   A. What types of nonverbal signals from your instructor or supervisor indicate to you that he or she is unhappy?
      (1)
      (2)
   B. What nonverbal cues indicate that you are getting angry?
      (1)
      (2)

C. List some of the nonverbal signals that you send when you are talking and someone interrupts you.

(1)

(2)

D. List some of the nonverbal signals that you send when you want to signal confidence or approval of the other person.

(1)

(2)

E. List changes you might make in the room where you are reading to alter its climate positively.

(1)

(2)

2. Write a two-paragraph description of a current interpersonal conflict you are experiencing. Be sure to indicate: (1) the behavior on the part of the other that has caused you a problem and (2) what "feelings" you are experiencing as a result of that behavior. Do not sign your name unless you want to be acknowledged. After the instructor has collected the descriptions, he or she may read them and either invite students to participate in role-playing of the situations using the guidelines for supportive verbal and nonverbal behavior or engage the class in a case study discussion of how the communication skills might be used to resolve the conflict.

3. You can increase your knowledge of nonverbal behavior by viewing others talking but not hearing what they are saying. Tune in the television channel to a soap opera or talk show; turn off the volume, watch the nonverbal behavior, and try to interpret it. After 3 to 5 minutes, turn the volume up. Then again, turn off the volume. Do this several times and attempt to grasp the verbal messages without the sound by merely interpreting the nonverbal behavior. Take notes and be prepared to share your experience in class.

4. As an in-class exercise, silently jot down the general "meanings" you derive from the nonverbal behaviors listed below. Compare answers with classmates. Is there general agreement on all, or is there a range of answers? Where answers vary, discuss the possible reasons why.

A. Lack of sustained eye contact

B. Lowering of eyes or looking away

C. Furrow on brow

D. Tight lips

E. Biting lip or quivering of lower lip

F. Nodding head up and down

G. Hanging head down

H. Shaking head right to left

I. Folding arms across chest

J. Unfolded arms

K. Leaning forward

L. Slouching, leaning back

M. Trembling hands

N. Flushed face

O. Holding hands tightly

P. Tapping foot continuously

Q. Sitting behind a desk

R. Sitting nearby without any intervening objects

5. The following is an exercise that you might try with friends. The first person expresses the message to the second person, who in turn expresses it to the third, and so on, until six people have heard it. Ordinarily, the message is audiotaped and played back. This allows the participants to see the many ways in which messages are altered as they pass from person to person.

MESSAGE: A child has hurt herself at the pool, and I must report it to the police. However, it is necessary for me to get to the hospital as soon as possible. She was walking up the diving board and getting ready to jump, when someone in a blue bathing suit pushed ahead. A boy in a red suit tried to stop her, but she fell off and landed on her back. The boy claims it was the young girl's fault, but she blames him.

CHAPTER 3

Interviewing

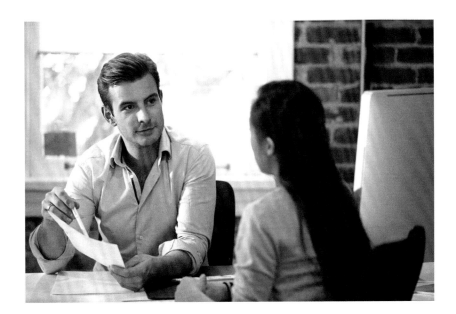

Objectives

- Discuss the purposes of different kinds of interviews, such as a food and nutrition interview and a pre-employment interview.
- Explain the conditions necessary for effective interviewing.
- Identify the parts of an interview and what should be included in each.
- Discuss the advantages and disadvantages of various types of questions.
- Develop a list of appropriate questions for a food and nutrition interview and sequence them.
- Identify the different types of responses to an interviewee's remarks.
- Use techniques of interviewing and conduct a food and nutrition interview.

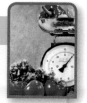

Delores Maynard is a 55-year-old woman who works in a corporate office. She visits the corporate wellness center and makes an appointment with Joan Stivers, a nutritionist. D.M is 5'2" tall and weighs 190 lb. She has mild hypertension. She is married with two grown children.

Nutritionist: "What brings you to today's appointment?"
D.M: "I need to lose some weight to help control my blood pressure."

Listening well is as powerful a means of communication and influence as to talk well.

—John Marshall

Introduction

Interviewing is a skill used by health professionals and managers. When was the last time you were interviewed? Was it when you were applying for college or for a job? Registered Dietitian Nutritionists (RDN), Nutrition and Dietetics Technicians, Registered (NDTR), and other health professionals use interviewing skills interacting with clients, patients, employees, and the public. Food and nutrition interviews and other communication techniques are used as part of an assessment of food intake and nutritional status in the prevention and treatment of obesity, chronic diseases, and in the maintenance of general health.[1]

Before beginning to counsel people, it is important to understand their lifestyle, cultural issues, and dietary and health practices. Using interviewing techniques, the professional questions the person to complete an assessment of current food choices, eating practices, and nutritional status. Along with other data, the Nutrition Assessment is a basis for a Nutrition Diagnosis and Nutrition Intervention in the Nutrition Care Process (NCP). During the final step, Nutrition Monitoring and Evaluation, the practitioner may take another food and nutrition history to check the person's understanding and to monitor progress toward goals and outcomes.[2]

Managing human resources is also a responsibility in many positions. These management capabilities frequently require interviewing skills.

A common misperception is that an interview involves two people having a conversation, with one asking questions and the other answering. Nothing could be further from the truth. Interviewing may be defined as a guided communication process between two people with the predetermined purpose of sharing, obtaining, and verifying specific information by the asking and answering of questions.[3]

The goal is to collect accurate information during the Nutrition Assessment as the basis for a Nutrition Diagnosis and Intervention, setting goals, and solving problems while maintaining an interpersonal environment conducive to full disclosure.[3] Professionals rely on interviewing skills to facilitate rapport as well as to gather information.

This chapter covers the basics of interviewing skills. Included are the principles and process of interviews, the conditions facilitating interviews, the three parts of an interview, the use of different types of questions, and the types of interviewee responses. One must be aware of variables including the impact of the environment, verbal and nonverbal communication interactions, perceptions and roles of the two parties, needs and interests, personalities, attitudes, beliefs, values, and feedback. Culture may impact how much is disclosed. To become a skilled interviewer takes time and practice until the principles and techniques come naturally.

An effective interviewer must be a good listener. The interviewer concentrates on both the verbal responses and the nonverbal behavior, or body language, of the respondent. To discover what is important to the person, one listens and notices not only facts, but also emotions, attitudes, feelings, and values. A person newly diagnosed with diabetes mellitus, for example, may be upset or anxious. These emotions need to be recognized and dealt with.

To illustrate the principles and process, two examples of interviews are presented in this chapter—the food and nutrition interview and the preemployment interview. Although a full explanation of the content of these types of interviews is beyond the scope of this book, more detailed information may be found in other sources.[3–8]

Nutrition Interviews

A food and nutrition interview, or diet history, is an account of a person's food habits, preferences, eating behaviors, and other factors influencing food choices. Some clients may have tracked their own dietary intake on the computer. Effective interviews depend on the client's memory and cooperation as well as the skill of the interviewer. An initial Nutrition Assessment interview serves one or more purposes.[2]

- Makes the professional and client aware of current dietary practices and their origins, influential lifestyle factors, and related information.
- Identifies any nutrition-related problems and screens for malnutrition so that an appropriate Nutrition Diagnosis and Intervention is planned.

- Contributes to defining the nutritional status of the client in conjunction with other data.
- Defines problems and issues so that realistic goals for change may be set.
- Helps the professional identify possible alternatives so that changes may be considered.
- Provides baseline data against which to monitor changes and progress.
- Enables the counselor to continue to develop rapport and a good relationship with the client.

The medical record is a source of information on height, weight, past and current health history, and psychosocial factors, such as age, occupation, family size, educational level, and the like. In completing the food and nutrition history, the professional may collect specific information to identify food and nutrition-related problems.[6–8]

1. The consumption of food (i.e., intake of foods, timing/location and patterns of meals and snacks, food portions, cues to eating, nutrition and herbal supplements, previous/current diets or restrictions, and intolerances).
2. Knowledge of nutrition and health (i.e., knowledge and beliefs about nutrition, self-monitoring and self-care practices, previous nutrition counseling and education, and readiness to learn).
3. Physical activity and exercise (i.e., activity patterns, sedentary time, and exercise frequency, intensity, and duration).
4. Food availability (i.e., family food planning, purchasing, and preparation abilities, food safety, food and nutrition assistance program utilization, and food insecurity).

CASE ANALYSIS 1

What specific questions would you ask Mrs. Maynard in obtaining her food and nutrition history? Why are they important?

Dietary Assessment

Methods of assessment include dietary records, spoken or printed dietary recalls, food frequency questionnaires, and computer applications to improve accuracy.[9] Because much is based on self-reporting, there is no gold standard method for obtaining information about a person's dietary intake, but approaches used frequently are the 24-hour recall, the food record of usual daily food intake, and the food-frequency questionnaire (FFQ).

In a 24-hour recall, the interviewer asks the client to recount the types and amounts of all foods and beverages consumed, including preparation methods, portion sizes, and dietary supplements in the previous 24-hour period.[10-12] It has the advantage of being based on short-term memory.

To enhance memory, one may prompt the individual to recall the day of the week, time of day, where the meal was eaten (home, work, restaurant), other events that happened during the day (watching television, exercising, e-mail, shopping), and others who were present (family, friends). Clients may be asked to bring food records to future appointments which will show day-to-day variations. Written instructions and recording forms may be provided. The National Cancer Institute (NCI) has an automatic self-administered 24-hour recall used in research as well as a Canadian Diet History Questionnaire.[13]

The second method, the usual daily food intake, asks clients to explain the types and amounts of foods and beverages usually consumed during one day's time. Responses show what the person typically eats and drinks during meals and snacks. In both approaches, the portion sizes, the methods of food preparation (frying versus baking), the between-meal snacks, the time and place food is consumed, the condiments, the use of vitamin and mineral supplements or alternative nutrition therapies, and any alcoholic beverages consumed require consideration.

A third method is a food frequency questionnaire. This food and beverage checklist identifies the daily, weekly, or monthly frequency of a client's consumption of basic foods and beverages, such as milk and dairy products, meats–fish–poultry, eggs, fruits and fruit juices, vegetables and salads, breads and cereals, desserts and sweets, butter–margarine–fats–oils, between-meal snacks, and beverages, including coffee, tea, soft drinks, and alcoholic beverages.[7] Another alternative is to ask the person to complete a 1- to 3-day food record as each item is consumed. Brand names, preparation methods, location where food is consumed, and portion sizes are noted.

No method is considered to have total accuracy in assessing the nutritional status of the client, and each has limitations and inherent inaccuracies, such as the following[7]:

- The previous 24-hour period may not have been typical or adequate to characterize a person's food intake.
- Weekends may differ from weekdays.
- There are seasonal variations.
- The person may be unable to judge portion sizes.
- The person may have memory lapses, lack motivation, or have literacy issues.
- There is underreporting, especially among the overweight.

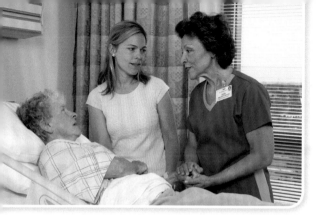

The professional interviews a client.

- Certain foods may be considered socially undesirable or unhealthy by clients, so they prefer not to reveal eating them.

The client's estimation of portion size is important. To overcome the problem of judging portion sizes, counselors may display three-dimensional food models, food pictures, serving utensils, dishes, measuring cups and spoons, and various sizes of beverage glasses. An 8-ounce glass is small, for example, compared with the large servings at convenience stores and fast-food restaurants.

CASE ANALYSIS 2

What questions would you ask Mrs. Maynard about food shopping and meal preparation?

The perception that large portions are appropriate to eat is called portion distortion. Consumers may have difficulty recognizing portions appropriate for their weight and activity level. Amorphous portions of foods such as potato chips, French fries, mashed potato, and popcorn may be difficult to visualize as are small portions such as spreads. A deck of cards, a baseball, or pieces of foam of various sizes can assist visualization. A selection of actual food packages, snack wrappers, food labels, and other resources may also be helpful.

Some reports indicate that clients may not volunteer information about foods they think others find less desirable. Examples of sensitive topics may include candy, desserts, alcoholic beverages, certain snacks, butter or margarine, take-out foods, binge eating, and others.[6] Underreporting of food intake is frequent. The client decides how sensitive the information is and what to provide.

New and future technologies when fully validated will improve practice as well as research. Self-reports of dietary intakes attained during interviews or keeping food records for 1 to 7 days are used. One study combined dietary recalls with pre- and postmeal digital photographs.[14] Innovations with mobile telephones capturing snacks and meals images and the use of wearable cameras provide image-based dietary records.[15] Image-assisted dietary assessments provide additional information.

Digital cameras, photographing meals and snacks, wearable cameras, and smartphones can record images of foods eaten. These supplement client data showing foods eaten, and portion sizes.[15-17] Wearable cameras have increased the accuracy of self-reports by showing unreported foods, such as snacks.[18] Using wearable cameras for 4 days when consuming food showed eating locations, portions, watching television, and environmental and social interactions.[19]

Digital camera photography was used to assess food intakes of adults and children using images of the foods selected and the plate waste as compared with standard portion sizes. In another study using a remote method, participants gathered information using apps downloaded to their smartphones. To estimate food intakes, they captured images of foods and leftovers which were sent wirelessly for analysis. Work will continue to improve on this method.[20]

Computer-administered FFQs or 24-hour recalls were found to improve the accuracy of paper-administered questionnaires. Recent technological and web-based methods for improving assessment in surveys and research are being used.[6] Other techniques are being tested.

To save time, a short dietary assessment using a diet history and/or FFQ can be narrowed to focus only on the person's health problem, such as emphasizing dietary sources of fat in heart disease, foods high in sodium in hypertension, or calcium and vitamin D in osteoporosis. One example is the MEDFICTS (**M**eats, **E**ggs, **D**airy, **F**ried foods, **I**n baked goods, **C**onvenience foods, **T**able fats, and **S**nacks) instrument used to evaluate adherence to Step 1 and 2 diets of the National Cholesterol Education Program. It concentrates on recording foods and portions contributing total fat, cholesterol, and saturated fat.[21,22]

Other short assessments include, for example, a 16-item questionnaire including photographs of foods being developed for Spanish speakers who are low-income and a lower-literate population.[23] Other examples are an online calcium quiz to screen for insufficient dietary calcium, a Brief Calcium Assessment Tool (BCAT) with 16 items,[23,24] and a FFQ to assess intake of n-3 polyunsaturated fatty acids.[25]

CASE ANALYSIS **3**

What questions would you ask related to Mrs. Maynard's family and lifestyle?

Preemployment Interviews

Interviewing skills are equally important in management positions where they are used to screen potential new employees, to obtain information from current employees, and to explore solutions to problems.[26] Managing human resources is a responsibility in many positions. An example is the preemployment interview used by a manager with prospective employees.

In preemployment interviews, several applicants are interviewed for a position to assess the person's credentials and skills for the job. After reviewing the application and resume, the interviewer communicates information about the job. A structured interview uses preplanned, standardized questions related to the job duties and requirements from the job description. Each applicant is asked the same questions.[4,5] This will decrease stereotypes and increase validity. Asking different questions of each applicant makes comparisons difficult.[4] A variation is to provide specific situations and ask how the person would respond.

One of the keys to finding out how a person will perform on a job is to analyze examples of past performance. A behavioral interview asks the person about actual situations from a previous job and how they were handled.[4] Competency-based hiring uses job descriptions emphasizing the knowledge, skills, and behaviors the person needs to perform the job, rather than a list of duties. In addition to knowledge and expertise needed to perform, behaviors may include, for example, computer and interpersonal skills. Other behaviors needed for success, such as initiative and collaboration with team members, are identified and discussed. Behavioral-based interviews focus on past job performances, challenges, and experiences as a measure of how a potential hire will perform on the job.[27]

Collecting previous examples expands on one's understanding of the candidate's work history, knowledge, previous experience, and motivation. The person may be asked to describe how a problem was solved or a decision was made, about a satisfying or challenging experience, or something learned in the past. Since Internet sites provide preemployment questions with answers, a behavioral interview specific to what the candidate has done and how it was done can be more helpful. For example, a person claiming computer skills needs to provide specific examples of what he or she has done.

Most interviews proceed in three stages or components: (1) introducing the process, (2) questioning by the interviewer as well as the interviewee, (3) with a closing including information on next steps and a timeline for each. At times a situational interview is presented, giving the candidate scenarios to explain what he or she would do.

The same interviewing principles and techniques are used, but for a different purpose. With potential employees, the interviewer wants to find the individual with the capability of performing the duties and responsibilities of the job according to the job-related knowledge, skills, abilities, and behaviors in the job description. Because federal legislation outlaws discrimination based on race, color, religion, gender, pregnancy, national origin, age 40 and over, and disability, questions about any of these are avoided as they may lead to costly lawsuits.[5] Those who need more information should consult additional resources.[4,5]

Conditions Facilitating Interviews

For best results, professionals need to increase their effectiveness as interviewers by doing the following[3]:

- Clearly define the purpose of the interview to the interviewee.
- Attend to verbal and nonverbal behaviors by listening and building rapport.
- Provide freedom from interruptions.
- Provide psychological privacy.
- Have appropriate physical surroundings.
- Have emotional objectivity.
- Consider the personal context of the respondent.
- Limit note taking or explain why notes are needed.

Purpose

The purpose distinguishes interviews from social conversations.[3] The interviewer needs to explain the purpose of the interview, or the respondent may be wondering why the questions are necessary. Without an answer, a person may be reluctant to respond. With healthcare clients, one can stress that the interview is necessary to provide assistance with healthcare recommendations. For example: "Let's do a careful evaluation of the foods you eat and see if we find any suggestions for improving your choices." With job applicants, note that it is important to find an employee who will be satisfied with the company and the position. If the purpose is clear and understood, better cooperation from the interviewee may be expected.

CASE ANALYSIS **4**

What is the purpose of the interview with Mrs. Maynard?

Attentiveness and Rapport

Professionals need skills in listening—an active, not a passive, process that requires a great deal of concentration. Listening attentively helps to build a collaborative relationship with the person and to create a climate in which the interviewee can communicate easily. The interviewer should listen carefully and assist respondents in communicating their thoughts, feelings, and information. The conversation includes both verbal and nonverbal behaviors. Periodically paraphrasing or summarizing confirms that you are listening and trying to understand.

Bear in mind that the interviewee is also observing you. Frequent looking at one's watch, using electronic devices, failure to maintain eye contact, sitting back in too relaxed a posture, frowning, yawning, and tone of voice all may convey a negative message and inhibit effective interviews. Attentiveness may be shown, for example, by appropriate nonverbal behaviors such as friendly eye contact, interested facial expression, good posture, smiling, and nodding.

It is normal for people to experience some discomfort or reluctance during interviews. Rapport is the personal relationship established between the interviewer and the respondent. Rapport should be established early and continue to be developed. It is important to build a friendly and supportive climate, to release stress, to put the person at ease, to build trust, and to provide nonjudgmental verbal and nonverbal responses no matter what the person says.[3] The person's disclosure should not be labeled "right" or "wrong."

The interviewer strives to create an environment of respect and trust by arranging conditions in which individuals perceive themselves as accepted, warmly received, valued, and understood. Trust must be earned; without it, vital self-disclosure on the part of the respondent may be limited. Setting oneself up as the "expert" and the respondent as the "receiver of one's expertise" inhibits relationships. "I've had a lot of experience with this and will be able to tell you what to do," is not a helpful approach. Respondents overwhelmed by the professional's expertise and position may reply with information they think is sought or acceptable instead of what is useful.

Rapport may be inhibited by addressing people by their first names. This may be interpreted as too informal or a lack of respect by some people and in certain cultures. A woman 72 years of age, for example, may not like being called "Martha" by someone who is 30 years old. When in doubt, use both names, such as "Martha Smith," "Mrs. Smith," or a query "Would you prefer to be addressed as Mrs. Smith or Martha?" Also tell how you wish to be addressed. Addressing yourself by your surname and the client by the first name creates a superior–subordinate relationship.

Freedom from Interruptions

To devote full attention to the interviewee, the professional should arrange to have phone calls held and turn off cell phones. If a call must be answered, the phone conversation should be brief, with apologies given to the interviewee. In the hospital setting, asking to turn off the television, closing the door, and selecting a time when staff and visitors are less likely to interrupt are advisable. The setting should be comfortable, quiet, and private.

Psychological Privacy

Since private matters will be discussed, the interviewer and interviewee should be alone. A quiet office without interruption is preferable. At the patient's hospital bedside, however, others may be present in the room. Whenever possible, arrange the setting so that the interview cannot be overheard and is not interrupted; this promotes the giving of undivided attention and that adheres to Health Insurance Portability and Accountability Act (HIPAA) requirements. Assure the interviewee that their information will be treated confidentially and shared only with pertinent healthcare providers.

Physical Surroundings

A comfortable environment with proper furniture, lighting, temperature, ventilation, and pleasant surroundings can enhance an interview. A setting should be arranged in which eye contact can be maintained. Since standing over a patient lying in a hospital bed may trigger deferential behavior, it is preferable to be at the same head level. The optimum distance between people involved in an interview is 2 to 4 ft (0.6 to 1.2 m), about an arm's length, but cultural practices differ.[3]

The most formal seating arrangement is for one person to sit across the desk from another, whereas a chair alongside the desk is less formal and makes people feel more equal. Two parties seated without a table is informal, but when viewing materials, a round table is less formal than a square or rectangle because it eliminates the head-of-the-table position. In general, the fewer the barriers in the line of sight, the better. A desk top with a computer, telephone, books, plants, and other materials between you and the client is a psychological barrier.

Emotional Objectivity

The patient should feel free to express all feelings, attitudes, and values. An attitude of acceptance and concern for the interviewee should be maintained, with a desire to understand behavior rather than pass judgment. A raised eyebrow, look of shock, surprise, or amusement, or an incredulous follow-up question (e.g., "You had three beers for lunch?" or "All you had for lunch was a box of cookies?") may cause the client to change or end the story.

Interviewers need to develop an awareness of their own conscious and unconscious values, biases, and prejudices. These include not only racial, ethnic, and religious preferences, but also exaggerated dislikes of people and their characteristics. Examples may include the poorly dressed, the less educated, aggressive women, meek men, highly pitched voices, or weak handshakes. Identifying your own intolerances may help to control any expression of them through nonverbal behaviors.

Personal Context

People bring with them their own personal contexts or systems of beliefs, attitudes, feelings, and values that must be recognized. Concerns about perceived threats to health can be so frightening, for example, that they preoccupy thoughts and block conversation. Interviewers need to recognize the respondent's situation and the subjective and objective aspects of it. After a heart attack, for example, a man may feel fear, resentment, anger, anxiety, dependence, or regression, which may interfere with concentration and cooperation. An understanding of the psychological reactions to illness and ways of dealing with them is helpful.

The professional relationship is most easily established with persons similar to ourselves, whereas barriers may arise with others. Interviews should be age-appropriate and population-specific with lists of foods based on the population's dietary habits.[7] A thorough understanding of the food choices and practices of various groups is important.

People from all socioeconomic groups, various cultural and ethnic groups, and ages from young to elderly participate differently in the professional relationship. Eye contact and other nonverbal behaviors should be culturally appropriate. Young children, for example, are not used to talking with adults other than family and friends. Knowing the child's vocabulary level is helpful.

The interviewer may need to facilitate the venting of feelings and to acknowledge them before proceeding with the interview. A job applicant, for example, may have been laid off recently from a long-time position. The way the person feels about the situation, however, is as important as the facts. Anxiety, nervousness, and other emotions may be evident. The manager should be alert to verbal and nonverbal clues as they give a frame of reference for understanding.

CASE ANALYSIS 5

What would you discuss with Mrs. Maynard about her previous attempts to lose weight?

Usually, the practitioner has some background information about the person in advance. In the hospital setting, the medical record is the source of information on the social, cultural, and economic circumstances, marital status, number in the household, age, employment, religion, level of education, physical health, medications, weight and height, medical history, and results of lab tests and X-rays. In preemployment interviews, the application form and resume

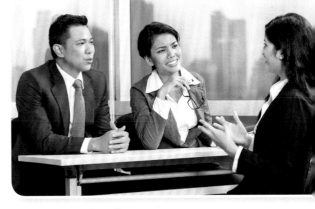

A preemployment interview.

should be examined before the interview, since they contain information on education and previous work experience.

Note Taking

Taking too many notes hampers the flow of conversation, inhibits rapport, and prevents the interviewer's concentration on the verbal and nonverbal answers of the respondent. In addition, the interviewee may be distracted or apprehensive about what is being written. An inexperienced interviewer, however, may find it necessary to take some notes. If so, they should be brief. To avoid concern, the individual should ask the interviewee's permission to jot down a few notes and should explain why they are necessary and how they will be used. The practitioner may say, for example: "Is it all right if I take a few notes so that I can review what we said later?"

While writing, try to maintain eye contact as much as possible. One needs to develop a few key words, phrases, or abbreviations to use. A breakfast of orange juice, cereal, toast, and coffee with cream and sugar, for example, may be abbreviated, "OJ, cer, tst, C-C-S," while a pineapple–cottage cheese salad may be noted as "P/A-CC sld."

Comprehensive notes should be dictated or recorded immediately after the person has departed. Waiting 15 minutes or longer, seeing another client or job applicant, or accepting phone calls may cause the interviewer to forget essential information.

During the interview, one can examine not only what the person says, but also what is not said. Are there gaps that the interviewer should be trying to fill? Also note nonverbal behaviors, such as tension, inability to maintain eye contact, hand movements, fidgeting, and facial expressions of discomfort, nervousness, anger, or lack of understanding. The nonverbal behaviors may be inconsistent with the verbal message, or may add to it.

Although practitioners adjust the pace of the interview to that of the respondent, they are also responsible for the direction of the interview. When the topics for discussion are inappropriate, the skilled interviewer brings the conversation back to appropriate ones. The client talking about his wife or children, for example, must be brought gently back to the nutrition history. A job applicant discussing a recent visit to Spain must be brought back to relevant topics. People who are especially talkative may ramble frequently, requiring more direction on the part of the interviewer. In these cases, restating or emphasizing the last thing said that was pertinent to the interview and asking a related question can be helpful.

Parts of the Interview

Each interview can be divided into three parts: (1) the opening, (2) exploration or body of the interview, and (3) closing.

The beginning of the interview, or opening, involves a greeting, introductions, and establishing rapport, a process of creating trust and goodwill between the parties.[3] The exploration phase includes the use of questions to obtain information while maintaining the personal relationship, as the interviewer guides and directs the interview with responses. In the final phase, the interview is closed and any future contacts are planned. Table 3-1 summarizes the interview process.

Opening

The opening sets the tone of the interview—friendly or unfriendly, professional or informal, relaxed or tense, leisurely or rushed—and influences how the interviewee perceives you. Practitioners should greet the client

Phases	Tasks
Opening	Introductions and overview
	Establish rapport
	Discuss purpose
Exploration or Body	Gather information with questions
	Explore problems
	Explore both thoughts and feelings
	Continue building rapport
Closing	Express appreciation
	Review purpose; ask for comments or questions. Plan future contacts.

Table 3-1 ■ The Interview Process

and state their name and job title, for example, "Good morning. I'm Judy Jones, a registered dietitian nutritionist." A smile, eye contact, a handshake or placing a hand on the other's hand or arm, with a friendly face and tone of voice are supporting nonverbal behaviors.[3]

In the hospital setting, the interviewer may ask, "Are you Mary Johnson?" If answered affirmatively, you may respond, "I'm glad to meet you. Do you prefer to be addressed as Mrs. Johnson or as Mary?" The professional may add how he or she prefers to be addressed, such as "Please call me Mike."

If the patient's physician has requested the contact, the interviewer may mention this. "Did Dr. Smith tell you that he asked me to visit you?" If the answer is "no," explain about the physician's request. A discussion of the nature and purpose of the interview may follow, along with how the individual will benefit. For example: "Dr. Smith mentioned that you have high blood pressure. He asked me to talk with you and see whether we can find a way to reduce the amount of salt and sodium in the foods you eat. This is one way to help you control your blood pressure."

Before unleashing a barrage of questions, a few minutes may be spent on other topics to develop some rapport. A dialogue, not a monologue, is appropriate. Discussion of known information from the medical record or from the application form or resume of job applicants may be appropriate. Alternatively, the weather, sporting events, holidays, a national or international event, traffic, parking, or any topic of joint interest may be helpful in opening the discussion. Although one has a task to complete, small talk is important in developing and building the relationship. It should not be prolonged, however, or the interviewee may be wondering when you will get to the purpose of the discussion. A time frame for the interview may be mentioned.

When interviewees initiate the appointment, it is preferable to let them state in their own words their problem or purpose for coming. The manager may ask, "What brought you to the Friendly Company to seek employment, Mr. Smithfield?" or for a client, "How have things been going since your last appointment when we talked about your goals for weight loss?" Or "When we talked on the phone, Mrs. Jones, you mentioned that your doctor told you that you have borderline diabetes. How can I help?" When interviewees are given the chance to express themselves first, the interview begins with their agenda, or what they think is important.

Although it may seem time-consuming, the opening exchange of either information or pleasantries is important and should not be omitted. It creates a positive climate for open communication.[26] Rapport, a degree of warmth, a supportive atmosphere, and a sense of mutual involvement are critical components in the interview. Willingness to disclose information about oneself is influenced by the level of trust established in the relationship, and cooperation and disclosure are crucial to success.

Interviewees quickly develop perceptions of the situation and make decisions about the amount and kind of information they will share. They form impressions of the interviewer just as the professional does of them. Before directing the conversation to the second stage, the purpose, goals, or nature of the interview, the length, and how the information will be used, should be clearly stated and understood so the person knows what to expect.[3]

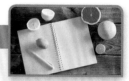

SELF-ASSESSMENT 1

How satisfactory are the following openings? How can they be improved?

Employee Interview:
1. "Come on in. I'm very busy today, but need to hire a new employee. Do you have any work experience?"
2. "Hi, I'm Steve Johnson (shaking hands). We're looking for a cook for early shift. Do you prefer early hours or late?"

Patient/Client Interview:
1. "Hi, Mr. Jones. I'm Mary, a nutritionist. Have you been on a diabetic diet before?"
2. Entering patient room: "Good morning, Julia. What's up? How are you guys doing today? I'm here to tell you what to eat on a sodium-restricted diet."

Exploration or Body

In the second stage, the exploration or body of the interview, the interviewee is asked a series of questions; these are the tools used to obtain information. They are not spur of the moment. A good interviewer has carefully preplanned these questions in a prepared "interview guide," an outline of the information desired or topics to be covered that are relevant to the clear purpose of the interview.[3] The guide should tell not only what questions will be asked, but also how questions will be phrased to gain the most information in the limited time available. With practice, a natural flow will occur. Effective interviewers speak extemporaneously rather than following a scripted, preplanned message.[26]

Topics should be arranged in a definite sequence. In a nutrition or diet history, for example, the interviewer may desire information about foods and beverages consumed, eating in restaurants, portion sizes, meals, methods of food preparation, and snacks. Put in sequence, the list includes meals, portion sizes, methods of food preparation, snacks, beverages, and eating in restaurants. See Box 3-1 for questions and directives for diet histories.

In a preemployment interview, the sequence may be examples of previous work experiences, career goals, education, present activities and interests that are job-related, and personal qualifications. Specific questions intended

1. "Who plans and prepares the meals at home? Who does the grocery shopping?"

2. "Are you currently restricting your food choices in any way?" (because of allergy, religion, intolerance, etc.)

3. "Please tell me about any questions or issues you have in making food choices; about the people in your family who eat together and any dietary problems they have."

4. "How physically active are you?"

5. "Now I am going to ask you to think of all the foods and beverages you consume in a typical day. Please tell me about the first food or drink you have after arising and the portion size of that food."

6. "That's good. Now tell me about what you eat and drink next including the amount."

7. "And then, what would you eat or drink next?"

8. "What types of seasonings do you use in cooking? Tell me about them."

9. "Snacks and beverages are often forgotten. What do you have between each of your meals and during the evening or before bed?"

10. "You haven't mentioned alcoholic beverages, including beer and wine. Please tell me about them?"

11. "How often do you take a vitamin–mineral supplement or use herbs or alternative therapies? Please describe the kinds and amounts."

12. "What time of day are your meals?"

13. "How many times a week do you eat a meal away from home? What would you have?"

14. "Would you say that the amounts of foods you have described are typical, more than usual, or less than usual?"

15. "To summarize what you have told me, can you tell me how many servings you eat daily or weekly of these foods?" (continue with a food-frequency checklist)

Box 3-1 ■ Examples of Questions and Directives for Diet Histories

to gain information about the applicant's qualifications, compared with those in the job description, should be planned in advance.

Although it ensures that information is gathered in a systematic manner, the interview guide should not be followed strictly. Questions should be adapted for age, region, and population group. Never read from the list of questions or try to follow a predetermined sequence. The interviewer should be thoroughly familiar with the questions and not have to refer to them constantly. When the interviewee brings up a topic or asks a question, this shows interest and should be pursued. Knowing the purpose and significance of each question is important so that questions are not asked in a perfunctory manner and so the interviewer does not accept superficial or inadequate answers.

Asking a job applicant about offices held in organizations, for example, is an attempt to seek information about leadership ability and the acceptance of responsibility. The technique of inquiring about career plans over the next 3 to 5 years attempts to learn about short- and long-range goals. To answer fully, interviewees must view the questions as relevant. With clients and patients, the professional can explain that the answers are a basis for a nutrition assessment, counseling, or education. See Box 3-2 for preemployment interview questions.

In general, questions asked in preemployment interviews should be job related or predictive of success on the job. They should elicit information to compare the individual's qualifications and interests with those of the job description for the vacant position. For example:

1. "Now I would like to ask you some questions about yourself and your previous work experience." Introduces the line of questioning.
2. "Tell me about your previous work experience and how it relates to the job you are interested in." Gives general impressions of whether the person is qualified.
3. "Please describe for me two important accomplishments in your previous job." Gives abilities.
4. "What were your responsibilities on your previous job?" Gives knowledge, skills, and abilities.
5. "What would you say are your greatest strengths as a worker? Areas to improve?" Gives skills and abilities.
6. "What kind of work interests you?" Tells interest and motivation.
7. "What organizations do you belong to that are relevant to the job you are applying for?" Shows interests and interpersonal skills.
8. "What offices have you held?" Shows leadership ability and acceptance of responsibility.
9. "What are your career goals? Where do you see yourself in 3 to 5 years?" Shows whether the person plans ahead and whether plans are congruent with those of the company.
10. "What hours do you prefer to work? How flexible is your schedule?"
11. "What brought you to our company to apply for work? Why would you like to work for us?" Tells whether the person is knowledgeable about the company.
12. "Do you prefer to work alone or in a group?" Tells if the person would work well in a team environment.
13. "Tell me about a time at your last job when teamwork was important."

Box 3-2 ■ Sample Preemployment Interview Questions

14. "Tell me about a problem you solved at work and how you solved it."
15. "Describe how you made an important decision at work."

Questions that *should not be* asked

Certain subjects can be the basis for complaints of discrimination on the basis of race, color, gender, marital status, national origin, religion, age, and disability. For this reason, the following questions are examples of ones that should be avoided in preemployment interviews. If the questions are not job related, do not ask.

1. "What is your nationality and native language?" "Place of birth?"
2. "What is your religious affiliation?"
3. "What is your marital status?" "Spouse's name?" "What is your maiden name?"
4. "Where does your spouse work?" "What does he/she think of your working?"
5. "Do you have a family or plans to start one?" "Who will baby-sit for you?"
6. "What is your date of birth?" "Date of graduation from school?" "Age?"

Box 3-2 ▪ (*continued*)

Using Questions

Questions play a major role in interviews as tools of the trade. The wording of questions is as important as one's manner and tone of voice. A friendly approach in asking the questions communicates the desire to understand and be of assistance. The kind of questions asked should require the other person to talk 60% to 70% of the time. Questions that are highly specific or may be answered with one word, such as "yes" or "no," should be avoided initially, but may be necessary to follow up on specific information. A skilled person listens and evaluates each answer and may probe further.

Questions may be classified in several ways: open or closed, primary or secondary, probing, and neutral or leading.[3]

Open and Closed Questions

Open questions are broad and give the interviewee great freedom in deciding what facts, thoughts, and feelings to express while giving the professional an opportunity to listen and observe. Open questions allow people to tell their story.[28] The following are examples of open questions:

"Will you tell me a little about yourself?"
"What are some foods you like to eat during the day?"
"What have you done in the past to try to lose weight?"
"What made you decide to seek employment here?"

At the beginning of an interview, open questions are less threatening and communicate more interest and trust; answers reveal what the interviewee thinks is most important.

Disadvantages are that they may involve a greater amount of time, the collection of unnecessary information, and lengthy, disorganized answers.[3]

The following are examples of open questions with moderate restrictions:

"Can you tell me about the types of meals you eat during the day?"

"What did the doctor tell you about your health and diet?"

"What were your job responsibilities in your previous position?"

"How did you become interested in this position?"

"What skills do you have that are important for this job?"

CASE ANALYSIS 6

What topics would you like to discuss with Mrs. Maynard about controlling her blood pressure?

In follow-up visits, open questions should be broad to allow the client to determine the focus of the interview. Examples are, "How are your dietary goals progressing?" or "What progress have you made since we last talked?" The counselor should begin discussion with whatever is of current concern to the client. For opening questions, the interviewer should also refer to the records regarding the client's background, problems, and previous counseling goals.

Closed questions are more restrictive; that is, they control the length of answers while obtaining a single fact or missing information. Some closed questions are more limiting than others, such as:

"Who cooks the food at home?"

"Do you salt your food?"

"Tell me about any snacks you eat between meals."

"What special diet or food restrictions, if any, do you follow?"

Closed questions give the interviewer more control, require less effort from the interviewee, and are less time consuming, which is of value when only a short screening is needed.[3] Disadvantages include the inhibition of communication, which might result if the interviewer shows little interest in the answers, and the need for additional questions to obtain information. Table 3-2 summarizes the advantages and disadvantages of the different kinds of questions.

Type of Questions	Advantages	Disadvantages
Open	Gives interviewee control	Time consuming
	Communicates trust/interest	Supplies unneeded information
	Less threatening	
	Tells what the person thinks is important	
Closed	Gives interviewer control	Provides incomplete answers
	Provides quick answers	Short answers force more questions
	Verifies information	
Primary	Introduces new topics	
Secondary	Elicits further information	
Leading		Directs person's answer
		Reveals bias of interviewer
Neutral	More accurate answers	

Table 3-2 ■ Advantages and Disadvantages of Questions

Primary and Secondary Questions

Questions may also be classified as primary or secondary. Primary questions or requests are used to introduce topics or new areas of discussion. The following are examples:

> "Now that we have discussed your most recent position, please tell me about your former job with Smith & Company."

> "Now that we have discussed the foods you eat at home, please tell me about what you eat when you go to restaurants."

Note that mentioning what was just said shows that you have been listening.

Secondary questions, also referred to as "follow-up" questions, are requests to obtain further information or explanation that primary questions have failed to elicit.[3] Interviewees may have given an inadequate response for many reasons, including poor memory, misunderstanding of the question or amount of detail needed, and the feeling that the question is too personal or irrelevant. Specific follow-up questions, such as the following, may be asked:

> "What do you have for dessert?"

"What other beverages do you drink?"

"In your previous position, how many people did you supervise?"

Probing

Although the client may not be able to answer the preceding questions on the spur of the moment, short-term memory of foods can be improved with some prompting. The client may be reminded of the day of the week, where he or she spent the day, whether meals were eaten at home or at a restaurant, whether others were present, and so on.

Probing questions are secondary questions that ask clients to clarify partial responses or to continue.[26] For example:

"Could you elaborate on. . ."

"Will you tell me more about. . ."

Neutral and Leading Questions

Neutral questions are preferred to leading questions. Neutral questions allow the respondent to decide the answer, whereas leading questions direct the respondent toward one answer, an effect that may be unintentional on the part of an inexperienced interviewer.[3] Leading questions suggest an expected answer, as in the following examples:

"You drink milk, don't you?" "Yes, of course." Instead, ask: "What beverages do you drink?"

"You aren't going to eat desserts anymore, are you?" "No." Instead ask: "What will you have for dessert?"

"Breakfast is SO important. What do you have? Cereal?" Instead ask: "What do you have to eat and drink first after you wake up in the morning?"

One of these questions assumes the client eats breakfast, and in these instances people may answer even if they usually omit the meal. Clients may change their answers on the basis of a nonverbal appearance of the practitioner of surprise, disgust, dislike, or disagreement with what clients are saying. To receive uninhibited responses from clients, the interviewer needs to avoid these appearances.

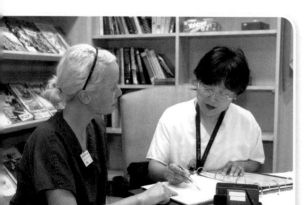

Discussing interview information.
Source: Photo by Joe Mitchell.

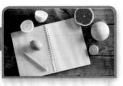

SELF-ASSESSMENT 2

Directions: Identify the following questions as open, closed, primary, secondary, or leading.

1. "You mentioned that the only meal you eat at home is dinner. Can you tell me where you eat your breakfast and lunch and what you are likely to have?"
2. "Do you put mustard on your hamburger?"
3. "What do you put on your salad?"
4. "How do you cook your meats?"

Directives

When you as the interviewer sense that too many questions are being asked and the respondent may be developing a feeling of interrogation, you may introduce some questions as a statement or directive. For example: "How has your diet been going?" may be changed to "I'd be interested in hearing how your diet has been going."

"How did you become interested in this position?" may be changed to "I'd be interested in some of the reasons you decided to apply for this position." This makes the interview more conversational. Questions should be asked one at a time and the interviewer should concentrate on listening carefully to the answers rather than thinking ahead to the next question.

Sequencing Questions

Questions can be arranged in a "funnel," "inverted funnel," or "tunnel" sequence. A funnel sequence begins with broad, open questions and proceeds to more restrictive or closed ones.[3,26] The funnel sequence is a series of questions, each covering a different topic to gain specific information. It may be an appropriate choice in a nutrition interview.

> **EXAMPLE** "Please tell me about the foods you eat during a day's time."
> "What do you have for snacks between meals?"
> "We haven't discussed beverages—what do you like to drink?"

Beginning the interview with open ended questions poses the least threat to the person and encourages a response.[28] The person then volunteers information, making it unnecessary to ask additional questions. An inverted funnel sequence may be preferable. In preemployment interviews, for example, an apprehensive applicant may feel more comfortable initially dealing with a specific closed question than with a broad, open one, such as "Tell me about yourself." As the meeting progresses, questions may become more open.[26]

In taking a food and nutrition history, questions or statements starting with "What" or "Tell me about" elicit better responses than "Do you . . .?" Review diet history examples in Box 3-1. Questions that do not require a sufficient answer or may be answered with one word or "yes" or "no" are less productive, as in the following examples:

> **EXAMPLE**   "Do you eat breakfast?" "Yes."
> "Do you like milk?" "No."
> "How often do you eat meat?" "Every day."

A series of short, sequential, dead-end questions from the professional's list of information to be gathered prevents people from telling their story and information may be omitted as a result. Instead, gather this information using a broad opening question or directives, as follows:

> **EXAMPLE**   "Please tell me about the first foods and drinks you have most days, what you eat, and the amount."

"Why" Questions

Some recommend avoiding questions beginning with why. "Why" may indicate one's disapproval, displeasure, or mistrust, thus provoking defensive feelings, as it appears to ask the person to justify or explain his or her behavior. For example:

> "Why don't you follow your diet more closely?"
> "Why don't you eat breakfast?"
> "Why don't you exercise more often?"
> "Why did you resign from your job?"

Clients may react defensively or explain their behavior in a manner they believe is acceptable.

> "I don't follow my diet because I don't like it. You wouldn't like it either."
> "I can eat breakfast if you think I should."
> "I don't exercise because I don't have time. Do you exercise?"
> "I resigned because there was no chance for advancement."

If threatened by a "why" question and unwilling to reveal the answer, the individual may answer in an evasive manner, in which case nothing is gained.

Responses

After the client answers, the interviewer may respond in one of several ways. Some responses are recommended and others are less helpful. They include the following: (1) Understanding responses, (2) Probing responses, (3) Confrontational responses, (4) Evaluative responses, (5) Hostile responses, and (6) Reassuring responses.

Understanding Responses

The understanding response is one of the best choices. With it, practitioners try to understand the person's message and recreate it within their own frame of reference. People have more rapport with those who try to understand them rather than judge them. This may lead to more cooperation on the part of the client.

> **EXAMPLE**   Mrs. Jones: "I haven't lost any weight this week. I ate just a few cookies. The diet doesn't work."
> Counselor, paraphrasing a feeling rather than a fact: "You are feeling concerned because you haven't lost any weight, Mrs. Jones, and you are wondering if it was something you ate, or a problem with the diet?"

The paraphrase in this understanding response helps the person feel accepted even if her behavior was not perfect. The client will feel safe in expressing her sentiments and exploring them further. Note that the professional should focus on Mrs. Jones's feelings and attitudes, rather than only on the content of what she said. She may be feeling guilty, concerned, or disappointed with the diet or with herself. The counselor has guessed "concerned," and if this is not correct, Mrs. Jones will correct the mistaken impression, thus furthering one's understanding and demonstrating that one is trying to understand.

The understanding response is most helpful in assisting clients to recognize problems and to devise their own solutions. The client may progress from initial negative feelings to more neutral ones and finally to more positive attitudes and solutions.

It is necessary to differentiate and understand both the content and the feelings of the client's remarks. To determine the content, you may ask yourself, "What is this person telling me or thinking?" Feelings may be classified as positive, negative, or ambivalent, and these may change as the interview progresses.

Paraphrasing, discussed in Chapter 2, checks your understanding. It is part of empathy which refers to the professional's attempt to accurately experience the person's world and communicate that understanding to the interviewee. It reflects the content of what the client said in your words to ensure that communication is understood. To verify understanding, use the following sentence in paraphrasing. The answer may be inserted into a format.

> **EXAMPLE**   "I think I hear you saying that you feel. . . because. . ."

To avoid overuse of the same phrase or sounding mechanistic, the phrase can be varied.

> **EXAMPLE**   "Do I understand correctly that you feel. . .?"
> "You seem to be saying that you are feeling. . ."
> "I gather that. . ."
> "You sound. . ."
> "In other words, you are feeling. . ."

Interviewee responses that suggest feelings about an event may provide an important key to the person's behavior. How clients feel about their lifestyles, food habits or choices, or their health is critical to dietary adherence. Food behaviors may be influenced by psychological, cultural, and environmental variables that are important to understand.

Job applicants may also express feelings about previous work experience, relationships with superiors and subordinates, and activities and interests. Preceding a statement with "I feel . . .," "I think . . .," or "I believe . . ." gives a signal that the statement expresses opinions, beliefs, attitudes, or values. Possible follow-up probes are included in the following examples:

> **EXAMPLE**   "Can you explain more about your feelings?"
> "What do you think about that?"
> "What do you think causes that?"

Some men may find exploring feelings and emotions difficult and some cultures may value restraint of feelings.

Probing Responses

The probing response is helpful in clarifying or in gaining additional information as people recall details. In dietary interviews, for example, details about food quantities, added ingredients, food preparation methods, and snacks are probed frequently. Probing implies that the person should give more information so that the counselor may understand.

> **EXAMPLE**   Mrs. Jones: "I haven't lost any weight this week. I ate just a few cookies. The diet doesn't work."
> Counselor: "You seem to think the diet doesn't work. I wonder if you could tell me a little more about that."

Rather than giving advice, which may be tempting or even an automatic response, this response helps the person tell her story, and further information can be obtained.

There are many probing techniques, which may be used in addition to secondary or follow-up questions. They should be nonthreatening, nonjudgmental, and nondirective to avoid leading people to specific answers. A brief silence may be effective, as may repetition of the last phrase spoken by the client, or a summary sentence. Probing further in the case of superficial and vague responses, as well as probing for feelings about events, is suggested in the following paragraphs.

When a more detailed response is desired in the case of superficial answers, the following may be asked:

> **EXAMPLE**   "Can you tell me more about that?"
> "What do you do next?"
> "Please explain a little more about . . ."
> "What else?"

To obtain clarification if the answer is vague, you may respond:

> **EXAMPLE**   "Could you clarify for me what you meant by. . .?" "I don't think I quite understand. . ."

Paraphrasing is another technique to ensure that the information is clear and correct. By repeating, summarizing, or rewording what was said, interviewers show that they are trying to understand.

When the person seems hesitant to go on, the interviewer may remain silent, pausing for the respondent to gather his or her thoughts and continue. The professional should appear attentive, with perhaps a thoughtful or expectant look, but should avoid eye contact for the moment. The inexperienced interviewer may find silence uncomfortable and push on

"Go on."

"I see."

"I understand, Mrs. Jones. Please continue."

"Uh huh."

"Hmmmm."

"And next."

"Oh?" or "Oh!"

"Really?"

"Very good!"

"That's interesting."

Box 3-3 ■ Other Probes

too quickly. If the respondent does not go on within 30 to 60 seconds, however, he or she may perceive the silence as disinterest or disapproval; the interviewer should commence before such an impression occurs. See Box 3-3 for other probes.

A technique useful in breaking a silence is to repeat or echo the last phrase or sentence the person has said, raising the tone of voice to a question.

> **EXAMPLE** "I follow my diet except when I eat out."
> "Except when you eat out?"
> "I especially enjoy doing special projects with coworkers."
> "Special projects with coworkers?"

Repetition, however, should not be overdone, or it has a parrot-like effect. If this is noticed, it will inhibit conversation.

A summary sentence stated as a question also elicits further elaboration.

> **EXAMPLE** "You say that you already know how to plan a diabetic diet?"
> "You think this company is the one you want to work for?"

"I see," "I understand," and "that's interesting" may give a feeling of acceptance and encourage conversation or elaboration of a point of view. "Very good" gives the person a pat on the back and is another kind of acceptance. Nonverbal probes include giving a quizzical look, leaning forward in the chair, and nodding of the head occasionally.[3]

Confrontational Responses

Confrontation is an authority-laden response in which the interviewer tactfully and tentatively calls to the person's attention some inconsistency or discrepancy in the client's story, words, or actions by pointing out the discrepancy to the client, such as claiming to follow the diet, but has not lost weight.

This response challenges and encourages the person to recognize and cope psychologically with some aspect of behavior that is self-defeating or to examine the consequences of some behavior. It should be said non-judgmentally as discussion centers on resolution of problems.

Confrontation is an advanced level skill that should seldom be used by an inexperienced interviewer or when good rapport, a trusting relationship, and a supportive atmosphere are lacking. Otherwise, such responses can be threatening and inhibit conversation.

Evaluative Responses

In an evaluative response, the interviewer makes a judgment about the person's behavior or responses or implies how the person ought to feel. The evaluative response leads to the offering of advice for the solution to the client's problem and is seldom helpful. The recipient of the advice has the choice of following the advice or not.

SELF-ASSESSMENT 1

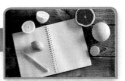

Directions: Identify the following types of responses as understanding, probing, confrontational, evaluative, hostile, or reassuring.

1. "The food does taste different without salt. Let's see if we can find some substitutes that you can try."
2. "I know you can do it. It just takes time."
3. "How do you expect to lose weight if you continue to eat fast foods every day?"
4. "That's interesting. Tell me more about that."
5. "You say that you watch your food choices weekdays, but eat whatever you want on weekends. Do you think that's why you haven't lost any weight?"
6. "When you're at a party, try to find someone to talk to instead of eating."

Hostile Responses

In the hostile response, the professional's anger or frustration is uncontrolled, and the response may lead to antagonism or humiliation of the client. The hostile response may result in the client retaliating. A vicious cycle of angry, hostile responses results, thus destroying the professional–client relationship.

Reassuring Responses

With a reassuring response, the client is prevented from working through her feelings because the interviewer suggests that there is nothing to worry about. Too frequently, a client's expressions of anxiety are followed by the counselor's reassuring response that things will improve and that the person should not worry. This response suggests that the problem does not exist, or that the counselor does not want to discuss it. Such responses make it difficult to discuss or solve the client's problem. Admission of failure with the diet may have been difficult for the client, but it indicated a desire to discuss the problem.

Closing the Interview

The third part or closing of the interview takes the shortest amount of time but should not be rushed or taken lightly. During the closing, end on a positive note, such as a word of appreciation sincerely expressed and thanking the person for his or her time and cooperation. Another suggestion is to review the purpose of the interview, summarize the points or goals, and declare the completion. "That's all the questions I have. Thank you for your time and information."

You may ask if there are any questions the person would like to ask or any other comments he or she wants to make, which may elicit important new information for which adequate time should be available. For example: "What else would you like to ask or tell me about?" You may ask the client to summarize points, goals, or next steps agreed on.

The time, place, and purpose of future contacts should be mentioned. To a hospitalized patient, the professional may say, "I'll stop by to see you tomorrow." With a client, arrangements for a future appointment may be made: "When can we meet again to discuss your progress and questions?" To make sure that each has understood the other, plans may be paraphrased. People tend to remember the last thing said.

For job applicants, one may inquire if here are questions and advocate for one's firm, if appropriate. For those who do not meet requirements, thank them, but mention that there are other candidates.[4] As a courtesy to job applicants, they should be told approximately when the employment decision will be made and how they will be notified if selected, as for example, "We are interviewing additional candidates for this position, but if you are selected, you'll hear from human resources in about a week or two. Thank you for coming and for your interest in our company."

One may signal the close of the interview nonverbally by breaking eye contact, pushing back the chair, standing up, offering to shake hands, smiling, and walking the interviewee to the door.[3]

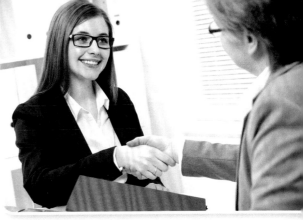
Closing the interview.

The interview session should be followed by a self-evaluation to determine areas that went well, as well as those that could be improved for the next interview. Questions one may ask include the following:

- How effective was the atmosphere? Was it relaxed and informal with good rapport?
- How effective was my interview opening?
- How effective were my questions in obtaining information I needed?
- How effective were my responses to the person's statements?
- How nonjudgmental and empathic was I?
- How effective was my interview closing?
- How much time did I listen versus talk?

Summary

In summary, interviewing is a skill and as with other skills, it takes practice to develop. The interviewer needs to plan in writing the topics to be covered. Various types of questions can be prepared in an appropriate sequence for the three parts of the interview. Physical surroundings and freedom from interruption should be planned. These conditions put the professional in a better position to concentrate on the interviewee and on the process of developing rapport, noting the verbal and nonverbal responses, and providing understanding responses with empathy.

Review and Discussion Questions

1. What are the possible purposes of a diet history or nutrition interview? Of a preemployment interview?
2. What conditions facilitate an interview?
3. Explain the three parts of an interview. What occurs in each part?
4. Differentiate between the following types of questions: open and closed; primary and secondary; and neutral and leading.
5. Explain the six types of responses.

Suggested Activities

1. Watch an interview on television noting the parts of the interview, techniques used, and verbal and nonverbal responses. Write up your reactions and analysis.
2. Make a list of what you consider to be the characteristics of a good interview. Then observe a television interview show, such as the *Tonight Show*, *Dr. Phil*, *Shark Tank*, or others. What types of questions are asked? What kinds of responses does the interviewer obtain? What was the level of rapport between the two parties? How well did the interview meet your criteria? Construct an interview guide from the questions asked with their sequence.
3. Plan an interview guide specifying the content and sequence of questions. Write examples of various kinds of questions, such as open and closed, primary and secondary, and neutral and leading. Which kinds of questions do you prefer to answer?
4. Divide into groups of two for role-playing using the 24-hour recall, with each person interviewing the other in turn. Use various types of responses, such as probing, paraphrasing, and understanding. If three people are available, the third may serve as an evaluator.

5. Using an interview guide, make an audiotape of a simulated or actual interview using the usual daily food intake, if the participant's permission is granted. Complete an evaluation.

6. Using an interview guide, make a videotape of a simulated or actual interview, if the participant's permission is granted. This will show both the verbal and nonverbal behaviors as well as any personal idiosyncrasies. Complete an evaluation.

7. Turn on the television set without the sound. Try to interpret the nonverbal behavior you are seeing.

8. Visit three offices and observe the physical surroundings. Which is most comfortable and conducive to communication? Why? Which is least comfortable? Why? Arrange the furniture in a room or office for an optimum interviewing setting.

9. Change the following technical words that are used by professionals into terms that will help a client to understand their meanings: fiber, nutrients, sodium, lipids, protein, serum glucose, carbohydrates, low-density lipoproteins, polyunsaturated fatty acids, saturated fatty acids, colitis, gastric ulcer, hypertension, fluid intake, osteoporosis.

10. **Directions:** Read the lettered statements below. Identify both the thought the person is expressing and the feelings the person may be experiencing. Write a paraphrased statement reflecting the thought or content of the message:

    A. "I've had diabetes for 6 years. They put me on a diet and insulin injections when I first found out about it, and I check my blood sugar sometimes. The diet isn't too bad."

    B. "I'm expecting my second baby. I never paid any attention to what I ate during my first pregnancy and my baby was healthy."

    C. "The doctor told me that I can go home tomorrow, but I live alone so I have no one to help me with a diet, and I'm in no hurry to leave."

    D. "Joan talks to people all day long and doesn't get her work done. The rest of us have to finish for her or we get yelled at."

    E. "I've been working here for 10 years. Now you come in as a new supervisor and want to change everything around. What's wrong with keeping things the way they are?"

    F. "How do you expect me to get all this work done? First, you tell me to do one thing, and then you tell me to do another."

    Directions: Write a second paraphrased statement reflecting the feelings in the preceding examples, such as:

    "You seem to be feeling (angry, depressed, lonely, etc.) because. . . ."

    "It sounds like you feel. . . ."

    "I hear you saying that you feel. . . . Tell me if I'm understanding you accurately."

EXAMPLE Client: "My friend and I are both dieting. She has lost weight, but I haven't even though I have been trying."

Counselor: "You seem to be feeling upset because your friend has lost weight and you haven't."

Discuss your paraphrases with others.

11. Obtain a copy of the mini nutrition assessment (available in 20 languages), available online (http://www.mna-elderly.com). Use it with an elderly person and evaluate the result.

12. Identify which of these preemployment questions are permissible and which are not.

    A. "Our floors are slippery when wet. Do you limp?"

    B. "Can you work weekends?"

    C. "Are you planning to have children?"

    D. "Can you work on religious holidays?"

    E. "What is your computer knowledge?"

    F. "What were your responsibilities on your previous job?"

13. Interview an experienced human resources recruiter about the questions asked, the degree of structure in the interview, and Equal Employment Opportunity (EEO) concerns.

Communication and Cultural Competence

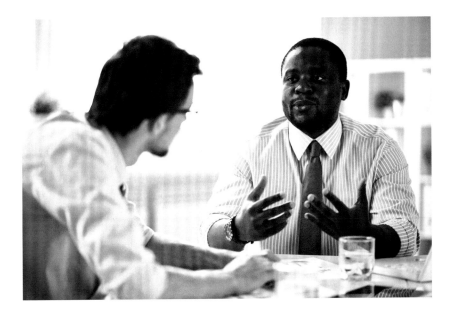

Objectives

- Describe aspects of cultural competence.
- Explain the differences between assimilation, enculturation, and acculturation.
- Discuss the dimensions of diversity in the workplace.
- Compare the cultural competence models.
- Identify key counseling strategies effective in culturally diverse populations.

Judy R. is a new registered dietitian nutritionist whose responsibilities at the medical center frequently involve nutrition interviewing, counseling, and community education. Many of her clients are from cultural and ethnic groups other than her own. They are mainly Mexican, Puerto Rican, Thai, and Korean. She is finding it somewhat overwhelming to understand the variety of unfamiliar foods that they eat. This also inhibits her ability to provide appropriate food alternatives as she counsels them on modifying their diets. She wants to increase her effectiveness as a counselor.

What we need to do is learn to respect and embrace our differences until our differences don't make a difference in how we are treated.

—*Yolanda King*

Introduction

The area of cultural communication, counseling, and quality healthcare is receiving increased attention. Our global society with changing demographics makes it common for food and nutrition professionals to be interacting with other healthcare professionals, employees, and clients with cultural backgrounds different from their own. Knowledge of food and food habits, the cultural influences of food, and the factors influencing lifestyle behaviors are fundamental for effective communication and education skills. The Academy of Nutrition and Dietetics prepares their members for the challenges of a multicultural society by integrating diversity and cultural competence into the Scope of Practice for both the Registered Dietitian Nutritionist (RDN) and Nutrition and Dietetic Technician, Registered (NDTR).[1,2] In the United States, the Joint Commission requires evidence of cultural and linguistic appropriate healthcare when accrediting healthcare facilities.[3]

The issue of culture and diversity is not new to America. The United States is continually evolving into an increasingly heterogeneous population.[4] Other countries are also experiencing new challenges in diversity due to global migration and mobility. The objectives of Healthy People 2020 reflect the health needs of a diverse population.[5] Because nutrition and dietetics professionals encounter diverse clients every day, they must make every effort to learn about customs and cultures different from their own. In this way, they can develop effective methods and strategies for serving all of their clients. Being alert to cultural diversity differences and similarities will enable the professional to better adapt and function in a multicultural environment.

Cultural competence is a broader term that attempts to encompass the multiple dimensions of an individual or group "core requirement for working effectively with culturally diverse people".[6] Competence infers a process, rather than an end point.[7] The challenge for health professionals is to be culturally competent in helping clients change their food choices without disturbing the sociocultural functions of food. For dietary changes to succeed, a combination of approaches—including behavioral and cognitive interventions, self-efficacy, relapse prevention, self-monitoring, stages of change, social support, and educational strategies—may be necessary to assist people to make changes in food choices.[8,9]

Food has been a cultural influence for centuries. Culture is the sum total of a group's learned and shared behavior. It is acquired by people living their everyday lives and provides a sense of identity, order, and security. As a group phenomenon, culture is learned from others and transmitted formally and informally to the next generation. These learned traditions are not static; they are dynamic with some changes accepted over time. All cultural and ethnic groups sustain their identities, in part, through their food practices, values, and beliefs. Family and culture determine what foods are appropriate and inappropriate.[8,9]

This chapter explores the effective strategies for use by nutrition and dietetics professionals in communicating with culturally diverse clients, employees, and other healthcare team members.

Cultural Diversity

What is cultural diversity? Cultural diversity and cultural identity have many components and definitions beyond ethnicity, nationality, and language. Cultural identity also includes race, age, gender, religion, disability, socioeconomic status, occupation, educational level, politics, physical ability, sexual orientation, and immigration status.[6] Diversity consists of the many ways in which individuals are unique or different while at the same time being similar in other ways. The United States is home to individuals and families of varied cultural and ethnic backgrounds who speak many different languages. The US Census Bureau reports that at least 350 languages are spoken in US homes (Figure 4-1).[4] The US population encompasses people of different races, religions, genders, sexual orientations, body sizes, physical abilities, health status, educational levels, ages, work experiences, lifestyles, values, marital status, socioeconomic status, and the like. It is important to value and understand all types of diversity and culture. Multicultural awareness can have a positive effect on policy, management, educational style, and overall success of an organization.

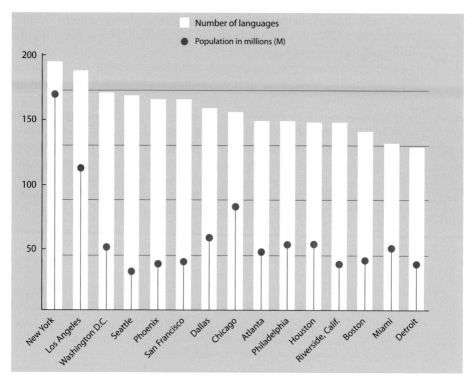

Figure 4-1 ■ Number of languages spoken in the 15 largest metro areas.
Source: US Census Bureau, 2009–2013 American Community Survey.

An old Asian saying notes that "All individuals, in many respects, are (a) like no other individuals, (b) like some individuals, and (c) like all other individuals."[8] It is true that we are all unique biologically and genetically and no two of us share the same experiences in society. But we have similarities to our social, ethnic, and cultural groups through shared experiences and characteristics. We also have similarities to others with common languages and life experiences such as love, marriage, gender, death, and emotions.

Thus, all people have individual, group, and universal levels of identity that make us unique. The health professional must recognize all dimensions and identities since culture determines how people view health and illness, where they seek treatment, and the relationship expected between client and health professionals.[9]

CASE ANALYSIS 1

What cultural diversity information would be beneficial for Judy?

Cultural Processes

Culture is the learned and shared knowledge that specific groups use to generate their behavior and interpret their experience in the world. It comprises beliefs about reality, how people should interact with each other, what they "know" about the world, and how they should respond to the social and material environments in which they find themselves. It is reflected in their religions, morals, customs, technologies, and survival strategies. It affects how they work, parent, love, marry, and understand health, mental health, wellness, illness, disability, and death.

Culture is a "framework that guides and bounds life's practices."[10] It enables a person to identify with a specific group or population. People begin to learn their culture at a very young age. By the time they are in school, they are already ingrained in their culture. As a deeply innate concept, cultural practices evolve gradually. They affect and guide the activities and daily behavior of specific groups.[10]

Culture influences many aspects of a person's identity; it shapes the foods served, methods of food preparation, meal patterns followed, the way holidays are celebrated, values, beliefs, spirituality, child-rearing practices, and expected family roles. Cultural roots influence attitudes and have a profound influence on behaviors.

Values differ related to cooperation versus competition, activity versus passivity, youth versus age, importance of family versus friends, and independence versus interdependence. For example, some cultures encourage competitiveness whereas others promote cooperation and teamwork.[8,9]

CASE ANALYSIS 2

What resources can you suggest for Judy to assist in her counseling? Where would she find them?

Enculturation and Intercultural Variation

Culture is learned, not inherited. It is passed from generation to generation in the home by a process called enculturation. Yet, within each culture, there exist different customs, practices, ideologies, and viewpoints. Many countries throughout the world have populations that comprise one major group as well as many subgroups that differ from one another in various ways. This is also called intracultural variation. For example, the Latino or Hispanic population is a major ethnic group in the Americas; yet within this community there are many subgroups, including Mexicans, Puerto Ricans, Cubans, and Central and South Americans. With these subgroups are further subcultures, and among these subcultures there are probably many similarities, but also distinct cultural differences. Another example is in the Asian culture. There are over 25 countries of origin that are classified under this one heading. Each country and region has its subcultures that have their own customs, lifestyles, traditions, foods, language, and dialects. We also see this in the African-American and many other cultures. Subgroups and variety in culture are the norm, rather than the typical stereotype.[8–10]

Acculturation and Assimilation

The process by which people from one cultural group modify their traditional behaviors, attitudes, and viewpoints as a result of contact with a new, dominant culture is termed acculturation.[11] Unlike the process of assimilation, in which members of a minority group adopt the practices and belief system of the dominant group, acculturation implies that both the traditional ethnic culture and the new, dominant culture play an important role in the process of cultural identity. As a result of this process, people may move toward the dominant culture, integrate the two cultures, reject the new culture while reaffirming their own traditional culture, or become alienated from both cultures.

The relationship between acculturation and dietary habits is well known. Longer exposure to a culture will result in higher acculturation. This can be observed with dietary recalls, food frequency questionnaires, and general dietary patterns. For example, Latinos residing in the United States for longer periods of time compared with new immigrants have been shown to increase sugar-sweetened beverage use while reducing their fiber intake from beans and fresh fruits. In addition, the globalization of the Western diet has also had an effect on the traditional diets consumed in many countries.[12] Newer immigrants were also less likely to shop with a written list of foods to purchase and tended to buy key familiar foods.[13,14]

As a nutrition practitioner, it is important to understand the concept of acculturation. One must understand acculturation so that they gain a better comprehension of the factors that hamper or enhance particular food choices. Practitioners must not assume that all dietary acculturation is healthy or unhealthy.[8] For example, an Asian who acculturates to the dominant American culture by eating fast food would be viewed as making unhealthy food choices, yet an Asian who maintains the minority group's traditional diet rich in whole grains and rice would be seen as healthy. Gender differences may also be seen. The nutrition and dietetics professionals must identify whether acculturation to the American culture is influencing chronic disease factors, and if so how.[7]

 CASE ANALYSIS   3

What activities can Judy plan in the community to educate these diverse groups? What advice would you share with Judy to make her efforts successful?

Diversity in the Workplace

There has always been diversity in the workplace, but government legislation mandating equal employment opportunities, affirmative action, and access for people with disabilities spurred changes in the 1960s and beyond.[15] Figure 4-2 shows the changing patterns of immigration from 2005 to 2010 from the US Census Bureau.[4] The annual influx of new immigrants, most recently people of Asian and Hispanic descent, has contributed to cultural diversity in the workplace. In earlier years, most immigrants came from Europe and Canada. More recently, immigrants have come from Asia, Mexico, Latin America, and Central America. By 2060, it is estimated that no racial or ethnic group will be traditionally classified as "minorities" but individuals under the age of 18 years will increase from 48% to 64%.[4,16]

Challenges of Diversity

Many immigrants who choose to make the United States their home face issues of assimilation. Generally, the first generation of immigrants has the most difficulty adapting to American culture. Many of them experience problems in speaking and interpreting the English language. Literacy can often be the biggest problem for nonnative learners or clients who must now read or write in English rather than in their native language. Thus, food and nutrition professionals may experience difficulty in communicating with their employees.

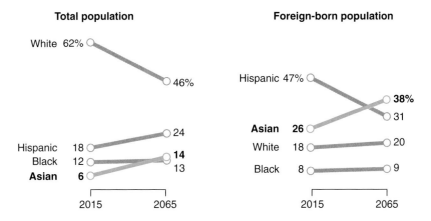

By 2065, No Racial or Ethnic Group Will Be a Majority

Note: Whites, blacks and Asians include only single-race non-Hispanics. Asians include Pacific Islanders. Hispanics are of any race. Other races included in totals but not shown.

Figure 4-2 ■ Foreign-born population by period of entry and world region of birth.
Source: Pew Research Center projections.

Food service departments employ a large proportion of immigrant populations and ethnic groups. As this pool of available employees continues to become more culturally diverse, supervisors are presented with numerous challenges. Nutrition professionals and managers are faced with integrating this diverse population into the workforce. They also must develop strategies and training programs that allow all workers to learn and communicate with one another. As many different types of immigrant populations are employed within the food industry, a non-English language barrier might also exist between managers and staff. Therefore, bilingual kitchens and cultural diversity are modern challenges faced by all healthcare employers and employees.[15,17]

Another area of diversity in the workplace is the culture of age. Lower-level workers are not always the youngest or the least experienced. The shortage of food service workers is often filled by immigrants and/or older employees. Many older adults are returning to the workforce looking for part-time jobs to supplement their income or stay involved with others. The projected percentage change in the labor force by age, from 2006 to 2016, shows the largest increase in the 65 years and older segment.[15,18]

Benefits of Diversity

There are many benefits to a diverse organization. First, organizations that are composed of diverse employees are better able to develop and implement a variety of ideas, policies, and programs.[15,19] An organization can better meet the needs and demands of the population at large by hiring people from a multitude of backgrounds who possess different viewpoints, experiences, and ideologies. A diverse staff can be essential for companies that serve diverse consumers or customer groups. Studies have shown that customers better identify with service providers whose gender and ethnic background are similar to their own. This finding may be attributed to embedded norms that enable the customer to better understand and relate to the service provider. An organization composed of diverse employees is also good for business because it enables the company to better understand a certain segment of the market that it is targeting for a product or service. If the organization reflects the community it serves, there is an increased chance that it will provide the goods and services that are needed or wanted.

Management professionals need to be committed to developing and supporting diverse groups and teams so they can effectively manage a culturally diverse workforce.[20] In an effort to create a culturally diverse organization, managers need to practice diversity every day. This includes job interviews, supervision of employees, staff development programs, and the creation of a fair and equal, harassment-free work environment. For example, in recruitment practices, managers should advertise job descriptions in places where minority groups might see them. All members of the organization, including those of the dominant culture, must not only accept diversity but also make a commitment to it and value it.[15,19,20]

Managing Diversity

The goal of an effective organization and operative workplace is to foster an environment in which all employees maximize their potential by contributing a variety of talents and abilities.[18,19] To do so, managers must harness cultural differences and create a productive environment where people feel their skill set is being efficiently utilized and valued. As such, all employees must be viewed as assets who work together toward achieving the universal goals and objectives of the organization, while prospering individually.

Although it is necessary to treat everyone within the organization with respect, some members of the organization may have difficulty developing cultural sensitivity and may inadvertently treat fellow employees differently. Moreover, when dealing with colleagues or clients who are different from themselves, some people may have a tendency to make assumptions or generalizations about the behaviors of these individuals. For example, in some environments, there is a tendency to label workers by their race, ethnicity, or sexual orientation.[15] Specifically, people might still refer to a colleague as being the Black supervisor, White waiter, Mexican cook, Japanese hostess, gay dishwasher, or Puerto Rican manager. In order to rectify this ethnic labeling, people must be made aware of their own biases, examine their prejudices, and work to overcome them. It is important not just to accept diversity but also to value it and demonstrate acceptance of it through words and actions. The leadership role in modeling cultural competence and diversity has been shown to be influential.[21]

In diversity-driven environments, individuality is nurtured and stressed. Thus, differences in ideas and experiences can lead to more creative solutions to problems and better decisions. Collaboration, consensus, and shared power, whereby professional authority is shared and determined by one's knowledge and skill set, make everyone feel more equal. In these types of work environments, the employees are more productive and the company is more competitive in achieving its objectives.[15,19-21]

The permanent change in how employees work together may take time. However, it is the responsibility of the management to establish a workplace where cultural acceptance is the norm.[20] The following are some questions to consider when evaluating workplace diversity:

- Are all employees viewed as assets?
- Are there lower expectations of any employees because of their ethnicity or literacy level?
- Is there an overall atmosphere of acceptance and encouragement for all workers?
- Do diverse workers have levels of responsibility comparable to the dominant group?
- Are managers' expectations lower for certain groups or individuals?
- Are certain ethnic groups overrepresented or underrepresented in some departments or areas?

- Are hiring and promotion opportunities open to all? What percent of management positions are filled by women and minorities? Are minorities or women regarded as "token" employees or are they respected? Are they resented?
- Are everyone's ideas, proposals, and suggestions taken seriously?
- Do all groups participate in the normal socialization and networking during work hours?
- Are English-speaking employees impatient with those who speak English slowly or poorly?
- Are different cultural mannerisms and body language accepted or misunderstood and ridiculed?
- Are all people treated with patience, tolerance, and understanding?
- Are training materials and sessions planned with the idea of being understood by all?

Cultural Competence Models

There are numerous definitions of cultural competence and ways for a person to achieve it. One model identifies three characteristics of a culturally competent professional as: (1) The professional is aware of his or her assumptions, values, and biases, such as ageism, sexism, or racism. (2) The professional understands the worldview of culturally diverse clients and their values and assumptions about human behaviors. (3) The professional develops appropriate intervention strategies and techniques for culturally different clients.[6] For example, self-disclosure may not be compatible with some groups such as Asian Americans, Hispanic Americans, and American Indians, gays, lesbians, bisexual, or transgender. Interpersonal communication may require different verbal and nonverbal approaches and responses. The above model defines cultural competence in terms of awareness, knowledge, and skills. To be effective, counselors must recognize their biases, develop knowledge of the groups that they work with, and develop culturally appropriate intervention strategies for different groups. While one cannot be knowledgeable of every possible group, professionals must become knowledgeable of those groups seen most often. As products of our own cultural conditioning, often Euro-American, we must guard against negative opinions of the lifestyles of other groups.

The ETHNIC model is another model of culturally competent care. It includes the six steps of (1) Explanation, (2) Treatment, (3) Healers, (4) Negotiation, (5) Intervention, and (6) Collaboration. Explanation asks the client to explain his or her illness to determine client understanding. Treatment inquires what treatment the client expects and what he or she may eat or avoid to stay healthy. Healers inquires whether the person has used nontraditional sources. In the Negotiation stage, one collaborates with the client to find acceptable treatment choices. Intervention asks for client feedback on the treatment choices and any concerns. Collaboration discusses the help from other healthcare team members or community and family resources.[6]

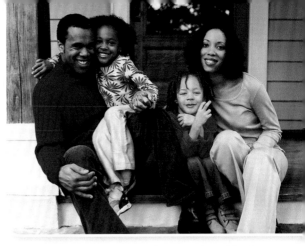

Professionals may inquire about foods purchased for the family.
Source: US Department of Agriculture.

The Campinha-Bacote model is a five-part framework for cultural competence in healthcare. It includes cultural awareness, cultural knowledge, cultural skill, cultural desire, and cultural encounter. In awareness, professionals think about their own beliefs and values. Cultural knowledge examines what cultural knowledge is needed by the professional. Cultural skill focuses on collecting cultural information from clients during assessments and interventions. Cultural desire is the desire of counselors to include cross-cultural care in the encounter and seek greater cultural competence. Finally, cultural encounter, which consists of the healthcare professionals' experiences with the client, includes interactions, motivation, and acceptance that advance the understanding of the culture. Verbal and nonverbal skills such as listening, observing, discussion, and nonjudgmental questions will enhance the cultural encounter.[22]

The Hand model of cultural sensitivity was developed by a nursing teacher in New Zealand where health professionals work with the Maori indigenous population. The thumb represents "awareness," with the other four fingers representing "connection, communication, negotiation, and advocacy." All fingers are connected to the palm, which represents the clasping and shaking of hands promoting shared meaning of health.[23] Nutrition counselors can experiment with different models to determine which approaches work for particular clients. Each model has the underlying premise of communication and respect.

Cultural Competence in Counseling

Frequently, nutrition and dietetics professionals communicate with diverse clients and population groups. It is important to be culturally competent, but one must be sure to work closely with the client and individualize the

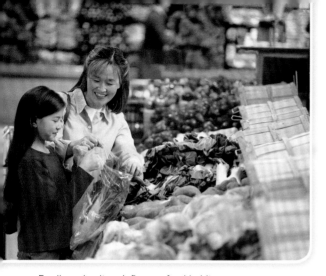

Family and culture influence food habits.
Source: US Department of Agriculture.

entire counseling experience. Numerous questions need to be asked and answered. One must never forget that the client is first and foremost an individual and not just a culture.

Cultural Assessment

To ensure that the diets of immigrants and minority groups are healthy, nutrition and dietetics professionals should begin with a cultural assessment including the degree of acculturation to American eating practices. This entails questions about traditional foods, the relationship of food to health, foods made or purchased, recipes, food preparation, and family and food interactions.[24–26]

The practitioner should consult and listen carefully to the client, because he or she is the best source of information about the types of foods consumed. Based on this assessment, the practitioner may determine that those who are more acculturated need more help in selecting healthy American foods. Similarly, those who are less acculturated may need help modifying their culture's traditional recipes if they are unhealthy.

Americans experiment with foods and mix the foods from a variety of cultural traditions, thus making eating practices a diverse cultural smorgasbord. Regional areas of the United States, such as Tex-Mex, New England, the Midwest, and the Southwest may also affect one's food choices. Examples of regional foods are New England clam chowder, Boston baked beans, Southern grits, New Orleans jambalaya, Texas chili, California sourdough bread, and Wisconsin fish boil. Similar regional differences are found within other countries as well.

The goal of nutrition counseling and education is to help clients modify and manage food choices and eating behaviors by creating individualized action plans. However, psychologists tell us that food and language are cultural traits humans learn first, and the ones that they change with the greatest reluctance. A major influence is the food eaten during childhood that forever defines what is familiar and brings comfort. Food preferences from childhood continue to be exhibited by adults, showing the profound role that early family experiences have in shaping food habits.[27] Changing one's dietary choices is possible but not easily accomplished, and some intervention strategies are more effective than others. One should remember that respect must always be shown for the client's choice of foods. Many times, these choices are based on family habits, traditions, or beliefs.

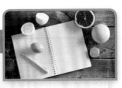

SELF-ASSESSMENT 1

Describe your own food preferences from childhood and their relationship with your current food and lifestyle choices.

Health Disparities in Diverse Population

The United States Department of Health and Human Services Office of Minority Health has developed practice recommendations to address racial and ethnic health disparities.[10] The overarching goals of Healthy People 2020 are to increase the quality years of life, create social and physical environments that promote health, and eliminate health disparities by promoting healthy development and behaviors for all population groups.[5] Two of the 10 leading health indicators that track and measure the health of our nation are physical activity and overweight/obesity. Nutrition has been linked to treatment or etiology of 5 out of 10 leading causes of death of Americans: cancer, diabetes, heart disease, kidney disease, and stroke, with obesity identified as a confounding factor. These objectives are tracked, monitored, and measured over time to determine if the targets have been met. Unfortunately, none of the objectives to achieve healthy weight and reduce incidence of overweight and obesity are currently being met.[5]

Health statistics also clearly indicate higher risk among many of the culturally diverse populations in the United States, particularly for obesity and diabetes. In fact, data show that the percentage of people outside of the United States who are overweight and obese is also increasing as well as global malnutrition.[28] These health disparity data are extremely helpful in planning community programs and counseling individuals of different ages and cultural or ethnic groups. An example is recent interventions to reduce the risk of diabetes in Pacific Islander communities that started with focus groups to assess needs. Successful family-centered education programs were implemented based on this community-focused process. Some of the educational content is shown in Table 4-1.[24,29]

Nutrition and dietetics professionals need to determine which groups are the most vulnerable and create nutrition messages targeted to those groups. Although all groups may benefit from nutrition education, it is important to focus on particular populations that are most at risk, based on available consumption data. For example, diabetes mellitus is higher in many diverse populations particularly Native Americans and Hispanics. Many opportunities exist to increase awareness of native food patterns and retention of healthy cultural foods in these populations to potentially reduce diabetes risk.[11,30] Culturally-appropriate health messages and treatment algorithms can further enhance adherence to medical nutrition therapy.[31]

Tailored	Standardized
Family eating history exercise	Review of general eating and exercise goals
Family meal planning exercise	Review of typical healthy eating pattern
Identify community resources to support family activities	Give standardized list of community resources
Identify healthy lifestyle values shared by family members	Give list of healthy lifestyle practices

Table 4-1 ■ Examples of Tailored versus Standardized Population Focus Delivered in the Pacific Islanders Lifestyle Intervention Community Education Program to Reduce Weight Regain.
Source: From Kaholokula JK, Mau MK, Efird JT, et al. A family and community focused lifestyle program prevents weight regain in Pacific Islanders: a pilot randomized controlled trial. Health Educ Behav. 2011;5:1–10.

Another example of a cultural group of concern nutritionally and newly mentioned in Healthy People 2020 is the Lesbian, Gay, Bisexual, and Transgender (LGBT) population. There are a number of issues that affect the health and nutrition status of this culture. Gay and bisexual men are at a higher risk for eating disorders. Lesbians and bisexual females are more likely to be overweight or obese, and the LGBT populations in general have the highest rates of tobacco, alcohol, and other drug use.[5]

In the diverse United States, healthcare professionals have the opportunity to serve clients from many different cultures. Thus, it is important that counselors recognize the influence of cultural factors on dietary patterns among various ethnic groups. Specifically, they must learn about each cultural group's traditional foods and food practices.[8,9] Transmission of this learning requires effective communication between the health professional and the audience.[16] Active learning environments like this promote exchange of information and collaborative conversation. Nutrition and dietetics professionals must recognize, respect, understand, and acknowledge the cultural differences or variations to eliminate disparities in the nutritional status of people from different cultural backgrounds. Otherwise, nutrition counseling and education will be ineffective.[8,9,15]

Sensitivity to Stereotype and Bias

As someone who serves diverse clients, it is also imperative that the nutrition and dietetics professional does not stereotype people based on their national origin or their appearance. India, for example, includes several cultural groups who practice different religions, have different customs, speak different languages, and eat a variety of different foods.

Although a healthcare professional may assume that all people from India practice Hinduism, he or she must recognize that this narrow-minded assumption is not true. Similarly, practitioners must recognize that all Arab people are not Muslim, while all Irish people are not Catholic. It is also important that nutrition professionals recognize the cultural divide that exists among various generations and groups within each culture. Individuals are unique in the degree to which they adhere to cultural patterns, with some identifying with the dominant culture more strongly than others. Generally, most first-generation immigrants cling closely to their cultural ways. Over time, the second- and third-generation off-spring of these immigrants tend to assimilate more completely into the dominant culture. They are more likely to adopt American customs and ideologies, yet they also keep some of their native cultural practices and food choices. Children, for example, adapt to new cultural patterns more easily than adults because they often interact with people of different cultures at school or in social activities.[7-9]

Nutrition professionals must also be prepared to combat and prevent ethnocentrism and be able to recognize their own bias. They must be able to look at their own culture and realize any biases they may have. Each professional must put all biases aside and place the benefit, education, and respect of the client first. Although culture creates harmony within ethnic groups, it can also create disharmony. Ethnocentrism is the innate belief that one's own values and practices are absolute truths. Ethnocentric people, in turn, have a tendency to judge all others based on their own established belief system. They believe that the norms and values of other cultures or ethnic populations are secondary to the norms and values of their own culture. To prevent ethnocentricity from penetrating the workplace, nutrition and dietetics professionals need to know that their opinions, viewpoints, and ideologies may differ from those of their colleagues or clients. They also must understand that their own culture and worldviews may not be inherently "right."[12] This realization requires that one knows one's own culture, its origins, its history, and its beliefs.

Nutrition and dietetics professionals need to develop cultural competence in order to treat clients with respect, understanding, care, and efficiency. Although cultural competence is similar to cultural understanding, there are key differences. Cultural competence consists of thinking and behaving that enable members of one cultural, ethnic, or linguistic group to work effectively with members of another.[6] Nutrition and dietetics professionals cannot be culturally competent in every culture, but they must be culturally competent about the various cultures they encounter on a regular basis. They also need to recognize and investigate unique differences with each particular culture and individual, so that they can determine the best way to treat their clients.

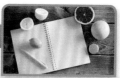

1. Describe your own culture, origins, history, and beliefs.
2. What cultural groups do you feel competent to counsel?

Understanding Health Practices

Culture determines how a person defines health, recognizes illness, and seeks treatment.[8,31,32] Each culture holds values, beliefs, and practices about good health and disease prevention, the care and treatment of the sick, whom to consult when ill, and the social roles and relationships between client and healthcare provider. Most Americans, for example, believe in westernized, scientific medicine. Many cultures, however, have food and health beliefs that are not grounded in evidence-based foundations. These practices need to be respected and do not necessarily need to be eliminated if they do not cause harm or exploit others. An example is the practice of intermittent fasting in many cultures or the use of integrative and complementary medicine.[33,34]

Americans typically make informed individual health decisions through informed consent and use the healthcare provider as the manager of care. Westernized healthcare also separates body, mind, and spirit in treatment programs. However, the healthcare orientation of other cultures may differ. For example, in numerous, non-American cultures, a family member or the community as a whole may have decision-making responsibility rather than the individual; emotional and psychological remedies may supersede scientific medicine; and body, mind, and spirit may be seen not as separate, but as joined.[10]

In Mexico, health is believed to be a matter of fate or God's will. Rather than believe in the power of science, medicine, or doctors to heal, many Mexicans believe that illnesses can be cured by folk healers or herbal remedies and teas. Similarly, they believe that particular medical conditions should be accompanied by particular food choices. These food choices are categorized as "hot" or "cold."[9] Specifically, pregnancy is considered to be a "hot" condition. As a result, pregnant Mexican women are urged to avoid foods

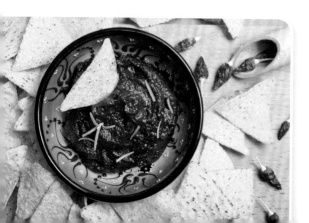

Counseling ethnic groups requires knowledge of their foods.
Source: US Department of Agriculture.

that are classified as "hot," such as garlic, grains, expensive meats, and alcohol. Instead, they are urged to eat "cold" foods, such as vegetables, dairy, inexpensive meats, and tropical fruits. In reviewing this list of "hot" versus "cold" foods, it is interesting to note that this health concept has nothing to do with the temperature or spiciness of the food (after all, breads or grains are not actually hot); instead, food is labeled according to traditions within the Mexican culture. In addition, in Mexican culture, men are often considered the dominant group, and the husband or his family is consulted and included in all decisions relating to a woman's pregnancy. Thus, a nutrition and dietetics professional who is working with a Hispanic pregnant woman may need to involve the father and his family in the decision-making sessions. The professional needs to always ask clients of their preference, if any, of who should be involved in the healthcare discussions. Also, the professional needs to inquire what, if any, alternative medicines, herbs, and supplements are used by the client.

Many other cultures also believe that diseases are caused by factors other than those identified by western scientific medicine. In India, disease is believed to be caused by an upset in the balance of the body. In some castes, the husband's dominance over his wife is quite pervasive, and unquestioned obedience to elders is expected. Conversely, Haitians believe that some illnesses originate supernaturally or magically and may be treated with voodoo medicine. The client should be asked what they believe may be causing their illness and the client's beliefs must always be respected. The nutrition dietetics professional must remain nonjudgmental. If these practices conflict with medical care, it should be discussed with the client and the primary healthcare provider.[9]

Understanding Nonverbal Behavior

Nonverbal behaviors also differ among cultural groups and have different connotations. Customs concerning personal contact, body gestures, eye contact, interpersonal space, public displays of affection, and punctuality vary greatly. In terms of personal contact, norms about touching another person are culturally determined. For example, in many Muslim communities, it is considered illicit to hug a married woman. Similar notions also apply to eye contact.

In American culture, it is considered disrespectful or suspicious to avoid meeting someone's eye. In some cultures, however, looking into a person's eyes is deemed disrespectful. Rules about touching and space are also culturally determined. Some cultures keep short distances between people, while others expect longer distances.[31,32] These spatial relationships also extend to signs of affection between men and women. In the United States, it is culturally acceptable to see partners exchange romantic gestures or tokens of affection; yet in other parts of the world, intimate partners do not even hold one another's hands.

Punctuality is also culturally determined. In the fast-paced United States, emphasis is placed on being on time and tardiness is frowned upon. Conversely, in parts of Asia as well as South and Central America, it is socially acceptable for a client to be late or miss an appointment without contacting the service provider. In these parts of the world, people's personal use of their own time is often considered to be a more important priority than the clock. Nutrition counselors need to be aware of these different customs so they can better serve and understand clients' behaviors and choices. Start each session by setting a neutral professional setting. Assess the situation by listening and observing mannerisms of your clients. Be cautious in shaking hands, touching a client, or making assumptions in the initial introduction phase of the counseling session.

Understanding Verbal Behaviors

In addition to understanding nonverbal behaviors, nutrition and dietetics professionals must also be privy to how verbal behaviors vary among different cultures. Slang is a verbal habit that professionals should be cautious about using in the workplace with employees or clients. In the American culture, people often greet each other informally by asking "How's it going?" or ask others to repeat what they just said by interjecting "What?" In many cultures, this level of familiarity would be considered improper and even disrespectful and condescending. Instead, dietetics professionals should greet clients by saying "Welcome" or another formal greeting. When they would like a client to repeat a statement, they should say "Excuse me" and then ask politely for the client to rephrase in their own words.

Similarly, nutrition and dietetics professionals should pay attention to how they address their clients. Americans are among the most informal people worldwide and frequently call both friends and strangers by their first names. Nutrition and dietetics professionals should ask how the client would like to be addressed. Nearly all other cultures expect a more formal and respectful approach, using the person's surname. [31,32] For example, if a client's full name is Diana Morales, the health professional should refer to her as Ms. Morales, not Diana.

Professionals should carefully craft the types of questions they ask their clients. Americans tend to be fairly direct and ask somewhat personal questions, yet in many cultures direct questions are deemed inappropriate. They may even cause people to feel uncomfortable.[10] Moreover, asking personal questions of a client in order to obtain personal health and nutrition data may be perceived as intrusive and disrespectful. Therefore, health professionals may want to try a formal approach rather than a quick, direct approach. Speak slowly and clearly. Listen first and seek to understand nonverbal behavior in conjunction with verbal conversation.[31,32]

Dietary managers and staff should try to understand the relationship that the client expects from them as a service provider.[15] In many cultures throughout the world, professionals are held in high regard for their expertise. Expecting individuals and families to be talkative and assertive may be unrealistic if they expect to have a dependent role in which they are told what types of foods they should be eating.

Understanding Family Relations

Another factor that nutrition and dietetic professionals must learn and understand is the various types of family compositions. Families may be patriarchal, matriarchal, nuclear, or extended. Because one's own culture generally determines the interactions and composition of one's family, the roles of each family member may vary by age or gender. In some non-American cultures, a woman may not be allowed to speak openly, may not be allowed to work outside the home, and may have to defer to her husband or mother-in-law. In these cultures, a woman may have an insignificant role in making decisions for both herself and her family. As a result, counseling sessions may need to include the woman's father, husband, or whomever is the family's decision maker.[8,9] Women may be more likely to breast-feed if they have strong family support.

Nutrition counseling must also identify whether the family is monocultural or bicultural. Monocultural families identify with one primary ethnic group; those that are bicultural identify with two or more groups. Clients may move back and forth among cultural groups easily. Consequently, the food choices made by clients may depend on situational factors or a diverse cultural identity.

Multicultural Awareness

To achieve multicultural competence in nutrition counseling, health professionals must first strive for multicultural awareness. A personal awareness of the various cultures within the United States first requires that the individual become aware of his or her own culture or heritage. Each individual has a cultural, ethnic, linguistic, and racial identity. Awareness of personal values, beliefs, assumptions, biases, and prejudices must be brought to the level of conscious awareness before one can become culturally competent. Therefore, professionals should learn about the customs and traditions of their own family and culture, identify the historical connections between their culture and those of others, and examine their worldviews and cultural assumptions.

Individuals may be unaware of the ways in which their own culture influences other people's behaviors, reactions, and interactions. This examination might begin by assessing all of the values, beliefs, or behaviors that shape one's self, including family and heritage, socioeconomic factors, politics,

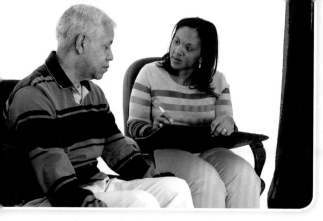

Counselors must be familiar with ethnic practices.
Source: CDC/Amanda Mills.

biases, religion, educational level, occupation, gestures, and terms of endearment. There are three key proficiencies that healthcare professionals must develop in order to be multiculturally competent. First, dietetics professionals must develop a multicultural competent attitude, that is, a mindset that respects cultural differences and similarities, while tolerating unclear intercultural communication due to language barriers. This attitude requires that healthcare professionals maintain a high level of patience for the additional time needed for effective communication. It also requires that the professional may need to modify usual training materials by making them easier to read and interpret (see Chapter 14). In some cases, use of visuals or pictures may have more success with certain clients. Second, dietetics professionals must develop multicultural competent practices. These practices should ensure that clients' traditional health beliefs and diet are being balanced with healthy American food choices. Third, nutrition professionals must develop multicultural counseling skills. These skills may include listening skills, bilingual communication skills, diet modification skills, or evaluation skills.[35]

Food and Nutrition Counseling Knowledge

To provide clients with effective counseling, nutrition professionals must have knowledge of multicultural foods and the cultural food practices of various groups. They should gather information regarding cultural food choices, food preparation methods within a cultural context, knowledge of cultural eating patterns, family dynamics, typical meal patterns, and traditions during celebrations. Information specific to each culture and community in which clients live is also needed. The counselor may determine the degree to which the family or each individual within the family follows these cultural traditions by consulting with each family member separately.[7-9]

How can we learn about cultures of clients and employees? One suggestion is to visit their neighborhoods and go to the various ethnic food stores and ethnic restaurants. If possible, attend religious ceremonies in their places of worship or other neighborhood events. Evaluate the presence of a food desert in your community. An audit of where the community secures their food helps define challenges, opportunities, and barriers. Another suggestion is to attend workshops or training sessions on cultural food practices. Nutrition and dietetics professionals can also learn about various cultures by reading about the role of foods in health and illness, approaches to health promotion, and treatment of disease and illness as well as beliefs about care and caregivers. Nutrition and dietetics professionals can also examine authentic recipe books and try cooking the characteristic foods of various cultures.

Focus groups can help nutrition professionals learn about their clients' culture and dietary habits.[23-25] During these sessions, the professional should explore the differences within cultural groups by talking about food preferences, recipes, ingredients, portion sizes, and how certain food items are prepared. If unfamiliar with eating a particular food, such as horse meat, Korean kimchi, Indian ghee, or hummus, the counselor should ask for a description of the food and cooking methods. It is important to gather all of this information so that one can respectfully incorporate family foods and cultural practices into proposed dietary changes.

While counseling people of different ethnic backgrounds, nutrition and dietetics professionals should use culturally appropriate education materials. There are many options available from government and private sources.[7-10] Figure 4-3 shows the Spanish myPlate version published by the United States Department of Agriculture.[36] The MyPlate is now also available in numerous other languages (Plate).[38] Some diet evaluation systems

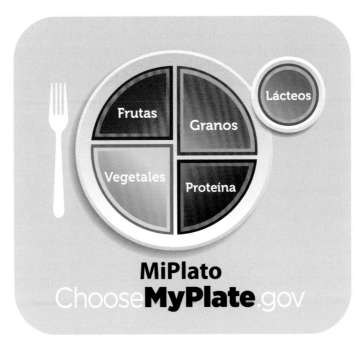

Figure 4-3 ■ The Spanish version of the US Department of Agriculture MyPlate.
Source: US Department of Agriculture.

may not meet the cultural or ethnic needs of their target population. An example of this would be cultures that consume numerous stews and soups.

The following phrases may be helpful in eliciting information about a client's cultural food practices:

"I am not familiar with the way you cook _____ (name of food). Will you please tell me about it?"

"When you celebrate a cultural holiday, what food items do you prepare? What types of snacks do you prefer?" (directs the focus to the whole group)

"That dinner dish you mentioned sounds interesting. Can you tell me how you prepare it?"

"You are the expert on your food choices. You can teach me a lot."

You should reinforce any client response with one of the following statements:

"Thank you for that information."

"You are helping me to understand."

"I appreciate your taking the time to explain your cultural foods to me."

Nutrition Counseling Skills

Multicultural nutrition counseling skills demonstrate one's ability to handle culturally appropriate interactions. These include conducting nutrition and cultural assessments, identifying nutrition-related problems, and planning and implementing relevant interventions.[8-10] Table 4-2 offers some suggestions for counseling in culturally diverse groups.

1. Assess prior knowledge by listening first. Focus on what is known and/or believed.

2. Reinforce correct knowledge, clarify misinformation.

3. Use simple language. Integrate visual media to "show" what you are teaching.

4. Talk in slow, clear words. Look for understanding. Repeat as necessary.

5. Encourage questions. Strive for interaction within cultural parameters.

6. Utilize the "teach-back" method. After each key concept is discussed, ask client to restate what was just presented in their own language.

Table 4-2 ■ Common Effective Strategies to Use When Delivering Culturally Diverse Nutrition Counseling

Source: Adapted from Academy of Nutrition and Dietetics. Practice tips: Cultural competence resources. http://www. eatrightpro.org/10877.pdf. Accessed January 10, 2016; Goody CM, Drago L, eds. Cultural Food Practices. Chicago, IL: American Dietetic Association; 2010; Duggan A, Street L. Interpersonal communication in health and illness. In: Glamz K, Rimer BK, Viswanath R, eds. Health Behavior: Theory, Research, and Practice. 5th ed. San Francisco, Jossey-Bass, 2015; and Kittler PG, Sucher KP, Nelms J. Food and Culture. 6th ed. Belmont, CA: Wadsworth, 2011.

Effective counseling skills require one to be aware of and knowledgeable about various cultures. Cultural healthcare beliefs must be acknowledged and respected. For example, some believe that a heavier body weight is preferable and favored.[10] Reason for this belief varies from culture to culture. The client's beliefs must be acknowledged and respected. The approach should be one of understanding. Instead of putting the emphasis of the counseling session on the weight numbers, using more of an "eating healthier" approach may be the technique to use in this situation.

Trust is an important counseling skill that all dietetics professionals must develop. One must be credible in the eyes of the client. Although the counselor may find that trust is difficult to develop, it is a necessary key to success.[8-10] The gap between the professional and the client must be bridged, whether the client comes voluntarily or by referral. One way to achieve this is to develop rapport through conversation on neutral subjects that are unrelated to health or nutrition. For example, you may want to develop a personal relationship with your clients first by asking questions such as "Where did you grow up?" In providing counseling, you may want to first inform clients of what you will be doing by saying "You are probably wondering what we are going to do. Let me explain." Then, you can explain the purpose, process, and the client's role as your guide. The client should take an active role in the session and decision-making process.

Finally, a counselor may want to call upon the services of a translator to assist with transmitting nutrition information. The translator may help rewriting written handouts or transmitting oral information into the client's language. An experienced translator should always be the first option. Although translating skills of the client's son or daughter are sufficient for these purposes, nutrition and dietetics professionals must be cautious about using a family member in this role. In many cultures, having a child act as the interpreter presents the problem of role reversal, which can lead to resentment and can change the family dynamics at home.[10] Regardless of the type of translator, remember to address questions directly to the client, not the interpreter, and focus on the client as answers are provided.

Limited Literacy

About 40 to 44 million people, or approximately 25% of the US adult population, cannot understand materials written at a basic proficiency level. Although individuals with limited literacy skills vary, most are of lower socioeconomic status, have dropped out of school, are learning disabled, or are older. They may be immigrants who do not yet know much English and may not read even in their native language.[4] It is important to identify these individuals, because poor reading skills are associated with poor health.

Practitioners probably encounter illiterate clients more often than they realize, as such individuals hide the fact that they cannot read. The nutrition professional should be aware of the following comments expressed by clients in an effort to hide their illiteracy: "I don't have my glasses with me and will read this later," or "I broke my glasses." Another technique to identify such individuals is to hand them written materials upside down. Readers normally turn the paper right-side up, whereas nonreaders may not. Another approach is to ask the person to select a food from a list on the paper and read the word aloud. If the client cannot read the word, then it is unlikely that he or she knows how to read.

The average reading level of US adults is around eighth-grade level, but among enrollees in Medicaid, it is only at the fifth-grade level. Typically, health education print materials are written at the tenth-grade level or higher instead of an appropriate level for the audience—generally fifth-grade level.[5] To rectify this imbalance, nutrition and dietetics professionals may need to test written materials for readability and incorporate more visuals (graphics and pictures) when educating people with low literacy. They should also keep language simple and repeat important information. "Dietary cholesterol" and "blood glucose," for example, are challenging terms to understand and are inappropriate for this audience. Another suggestion is to keep sentences short (10–15 words) and use one- and two-syllable words when possible (see Chapter 14). Paragraphs should also be limited to three or four sentences. To ensure that clients understand the words, the counselor should ask them to repeat what was said. This is called the "teach-back" method. Actual practice, such as planning a menu or a grocery shopping list, and role-playing are helpful activities in helping clients connect words to language. Literacy assessment tools are available for evaluation of written materials. These and other tools can help professionals promote nutritional literacy among their clients who are illiterate or have limited literacy (see Chapter 14 for more suggestions on how to develop lower literacy materials).

The principle to remember is to be sensitive to the fact that many clients may have literacy problems that they may attempt to hide during the assessment process. If the issue of literacy is not properly diagnosed, addressed, and remedied, the chances of successfully counseling the individual will be greatly reduced. You also must not assume that clients of a specific culture can read the language commonly used in that culture. The clients may be nonreaders in their native language, thus requiring the use of more visuals and examples than written materials.

Summary

This chapter examined the challenges and importance of dealing with a diverse workforce as well as the counseling and education of culturally diverse clients. As the United States and the world become increasingly heterogeneous, the need to be cross-culturally competent is critical. Food and nutrition professionals must develop awareness, knowledge, communication skills, and respect for all cultures in order to be successful. This requires one to perceive and recognize the value and uniqueness of people of all cultures, whether a minority or a majority.

Review and Discussion Questions

1. What is cultural diversity? What are some of the ways in which people differ?
2. As a manager, what would you see as the goals and benefits of workplace diversity?
3. What activities can be planned to address workplace diversity? How can they be evaluated?
4. Compare and contrast several models of cultural competence.
5. Define assimilation, ethnocentrism, enculturation, and acculturation.
6. How does culture influence people's daily practices, including food choices?
7. Think about your own food practices. What influences them? To what extent are social and cultural factors involved?
8. Discuss with peers the family and cultural origin of your food habits.
9. What is cultural competence? What steps can a professional take to develop it?

Suggested Activities

1. At your place of employment, identify which cultural and ethnic groups are represented. Do you believe that the talents of the diverse workers are being recognized?
2. List the cultural and traditional foods that you and your family members prepare. Share your cultural foods with neighbors and friends and inform them about your cultural customs.
3. Select one cultural or ethnic group with which you are unfamiliar. Research the food choices and practices of this culture.
4. Find someone from a culture you would like to learn more about. Ask the person to be your cultural guide or teacher. After developing a list of

questions to ask in advance, interview the person to gather information on their food choices, practices, recipes, cooking methods, and foods for special occasions such as holidays. Include spiritual beliefs and practices that influence food choices and overall health.

5. Interview a nutrition and dietetics professional who counsels culturally diverse populations. Ask questions about the counseling challenges and opportunities working with this group.

6. Visit a grocery store specialized in culturally diverse foods. Compare the price, packaging, and nutritional label information on two products that you can also find in a local grocery store chain.

7. Search the Internet for four culturally-appropriate education materials. Critique them for messages found in Table 4-2.

8. Locate the nearest food desert to your home or school. If possible, use the area to understand the opportunities and barriers for healthy food purchase.

Counseling for Health Behavior Change

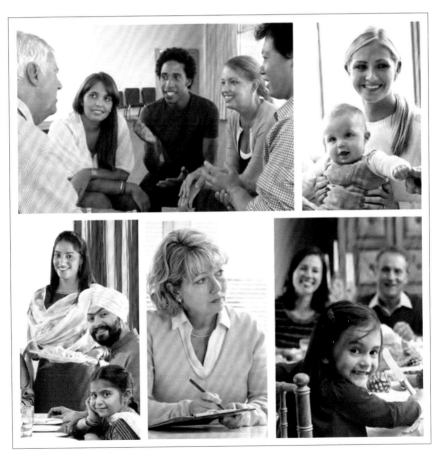

Stages and Processes of Health Behavior Change

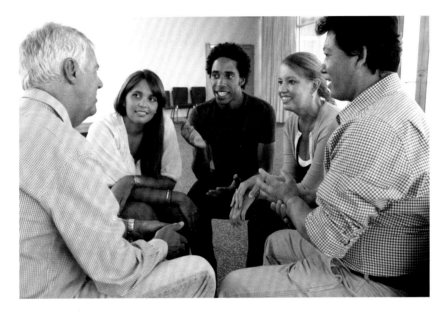

Objectives

- Explain the six stages of change.
- Identify one or more processes appropriate for each stage of change.
- Discuss the decisional balance and how should it be used.
- Describe the impact of self-efficacy on behavior change.
- Explain the steps in goal-setting process and practice them with a client.
- Describe Nutrition Monitoring and Evaluation in the Nutrition Care Process (NCP).
- Explain the requirements of the Health Insurance Portability and Accountability Act (HIPAA).

Len Howard is a 48-year-old male executive in a Fortune 500 company. In a recent physical exam, he was 5'11" tall and weighed 175 lb. His serum cholesterol was 290 (desirable less than 200 mg/dL) with HDL of 40 (desirable, 40 mg/dL or higher) and LDL of 160 (desirable less than 130 mg/dL.) His family history revealed that his father and older brother both died of heart disease. His wife is employed as an attorney, and they have a 15-year-old son.

Nutritionist: "You mentioned that the doctor wants you to try modifying your diet. Let's talk about what you are eating now. Then we can identify what you are eating that is OK and what, if any, changes you may be willing to make."

Mr. Howard's food intake revealed the following:

Breakfast: Orange juice, bacon, two slices of toast with peanut butter, and coffee.

Mid-AM Snack: Coffee and doughnut.

Lunch: Beef sandwich or bacon cheeseburger, French fries, and cola.

Dinner: 8 oz steak, baked potato with butter and sour cream, green vegetable, salad with blue cheese dressing, cookies, and wine.

Evening snack: Beer and pretzels.

One change leaves the way open for others.

—Niccolo Machiavelli

Introduction

There is no single gold standard method or unifying theory of counseling patients and clients that can account for all of the complexities of behavioral change and ensure success in changing people's food choices, eating, and exercise behaviors. Instead, the nutrition and dietetics counselor needs to be proficient in using several approaches and interventions yet adapting them to the person being counseled. Food and health behaviors are influenced by many factors including family, culture, physical, and social environments.[1]

This chapter explores the Transtheoretical Model of behavior change and the goal-setting process. The model emphasizes that people progress through various stages in modifying diet, exercise, and other health behaviors and that the counseling intervention strategies should be modified according to the client's Stage of Change.[2] Later chapters emphasize other counseling approaches, including motivational interviewing, the Health

Belief Model, behavior modification, counseling for cognitive change, the role of self-efficacy in making lifestyle changes, and preventing or dealing with lapses and relapse.

Transtheoretical Model/Stages of Change

Prochaska and colleagues developed the Transtheoretical Model (TTM), also referred to as Stages of Change (SOC).[3,4] (See Figure 5-1.) The purpose of the TTM is to guide the timing and content of interventions for better health. It is composed of four constructs: (1) Stages of Change, (2) processes of change or how people change, (3) decisional balance, and (4) situational self-efficacy. The model has guided interventions for a variety of health behaviors.[2]

CASE ANALYSIS 1

What is Mr. Howard eating that is desirable and that you can encourage him to continue doing? (foods reduced in cholesterol and saturated fatty acids)

The TTM is used to promote behavior change to improve health. After understanding the client's continuum of motivation to change, the framework helps the counselor with planning and implementing an appropriate intervention. Individuals progress through the six stages, often making many attempts to change problem health behaviors, such as eating too much, consuming less desirable foods, or not exercising. Within different stages, the various constructs and processes are used, to a greater or lesser extent, to promote movement through the stages.

Many health interventions and educational programs are action oriented, assuming that people who arrive for counseling are ready to make changes. However, a large number of people are in denial or resistant to change. Others may be thinking about it, and a few may be ready to change. Assuming that the client is prepared to change eating and exercise behaviors can be counterproductive.

People do not change their food choices because they know they have a health problem that requires change. It is a challenge to help people make positive dietary changes and motivate them to continue healthful choices for a lifetime. The key to successful nutrition counseling and education is to assess and identify the person's stage or readiness for change and match the interventions to it. Different counseling strategies are needed, for example, for those resisting efforts to change. Using the appropriate

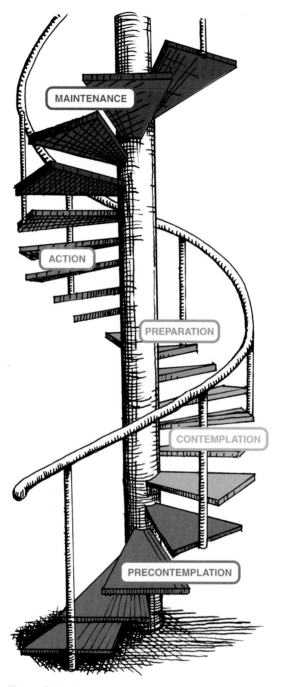

Figure 5-1 ■ Clients progress through Stages of Change.

intervention should increase the effectiveness, assist the client in progressing to the next SOC because of enhanced motivation and readiness, and reduce the likelihood of dropping out of treatment because the intervention was not appropriate.

Stages of Change

Change is *not* viewed as a single event, such as "I will eat less sodium starting today," but as an unfolding process over time requiring more than one attempt. The model in Table 5-1 shows the how, not the why, people change either with counseling or without it on their own. To make changes, people progress through six identified stages. The tasks at each stage vary, and movement through the stages represents personal progress for the client.

Precontemplation

In stage 1, *Precontemplation*, a person is unaware or underaware that a health problem exists, denies that there is a problem, or has no intention to take action to change. Thus, the individual has no plans, for example, to modify eating practices to lose weight or start exercising in the next 6 months.[3,4] The person may have tried a change previously and failed, such as to lose weight, and may be resistant to the health professional's efforts to suggest possible changes. Perhaps a visit to the doctor initiated a referral to see the nutrition and dietetics counselor for weight loss, even if the patient was not concerned with his or her weight.

Because these clients are unaware, uninformed, or unconcerned about the health problem, the counselor needs to assess the client's views on making a change and address the reasons for not wanting to change rather than providing dietary information.[3] Educating the client about food changes is not appropriate at this stage. To identify this stage, the counselor may ask: "Are you seriously intending to change (name the problem behavior) in the next 6 months?"

1. Precontemplation	No intention of changing in the next 6 mo.
2. Contemplation	Intending to change, but not soon.
3. Preparation	Small changes are made, intending to change in 30 d.
4. Action	Changes are made in food choices regularly
5. Maintenance	Behavior changes maintained for 6 mo.
6. Termination	Occurs only if changes are maintained for a year or more.

Table 5-1 ■ Stages of Change

For people ignoring the relationship between a high-fat diet and coronary heart disease, for example, one may ask: "Have you thought about eating less fat (or more fruits and vegetables) in the near future?" At this stage, a person with a heart problem may need to know the health benefits of change as well as the risks of not addressing the problem.

The client needs to "own" or acknowledge the health problem and its negative aspects.[3,4] These individuals are not ready for action-oriented interventions. Knowing the person's SOC helps the counselor identify the appropriate type of intervention. Table 5-2 lists sample questions and interventions at each stage.

Stage	Question for Client	Intervention
Precontemplation	"What can I do to help?"	Consciousness raising
	"Do you ever read articles about. . .?"	Assess knowledge
	"What do you know about the relationship between. . ."	Increase self-awareness, give written and oral information
	"Does anyone in your family have this problem?"	Assess values, beliefs
	"Are you aware of the consequences?"	Cognitive restructuring
	"How do you feel about making a change?"	Discuss risks and benefits
Contemplation	"What changes have you been thinking about?"	Assess knowledge
	"What are the pros and cons?"	Assess values, beliefs
	"How do you feel about it?"	Assess thoughts, feelings
	"What would make it easier or harder?"	Increase pros, decrease barriers
	"What would be the results of the change?"	Self-evaluation
	"How can I help?"	Cognitive restructuring
Preparation	"Are you intending to act in the next 1–6 mo?"	Self-efficacy, commitment
	"How will you do it?"	Decision making
	"What changes have you made already?"	Discuss beliefs about ability
	"How will your life be improved?"	Plan goals

Table 5-2 ■ Stages of Change Interventions

Action	"What are you doing differently?"	Stimulus control
	"What problems are you having?"	Self-reinforcement
	"Who can help you?"	Social support
	"How can I help?"	Self-management
	"What do you do instead of (former behavior)?"	Goal setting, group sessions, self-monitoring, relapse prevention
Maintenance	"How do you handle times when you slip up?"	Coping responses
	"What obstacles are you facing?"	Relapse prevention
	"What are your future plans?"	Self-management
	"What issues have you solved?"	Commitment, goal setting, control environment
Termination		Self-management, self-efficacy

Table 5-2 ■ (continued)

Contemplation

In stage 2, *Contemplation*, a person is aware that the health problem exists and intends to do better eventually, such as eating differently or exercising more. He or she has no serious thought of or commitment to making a change, however, and keeps putting it off.[3,4] The person may be mentally struggling with the amount of time, energy, effort, and cost of overcoming a health problem or may be discouraged by previous failures. When the cons of changing a behavior are large and the pros are small, the result may be ambivalence that keeps people stuck at this stage for long periods of time, even months or years.[3] The person needs to make a decision.

The counselor may ask, for example:

"What have you been thinking about in terms of making a change?"
"What are the pros and cons of doing it?"
"How can you change your environment?"
"What do you think about eating less fat? What are the barriers or obstacles to doing it?"

Preparation

In stage 3, *Preparation*, a person is more determined to make a change and intends to take initial action soon, perhaps in about 30 days.[4] He or she may report small changes in addressing the problem behavior, such as reading a few food labels or buying low-fat foods. Clients need to make a commitment to change, set priorities or goals, and develop a plan of action.[3,4]

The counselor may inquire about possible interest in losing weight, becoming more physically active, making healthier choices, and keeping records of food intakes. A study of parents of obese children needing weight loss found that about 62% of parents were in the action SOC for child dietary behaviors, but only 41% were for physical activity child behaviors. Parents who thought their own weight was a problem were less likely to make changes in their overweight children's behaviors.[5]

Action

In stage 4, *Action*, a person takes action to implement a plan and overcome the health problem by actively modifying food choices, behaviors, environments, and experiences.[3] Keep in mind that most clients are *not* in the action stage when first referred for counseling. People are classified in this stage if they have altered a behavior successfully for a certain period or up to 6 months, such as purchasing different groceries or exercising three times a week.

Considerable commitment of time and energy is required in the action stage when people are trying to change.[3] The counselor may ask: "What are you doing differently already?" At this stage, clients need knowledge and skills and should know how to respond to a lapse or relapse.[3] New behaviors are not firmly established in a week or a month, and old patterns may resurface.

With overweight adults using TTM with SOC, there was some evidence in an intervention that there were improvements in dietary habits and in physical activity. Examples were increased exercise frequency and duration, increased fruit and vegetable consumption, and reduced dietary fat intake.[6]

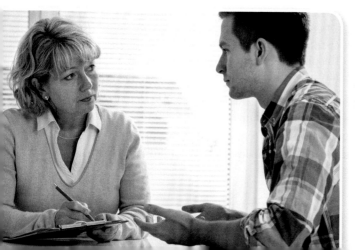

The counselor develops a relationship with the client.

Maintenance

In stage 5, *Maintenance,* a person consolidates and integrates new health behaviors into his or her lifestyle made over several months. With time, new behaviors need to become automatic. The client has to maintain the new, healthier habits and work to prevent relapse.[3,7] Maintaining weight loss, for example, takes continuing effort. For some people, this stage continues for months, years, or a lifetime, or until the behavior becomes a pattern and is incorporated into one's lifestyle.[3] The counselor may ask: "How do you handle small lapses?" Additional information on counseling about lapses and relapse is found in Chapter 8.

Termination

The ultimate goal is the *Termination* stage, in which changes have been maintained for years. The termination of a behavioral problem occurs if the client reacts automatically, is no longer tempted by the former behavior, and is no longer lapsing or relapsing. Some people never reach this stage, but periodically struggle with the health problem. In situations like weight control, a lifetime of maintenance may be the realistic goal.[4]

Recycling

Most people do not maintain changes in behaviors successfully on the first attempt. How long do your New Year's Eve resolutions last, for example? Prochaska proposed that most people proceed through the stages in a spiral, rather than a linear fashion.[3] Because lapses and relapse are common problems, recycling to an earlier stage, such as from action back to preparation or from preparation back to contemplation, may be expected several times as people struggle to modify or cease behaviors.[3]

People may avoid high fat and fried foods, for example, and then start eating them again. Moving back and forth through the stages represents a learning process for the client. Lapse and relapse and the negative emotional reactions (guilt, shame, failure) that may result are discussed along with the skills to recover in Chapter 8. People can learn from their mistakes with the help of the counselor and continue trying.

Processes of Change

A second dimension of the model examines 10 processes of change or the activities people use to progress through the SOC when there are shifts in behaviors, thoughts, and intentions. The 10 processes are cognitive and behavioral activities that clients use at different stages to promote changes in behaviors.[3,4] At each stage, there are specific, appropriate tasks and goals to be accomplished in moving on to the next stage.[3]

The 10 processes should be integrated into the SOC so that the treatment intervention matches the client's current stage. These are the ways that people adopt or modify new health promoting behaviors, eliminate risky behaviors, or change individual environments, either by themselves or with counseling.[3,7]

1. *Consciousness raising* increases the client's awareness of the health risks and insight into the consequences of the problem health behavior. It is the change process with the greatest focus and agreement.[3] It is most effective in helping people process information outside of their consciousness.

   Because people notice the positive information about themselves and ignore the negative, an outside party can provide feedback and education about the health behavior. Possible interventions are feedback from the counselor or others, confrontations, providing educational reading materials, media, and motivational interviewing approaches discussed in Chapter 6. Precontemplaters and contemplaters in stages 1 and 2 become more aware of the negative consequences of their behaviors, such as overeating and weight gain.

2. *Dramatic relief or catharsis* increases emotional awareness and feelings about the unhealthy behavior that may be relieved if appropriate action is taken. Techniques to use include role playing, personal testimonies, feedback, media, and motivational interviewing approaches.

3. *Self-reevaluation* includes both cognitive (thoughts) and affective (feelings) reassessments of the client's self-image either with or without the unhealthy eating, such as one's image as an obese person or a thinner person. Healthy role models, clarifying personal core values about health, and imagery may be useful. Changes are needed in how a person thinks and feels in the contemplation stage.[3]

4. *Environmental reevaluation* includes both cognitive (thoughts) and affective (feelings) assessment of how the personal behavior or health problem affects the client's social environment, especially family members. The client becomes aware that he or she may be a positive or negative role model for others. Reassessment may come from empathy training, testimonials, documentaries, or family interventions.

5. *Self-liberation* is the belief that one can change and the commitment to act on that belief. Public testimonies, New Year's resolutions, and

having multiple choices and alternatives may enhance willpower and belief in oneself.

6. *Social liberation* increases social alternatives and opportunities that support healthy behaviors for those who lack them. Empowerment and advocacy may be helpful.[7]

7. *Counterconditioning* entails changing the behavior in response to activities, such as substituting healthier coping strategies for unhealthy ones. Positive self-statements ("I can do it."), relaxation, and assertion are other strategies in the action stage.

8. *Stimulus control* removes environmental cues for unhealthy eating behavior and adds healthy ones instead; this is discussed further in Chapter 7. Avoidance of unhealthy foods, removing these cues to eating, choosing healthier food choices, and self-help groups can support change in eating practices in the action stage.

9. *Reinforcement management* includes positive reinforcement and rewards for healthy behaviors, as discussed in Chapter 7, and is helpful in the action stage. Behaviors are controlled by their consequences. When reinforcement is contingent on a certain response, that behavior may increase. Incentives, written contracts, reinforcement from others, and group recognition are strategies.[4]

10. *Helping relationships* provide caring, openness, acceptance, and support for healthy food choices and behavior change. Counselor phone calls or emails, having a buddy, attending a support group, and rapport with others can give social support.[3,4]

CASE ANALYSIS 3

What processes of change are appropriate for Mr. Howard's SOC?

Matching Processes to Stages of Change

The 10 processes are more effective during certain of the six SOC. Each stage has its own challenges. As a result, the counselor needs to match the processes with the person's identified SOC. In earlier stages, such as precontemplation, focusing on the benefits of making a change and how that change can improve the individual's life or health is suggested. The goal is for the client to think about the health problem. Clients may, however, doubt their ability to change and have decreased self-efficacy.

During precontemplation, clients are not thinking about making a change, are resistant, and have no plans to change. *Consciousness raising* methods can help clients become more aware of the negative consequences of their behaviors and possible changes that could help. The disease or death of a friend with the same or similar medical problem may raise consciousness also.[3]

In precontemplation, *consciousness raising* by providing nutrition information (oral, written, web addresses) about the benefits of healthy food choices, about the individual's risk of chronic disease based on dietary habits, and about the advantages of change is suggested. *Self-reevaluation* of thoughts, feelings, values, problems, self, and the environment is appropriate. The client needs to weigh the pros and cons of change, with the pros ("I'll see my grandchildren grow up.") outweighing the cons ("I can't eat whatever I want anymore."). Cons outweigh the pros at this stage.

Consciousness raising continues in the contemplation stage as clients note the nature of their health problems and reevaluate themselves. The *self-reevaluation* of the client's values and *environmental reevaluation* will consider the effects of the behaviors on the people they care about. Changes are required in how people think and feel about their health problems and lifestyle.[3] *Cognitive and affective self-reevaluation*, in addition to raising awareness, is suggested in the contemplation stage.

The preparation stage shows a readiness to change and may include learning from past attempts to make changes. Setting specific goals, priorities, and developing an action plan with a commitment to follow it is helpful. Because some small changes have been made, clients are already involved in self-regulation of their health behaviors.[3] They are taking small steps, may use *stimulus control* and *reinforcement control*, and need to believe that they can change.

Self-liberation, a belief that one can change, the actual making of a commitment to it, and using behavioral techniques are important in the preparation stage. *Self-liberation* is partly based on *self-efficacy* or the belief that one can succeed.[3] In the client's assessment, the benefits or pros of making changes must outweigh the cons.

The action stage requires *stimulus control, counterconditioning*, and *reinforcement management* to cope with conditions that may lead to lapsing. In the action and maintenance stages, behavioral techniques, such as those discussed in Chapter 7, namely, *stimulus control, reinforcement management, self-monitoring*, as well as recipe modification, and learning coping responses during conditions when relapse is likely, are helpful. Developing a social support system of significant others is useful.[3] Skills for controlling lapses and relapse are discussed in Chapter 8.

In sum, the client's effective health behavior change depends

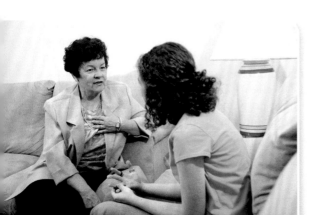

It is important to identify the client's SOC.

on doing the right things (processes) at the right time (stages). The best strategies at one stage may be ineffective at another. After identifying the person's health, dietary problems, and need for change, integrating the stage levels with the processes of change provides intervention suggestions for the counselor.[3] Keep in mind that the client may be at an early stage for one type of change, such as increasing fruit and vegetable intake, but at another stage for a different behavior, such as increasing exercise or decreasing portion sizes.

The counselor needs to be collaborative, empathic, and supportive in encouraging the client to develop insight into the health problem. By the action stage, the counselor is more like a coach and consultant available to provide expert advice and support.[3]

Decisional Balance

Decisional balance is a process of weighing the client's pros or advantages of changing with the cons or barriers to changing. The counselor may ask the client to make a written list of the pros and the cons. Clients who are unwilling to discuss the cons need to be encouraged to do so because they must be recognized and addressed. The balance between pros and cons varies by stage, with the cons outweighing the pros in the earlier stages. By the contemplation stage, the pros need to start outweighing the cons. See Table 5-3 for an example of a cost–benefit of change.

Whether dealing with weight control, reducing dietary fat or sodium, or increasing exercise, daily temptations and urges to eat unhealthy foods may arise when one is emotionally upset, in social situations with others, or craving a favorite food.[4] One may or may not be able to cope in high-risk situations when decisions are made about what to eat.

Across the stages, changes in pros need to occur more frequently than changes in cons. The pros may change more easily because the benefits are more immediate, such as feeling better about oneself for losing weight.

Continue to Eat as Before		Change Eating Behavior	
Pros	**Cons**	**Pros**	**Cons**
Pleasurable	Damages health	Better health	Change is difficult
Comfortable	Bad example for family	Feel better	Can't party with friends
Easy		Loses weight	Requires effort
Decreases loneliness			

Table 5-3 ■ Cost–Benefit Analysis for Change

Some of the cons may be beyond the individual's control, such as the cost and availability of healthful foods, yet others may be strongly held preexisting beliefs. It may be easier to increase the pros of the client by promoting awareness of the benefits of change, some of which may be unrecognized by the client.

SELF-ASSESSMENT 1

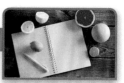

1. Think of a health problem or food behavior you would like to change.
2. Identify your SOC.
3. What processes or interventions are recommended for your SOC?
4. List the pros and cons of making the change.
5. On a scale of 1 to 10, with 10 the highest, how important is the change to you?

Self-efficacy

Self-efficacy is the belief that one can cope with temptations in high-risk situations without giving in or relapsing to former behaviors.[4] Based on Bandura's theory, self-efficacy refers to the confidence that the client has in adopting the new healthful behaviors. Because temptations are likely to occur, the client has to strive to avoid lapses and relapse. Examples of temptations to lapse are negative feelings and moods, holidays, emotional problems, cravings for food, and attending social events where food is served. A person with strong self-efficacy will perform healthy behaviors even when conditions are not ideal.

Self-efficacy affects one's motivation and the coping the client deals with. More than one change may be recommended, such as to consume a low-fat, low-calorie diet; add more fruits and vegetables; exercise daily; and stop smoking. These factors may be influenced by a person's age, sex, economic status, income, cultural group, educational level, and the like. Chapter 8 examines self-efficacy and relapse prevention.

In using personal stories of health behavior change from the Internet, one study selected and used those having the greatest impact on client attitudes toward weight loss. Outcomes indicated a change in self-efficacy and decisional balance for weight loss before and after personal stories were read.[8]

The key is not to prioritize what's on your schedule, but to schedule your priorities.

—Stephen Covey

Goal Setting

If the assessment of the client's SOC indicates a readiness to change, goal setting is one approach to use in counseling.[9] A client's new behaviors may be enhanced by deciding upon and making a commitment to specific goals. Nutrition counselors can assist individuals in establishing goals and action plans. Because clients are responsible for their own care, the nutrition interventions should be based on what the client is willing to change. This involves clients in their own health care and has them take an active part in their self-care and treatment.

In diabetes, for example, managing the disease is a daily event. Client-defined behavioral goals are effective in supporting self-management behaviors. Self-management and self-care goals and action plans for diabetes or pre-diabetes management, for example, may lead to improvements in diet, physical exercise, and self-efficacy.[10-12]

Before problems are explored and goals are set, it is advisable to discuss with the client, show approval for, and reinforce those current food choices that do not need changing, that is, what the individual is already doing right according to the Nutrition Assessment. After problems are identified, talk should turn to possible solutions.[3] Foods that should be limited and foods, or cooking practices, that should be changed may be discussed next, perhaps starting with what the client is willing to consider.

Goals should be mutually negotiated based on the Nutrition Intervention and desired clinical outcomes. In the case of normal nutrition, the Dietary Guidelines for Americans (DGA), which uses science-based advice to promote health and reduce the risk of disease, is appropriate. The DGA provides recommendations for the prevention of disease and for people who are at increased risk of a chronic disease, as seen in Box 5-1.[13,14] After conditions and circumstances surrounding food behaviors are explored, clients need to find solutions to their problems and develop goals and plans of action with the help of the counselor.

By law, every 5 years an advisory committee of recognized experts in the fields of nutrition and health review scientific and medical knowledge in providing recommendations for updating the Guidelines. They provide evidence-based nutrition and physical activity strategies for health promotion and disease prevention.[14]

Nutrition counseling should be directed not solely at the client's knowledge, but also at feelings, attitudes, beliefs, and values, which have strong and powerful influences on dietary behaviors. Knowledge is a tool only if and when a person is ready to change and is motivated to change. The counselor may ask any of the following types of questions:

For example

"Is this the right time to make changes?"

- Follow a healthy eating pattern across the life span.
- Focus on variety, nutrient density, and amount across all food groups.
- Limit calories from added sugars and saturated fats, and reduce sodium intake.
- Shift to healthier food and beverage choices within all food groups.
- Support healthy eating patterns for all: at home, school, and work.
- Meet physical guidelines for Americans.

Key Recommendations A Healthy Eating Pattern Includes:

- A variety of vegetables—dark green, red, and orange, legumes (beans/peas), starchy, and others.
- Fruits—especially whole fruits.
- Grains—at least half of which are whole grains.
- Fat-free or low-fat dairy, including milk, yogurt, cheese, and/or fortified soy beverages.
- A variety of protein foods, including seafood, lean meats and poultry, eggs, legumes (beans/peas); and nuts, seeds, and soy products.
- Oils

Limitations

- Saturated fats and trans fats, added sugars, and sodium.
- Consume less than 10% of calories per day from saturated fats.
- Consume less than 2,300 mg/day of sodium.
- If alcohol is consumed, it should be consumed in moderation—up to one drink per day for women and up to two drinks per day for men—and only by adults of drinking age.

Box 5-1 ■ Dietary Guidelines for Americans, 2015 to 2020: Guidelines.

"What was your goal in coming today?

"Which of these alternatives or changes do you think you could try?"

"What would be the easiest?" "The hardest?"

"What foods could you substitute?"

"How will things be better or worse after you make the change?"

"How do you feel about making this change?"

"Do you think you can succeed?"

The client weighs the pros and cons of the options.

The goals we choose determine how we will live. Clients (not the counselor) at the Preparation, Action, and Maintenance SOC should select one or two priorities or goals for change for the next week or so. An obesity intervention group, for example, received health information and goal-setting support through group meetings and newsletters. Results showed participants moving from Contemplation to Action/Maintenance for the goals of improving diet and physical activity.[15]

Those who are enthusiastic or unrealistic about making total changes immediately, such as losing 20 lb in a month, are setting themselves up for frustration and possible failure, which may lead to abandoning the dietary changes altogether.[16] The counselor should guard against this and use other interventions instead. Slow, steady changes that will persist over time are preferable. Rather than focusing on long-term goals, the focus should be on achieving short-term behavioral goals of meeting daily food and exercise goals.[17]

The session with a client needing a meal pattern limited in sodium, for example, may uncover the following obstacles:

1. Uses salt in cooking and at the table.
2. Snacks include crackers and potato chips.
3. Uses some high-sodium spices and flavorings.
4. Likes bacon, ham, and salami.
5. Eats lunch in a restaurant.
6. Is the only one in the family on a limited sodium diet.
7. Grocery shopping is done by the wife, who does not read labels.

Four steps may be used in setting goals with clients. They include (1) goal identification, (2) goal importance and acceptance, (3) goal analysis and overcoming obstacles, and (4) goal implementation.

Step 1: Goal Identification

The first step in goal setting is identification of what the client finds is appropriate and feasible. Personal goals can spur clients to new achievements and changes because they give people something to strive for as well as a standard against which to judge one's progress. Because clients are more committed to changes that they select, the counselor may inquire which one or more potential changes the person wants to address first by saying, "Which one or two changes do you think that you can work on this week?" When people play a significant role in selecting goals, they hold themselves responsible for progress. If goals are imposed by the counselor, people may not accept them or feel personally responsible for fulfilling them.

What are some possible short-term goals for change for Mr. Howard to consider with you?

The goals should meet each of the elements of the S.M.A.R.T System, which stands for Specific, Measurable, Attainable, Realistic, and Time Specific.[18] Goals selected by the client should be positively stated as concrete behaviors. A goal should specify what the person will do or is trying to achieve. The following are examples of specific goals:

> **EXAMPLE**   "I will eat fruit instead of baked desserts 5 days this week."
> "I will lose 1 to 2 lb each week for the next 4 weeks."
> "I will walk for 20 minutes on Monday, Wednesday, and Friday this week."

Specific, clear, attainable goals produce higher levels of performance than do general intentions to do the best one can, which may have little or no effect. An example of the latter is a statement such as "I'll look for low-sodium foods the next time I am at the grocery store." When goals are set unrealistically high, performance may prove disappointing. If the client selects problems numbered 1 and 2 from the earlier sodium list, for example, these can be reinterpreted into achievable goals for change as follows:

> **EXAMPLE**   "I will use low-sodium seasonings in cooking and pepper at the table starting today."
> "I will eat fruits and low-sodium crackers for snacks 4 days this week."

Note that the positive statement of using low-sodium seasonings is preferable to the negative goal of avoiding salt. It is easier to do something positive than to avoid doing something. A plan for reaching each goal can be explored by asking the question, "How will you do that?"[19]

Setting specific goals can be motivating and result in positive outcomes. For example: "I will walk for 30 minutes every day." Measurable goals should be written down with a frequency and time frame and referred to regularly to serve as a constant reminder of the plan of fulfilling them.[19] One should keep a log daily or weekly of what was done to fulfill the goals.

To be realistic and reasonable, goals should be based on the person's past and current behavior. The first challenge should be only a small step away, not a major change from the current behavior, and should be matched with the client's perceived capabilities for achieving it. The counselor should guide people toward those goals that they believe can realistically be accomplished. A brief discussion as to "why" the person decided on a goal may add to motivation, as in "Tell me about the reasons that you are interested in losing 10 lb."

A distinction must be made between short-term goals and distal or end goals. Short-term goals that are challenging, but attainable with effort, are likely to be more motivating and self-satisfying. Self-motivation can be increased by progressively achieving short-term goals, even though a long-range goal of losing 20 lb is difficult to realize. For example, people need to commit themselves to the goal of following the dietary changes or goals today, rather than a long-term goal of never eating high-fat foods again. When the distant future is the focus, such as losing 20 lb, it is easy to put off the goal and decide to start some other day. Persistence that leads to eventual mastery of an activity is thus ensured through a progression of short-term goals, each with a high probability of success.

Step 2: Goal Importance and Acceptance

After identifying one or two goals, the counselor assesses the importance of the goal by asking, for example: "On a scale of 1 to 10, with 10 being the highest, how important is that goal to you?" If the answer is "5," a different goal should be found. Goals that are not perceived as important by the client are unlikely to be achieved.

CASE ANALYSIS   5

How would you ask Mr. Howard to assess the importance of a choice of goals?

The strength of a person's goal commitment and priorities is affected by several factors.[19] The counselor may inquire about these:

"How will you do it?"
"What makes this important to you?"
"What are the benefits of reaching the goal?"
"Is there someone else with whom you can share your plans?"

Step 3: Goal Analysis and Overcoming Obstacles

It is important to discuss how the impact of physical, cultural, social, and cognitive environments will affect goals. The counselor may ask: "What problems do you see in achieving this goal?" "What may interfere?" "How do you feel about this change?" It is advisable to tell the client to expect some problems, since obstacles may come up that were not considered during the counseling session. When the client is aware of the possibility of problems, he or she may avoid abandoning the dietary changes with the first lapse or obstacle. After all, basketball players do not make a basket every time they shoot the ball. But they keep on trying.

CASE ANALYSIS 6

How would you discuss any obstacles Mr. Howard sees to reaching the goals?

Step 4: Goal Implementation

In the final step in the intervention process, clients can discuss what specific action steps they plan to take to reach the goals.[18,19] For example, the goal of using low-sodium seasonings may require identifying and purchasing them, acquiring new recipes for using them, and modifying favorite recipes to replace salt.

CASE ANALYSIS 7

What are some possible steps Mr. Howard could take to reach his goals? What key discussion points would you identify?

By selecting a level of performance, people create their own incentives to persist in their efforts until they match the standards of the goals. Clients compare results against the goals continually so that they know when they are succeeding. The personal standards against which performance attainments are compared affect how much self-satisfaction or self-efficacy the client derives from the goal. Feedback on progress is provided by mental comparison with the goal and a self-evaluation. Clients' active participation in selecting and setting goals for diet and physical exercise resulted in successful

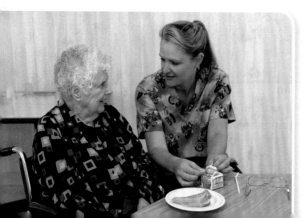

Goals for change are developed.

outcomes.[20] The counselor should also provide positive feedback no matter how small the change.

The attainment of short-term goals builds motivation, competencies, interest, and self-perceptions of efficacy. Motivational effects do not derive from the goals themselves, but from accomplishing them. When individuals commit themselves to goals, negative discrepancies between what they are doing and what they seek to achieve create self-dissatisfactions that may serve as incentives motivating enhanced effort.

Without standards against which to measure performance, people have little basis for judging how well they are doing, nor do they have a basis for judging their capabilities. Short-term attainments increase self-efficacy, and self-satisfaction sustains one's efforts. Accomplishments may be positively reinforced verbally or rewarded with something the client desires.[18,19] Attainments falling short of the goals lower perceived self-efficacy and the way one feels about oneself.

CASE ANALYSIS **8**

What type of follow-up would you recommend with Mr. Howard?

Nutrition Intervention

The nutrition intervention is determined based on the nutrition assessment, nutrition diagnosis, and the client's goals. The goals suggest the information, knowledge, and skills the client needs to make dietary changes. The counselor judges what information to provide, how much information can be absorbed at each session, at what educational or literacy level, and what handouts and media to use as supplements. The amount of information to provide and the best method of doing so must be individualized and matched to the client's SOC and cultural influences.

The intervention may include nutrition education, for example, about the following topics and activities: reading food labels; adapting recipes; menu planning; restaurant or carry-out meals; principles of healthful eating; food safety; nutrients in selected foods; nutritional supplements; nutrition misinformation; fat, carbohydrate, sodium, or calorie counting; nutrient–drug interactions; managing appetite; and the relationship of nutrition to the health problem. In addition, clients need to know about exercise, self-monitoring, and self-management. Problem-solving interventions for meal planning, food preparation, and food purchasing may be needed. Culturally sensitive interventions are important in meeting the needs, desires, and lifestyles of ethnic clients.

By the end of the counseling session, the client should not only know what to do and how to do it, but also be committed to doing it. Clients should be asked to summarize their plans to check for understanding and commitment. To succeed, the client has to perceive and accept the need for change. Motivation for change should be explored, as well as the health dangers in continuing the current dietary patterns. Solely providing information about a dietary regimen is not usually enough to interest or enable people to improve their eating practices.

The counselor obtains and documents the client's commitment to specific action behaviors at specific times. Practitioners frequently ask clients to keep self-monitoring records of food intakes, exercise, and environments. They may be submitted in advance or brought to the next appointment as a way to learn about factors affecting eating behaviors and as a demonstration of a commitment to change.

Self-monitoring is a process in which the person observes and records information about dietary intake, physical activity, and body weight. It is often coupled with goal setting and is helpful in weight management.[21] Clients' personal records, observations, and analyses of their environment contribute to their personal awareness and understanding. There is some evidence in overweight adult women that self-monitoring of diet, weight, or both in a program incorporating goal setting was associated with better weight loss outcomes.[21] Self-monitoring of food intake improved nutrition outcomes related to weight loss.[20]

Nutrition Monitoring and Evaluation

Nutrition monitoring and evaluation together comprise the fourth step in the nutrition care process (NCP).[22] Monitoring is the follow-up step and evaluation is the comparison step, whether it is comparison with the previous client visit or with a standard or goal. The purpose of monitoring and evaluation is to ascertain progress and modify recommendations as needed to promote progress toward goals. The determination of what the intervention should be and the evaluation mechanisms are individualized.

An outcome is the measured result of the counseling process. Outcome data identify the benefits of medical nutrition therapy in patient and client care. In using these systems of quality control, nutrition and dietetics counselors may wish to evaluate several things: (1) the success of the client in following the goals set and in implementing new eating behaviors; (2) the degree of success of the nutrition intervention, including its strengths and weaknesses; and (3) their own personal skills as counselors.

The counselor should keep records of the client's issues and goals, the factors influencing them, and the intervention for future measurement of client change. Some examples of outcomes are changes in weight, glycemic control, blood pressure, lipid, and other laboratory values; patient acceptance and progress at self-care and self-management; improvements in knowledge and dietary changes; and lifestyle changes. These indicate the impact of the intervention and can be used to evaluate the effectiveness of the treatment. The counselor and client should engage in evaluation together.

Some measures of success are obvious, such as an overweight person who is now eating differently. Other outcome measures may be indicators of quality of care. Some tools or data sources for monitoring and evaluation are questionnaires, interviews, anthropometric assessments, biochemical and medical tests, and food and nutrition intake records. The blood pressure and lipid levels of cardiovascular patients can be monitored, for example, although they are more difficult to evaluate because they may depend on factors beyond dietary adherence. Despite the client's commitment to dietary change, results may not reflect adherence to the regimen. These outcomes can be used by the health care team working together to adjust the treatment to achieve or maintain treatment goals.

Frequent follow-up for reassessment, further intervention, coaching, and support is essential until the client is self-sufficient. Discussion at subsequent sessions should focus first on what went well, that is, the successful experiences and short-term goals reached, no matter how small. Such a positive focus helps clients feel that they can have some control over their eating, health, and life, and builds a sense of personal mastery and coping ability.

Self-monitoring records kept by the client should be examined jointly, discussed, and difficulties identified and resolved. Overlooking the records indicates to clients that they were not considered important. If progress is made, new short-term goals for change may be established jointly for the appropriate SOC. Support and reinforcement to strengthen desirable habits along with gradual, planned changes should continue as long as necessary until the client is successful at self-management.

Enthusiasm for change may decline during the first week and even more during the second week, as obstacles develop. Therefore, frequent follow-up appointments should be scheduled if possible. Counselors in acute care settings who do not have the opportunity for follow-up may need to refer patients to nutrition and dietetics counselors in outpatient settings or in private practice, because one session with a client is insufficient to promote long-term change in health practices.

Documentation

The Joint Commission sets standards that are required to address quality-of-care issues in the health care environment. Documentation is essential to quality patient care and reimbursement, and health care professionals need to meet the provisions in the Joint Commission standards.

A summary of the professionals' interventions with the patient or client should be communicated to the medical team or other referral source in the medical record using the NCP.[22] Documentation is ongoing and supports all of the steps in the NCP. Hospital discharge instructions must be documented and provided to the organization or individual responsible for the person's continuing care.

As the client returns for follow-up appointments, results of health outcomes and goals achieved should be noted. Changes in weight, meal intake, tolerance problems, results of new laboratory values, medications, and skills in self-management may be assessed. Follow-up reassessment with new goals and interventions should be recorded.

Electronic Communication

Traditional counseling roles are changing. With advances in technology, nutrition and dietetics professionals can communicate with clients in more ways, such as the Internet, email, and telephone. Some have their own web sites. Our clients have access to computers, email, and may have searched the Internet for health and nutrition information.

Some professionals are counseling over the telephone, on email, or via the web. A recent evaluation of client monitoring of dietary intake assessed using computer, smartphone, and/or paper based options reported that online computer smartphone records were as accurate as paper records.[23] A computer-administered food frequency questionnaire (FFQ) was evaluated and reported to be as good as reported on paper FFQs.[24] Clients may be asked to submit their food records before the appointment or bring them with them.

Nutrition counselors in private practice need to maintain written policies and procedures for handling private health information (PHI). The Health Insurance Portability and Accountability Act (HIPAA) requires compliance with their standards and regulations for safeguarding the PHI of clients and patients.[25] This includes any health care information that can identify the person in oral conversations, paper, or electronic form.[26]

In offering remote health care, video conferencing has been used for delivering telehealth service in the United States and Australia. When information is transmitted electronically by telehealth or video services, the HIPAA requirements for protection of patient information are still necessary. HIPAA requires maintaining safeguards to protect the security and confidentiality of PHI including personal information transmitted electronically.[27]

The standards on Privacy of Identifiable Health Information guarantees privacy and confidentiality of patient medical records and information.[25] In private practice, one is considered a Covered Entity (CE) who may access and transmit PHI and thus must follow HIPAA regulations. Any Business

Associates (BA) of CEs who may access or transmit PHI must also follow HIPPA and need a written Business Associate Agreement (BAA) or contract to handle client health information safely and securely.[25]

The professional in private practice is required to have a Notice of Privacy Practices (NPP) and is responsible for giving one to clients.[26] Online resources for documents and explanations can be found at web sites of the Department of Health and Human Services (HHS) and the American Medical Association.[26,28] One's laptop computer that contains PHI should be password protected or encrypted to secure health information. This will allow sending clients their health information in secure form. Because of the complexity of government regulations and changes in the rules and information, other resources should be examined by those who are affected.[26,28,29]

Patient/client information must be safeguarded. There should be policies that restrict use and disclosure of information without authorization. The client's informed consent and agreement for the use and disclosure of PHI for electronic or phone treatment and for payment purposes is needed.[28] Forms should be signed by the client and documented with a copy to the client. Electronic policies should protect both the client and the practitioner. Professionals should retain in long-term storage electronic or paper copies of electronic communications with clients in a way that maintains confidentiality.

It is important to know whether or not your incoming and outgoing email messages are encrypted. If not, email messages are not secure and are unprotected traveling over the Internet. Some configure an automatic reply to acknowledge the receipt of email messages with an added standard text with the practitioner's name, contact information, and security reminders. Others use email for follow-up because written copies of electronic communications with clients may be subject to less distortion or misunderstanding than verbal follow-up by telephone. Electronic or paper copies of electronic communications with clients should be retained in secure, protected, long-term storage.[28]

Summary

All nutrition and dietetics professionals need to be knowledgeable about the theories, models, concepts, processes, and techniques of counseling. A comprehensive approach to counseling that considers lifestyle, environments, culture, and psychological and social factors is needed. The SOC construct from the TTM identifies clients' readiness and motivation to change health behaviors whereas the processes of change identify a number of choices of interventions that are appropriate at the different SOC. Counselors assist clients in formulating one or more realistic, behavioral goals for change as an incentive to measure performance. The following chapters discuss other approaches to counseling.

Review and Discussion Questions

1. Explain the six steps in the SOC.
2. Compare the processes of change at the precontemplation stage with those at the action SOC.
3. Explain the decisional balance and how it may be used with clients.
4. Explain the steps in the process of goal setting.

Suggested Activities

1. During the next week, make arrangements to observe a nutritionist's counseling session. Afterward, discuss the approaches and theories of nutrition counseling.
2. Interview someone who would like to modify his or her food behaviors. Identify the person's SOC. Determine which processes of change are appropriate to the identified SOC, and implement them.
3. Form triads consisting of a counselor, counselee, and observer. Each person should take a turn in each of the roles for 7 minutes. The counselee should play the role of a client with hypertension or obesity, and the counselor should use paraphrasing and empathizing along with open and closed questions to determine the person's SOC and facilitate disclosure and problem solving. After each round, the observer should share reactions to the counselor's approach and encourage feedback from the counselee to the counselor. From the counselee's perspective, what did the counselor do that helped their interaction; what did he or she do that hindered it?

4. In groups of two, take turns discussing a lifestyle problem and restating it as a goal for change.

   A. Think of a lifestyle problem the counselee would like to change, such as eating too much; eating the wrong foods; needing to eat more fruits and vegetables, more fiber, or less fat; exercising too little; needing to budget better; drinking too much; smoking too much; or the like.

   B. Help the person discuss the problem and the conditions and circumstances surrounding it. Then have the counselee restate the problem as a positive goal for change, that is, "I will. . ."

   C. Assess the importance of the goal on a scale of 1 to 10, with 10 representing the highest importance. Revise the goal if necessary.

   D. Ask about and discuss the obstacles and barriers to accomplishing the goal, and try to have the person resolve these.

   E. Have the person list the steps toward achieving the goal. What will the person do, and when will it be done?

5. Visit one or more web sites to determine what clients may find and how it may or may not help them change their food choices. Share your results with the class.

6. In groups of two, discuss the following client statements to determine what SOC the person is in.

   A. "I have made some changes in my food choices over the past 6 months."

   B. "I am intending to change the foods I eat in a few weeks."

   C. "I intend to make some changes in the next 6 months."

   D. "I don't eat high-fat foods anymore."

   E. "Maybe I'll make some changes."

   F. "I think my food choices are OK."

Person-Centered Counseling

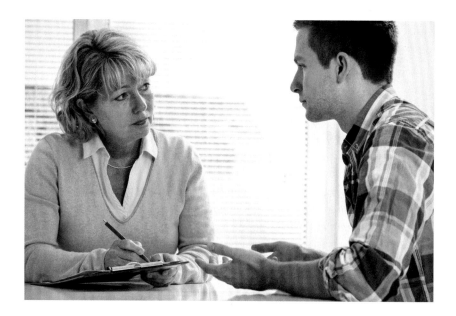

Objectives

- List Rogers' six conditions in a client relationship.
- List and explain the principles of motivational interviewing.
- Explain the communication methods used in motivational interviewing.
- Explain how reflective listening is used.
- Explain the Health Belief Theory.
- Describe the guidelines for directive counseling.

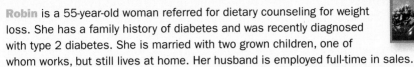

Robin is a 55-year-old woman referred for dietary counseling for weight loss. She has a family history of diabetes and was recently diagnosed with type 2 diabetes. She is married with two grown children, one of whom works, but still lives at home. Her husband is employed full-time in sales.

Robin works half-time at a retail store. She is 5'4" tall and weighs 185 lb. Her doctor suggested that she lose some weight to improve her blood sugar level. She indicated that she lost weight before, but gained it all back. She is ambivalent about changing her food habits or family food preferences.

Counseling—the art of providing listening, advice, guidance, or direction regarding an action or decision to help a person change.

Introduction

One of the key roles of nutrition and dietetics professionals is to promote the optimal health of the public. The practitioner translates the science of nutrition into healthful foods and nutrient intake for individuals or groups. To achieve appropriate food intake, often health behaviors and lifestyles must change.

Many factors influence the health behaviors we engage in, whether beneficial or harmful to our health, such as failure to exercise or to eat healthfully. Some of these factors include socioeconomic status, environment, culture, skills, attitudes, values, beliefs, and religion. Nutrition counseling focuses on helping clients accomplish changes. Counseling also comes into play in the managerial aspects of dietetics in the form of staff counseling for development or remediation.

In this chapter, counseling approaches, theories, and models are considered as approaches to implementing a nutrition care plan and intervention. Strategies selected should be based on the best current knowledge and evidence available. If the intervention, whether education or counseling, does not produce a change in knowledge, skills, behavior, or health outcome, the continuation of the intervention will be questioned.

Using Theories and Models

Theory is a foundation of professional practice providing interrelated constructs, concepts, propositions, and definitions with the purpose of understanding, explaining, and predicting relationships and health behaviors.[1,2] One selects the theory and intervention to use to achieve behavior change.

After identifying the person's health issues and current behaviors, one's professional experience is a guide in implementing a theory-based intervention. Because no one theory is appropriate in every situation, it is not unusual to combine constructs from different models and theories.[1] If the theory or model helps explain a behavior, it may suggest ways to design interventions that achieve behavior change and improve a person's health.

Nutrition counseling is a collaborative counselor–patient/client relationship to set priorities, establish goals, and create individualized action plans that acknowledge and foster responsibility for self-care and self-management. Nutrition counseling strategies are designed to achieve behavior change toward a particular client goal.

Counseling assists people in learning about themselves and their environments. Counselors aid individuals with the decision-making process, resolving interpersonal concerns, and helping them learn new skills and ways of dealing with life situations. Counseling is a science as well as an art. The skills of the counselor allow for customizing the counseling for the individual client.

This chapter views the counseling process as one that involves the development of a trusting, collaborative relationship between counselor and client, includes the evaluation of client issues, and the use of various techniques of problem solving. The approaches to counseling may be classified as nondirective or directive. The nondirective or "client-centered" approach may be applied to the nutrition counseling of clients. It includes active listening and helping the person determine how to proceed. Directive counseling is applied more often to staff regarding job-related issues.

Counseling is an individualized process that involves suggesting constructive alternatives based on what is important to and manageable for the client. Several theories, models, and approaches are described in this chapter, including nondirective and directive counseling, Motivational Interviewing, and the Health Belief Model. Chapters 7, 8, and 9 expand the discussion of counseling to include other theories and models of counseling for behavior change.

Nondirective Counseling

The nondirective approach to counseling is often called "client-centered," "person-centered," or "Rogerian counseling" and is best represented by the writings of its originator, Carl Ransom Rogers. Rogers used the term "nondirective" as the client directs the flow of conversation. The theory is one of the more detailed and consistent.

A basic assumption in the Rogerian client-centered point of view is that people are rational and realistic. Individuals possess an inherent tendency toward realizing their potential for growth and self-actualization, if their needs for positive regard from others and for positive self-regard or self-esteem are satisfied.

One of the most important characteristics of the Rogerian theory is the therapeutic relationship between the counselor and the client. The underlying assumption is that the client cannot be helped simply by listening to the knowledge the counselor possesses or to the counselor's explanation of the client's behavior.[3-5] Prescribing "cures" and corrective behaviors are seen as being of little lasting value. The relationship that is most helpful to clients enables them to discover within themselves the capacity to use the relationship to change and grow. One of the phrases that is used to describe Rogers' therapy is supportive, not reconstructive.

Rogers' approach suggests six conditions that are necessary in the relationship with the client.[3-5]

1. *Relationship.* The counselor and client have a relationship in which each makes a difference to the other. The counselor needs to be *accepting* of and respect the clients as individuals as they are, with their good and bad points, their conflicts and inconsistencies without judgment or disapproval. Only after clients are convinced that they are accepted with unconditional positive regard can they begin to trust the counselor.

2. *Vulnerability.* The client is vulnerable to anxiety in the relationship, but is motivated to continue the counseling relationship.

3. *Genuineness.* In the counseling relationship, the counselor is willing to express his or her own feelings. Exceptional counselors are characterized by *congruence or genuine*ness within the counseling relationship. They are honest, integrated, and consistent, with no contradictions between what they are and what they say. These counselors are able to express outwardly to their clients what they are feeling within themselves. Their verbal and nonverbal behaviors are consistent.

4. *Unconditional positive regard.* The counselor experiences unconditional positive regard for the client. The counselor cares about the client and this is perceived by the client. The client's positive self-regard is strengthened.

5. *Accurate empathy.* The counselor experiences the client's world through empathy and communicates the understanding to the client. The counselor must experience an accurate, *empathic understanding* of the client's world as seen from the inside, sensing the client's world as if it were his or her own. This understanding enables clients to explore freely and deeply and develop a better comprehension of themselves. It is of no value for the counselor to be accepting, genuine, and understanding if the client does not perceive or experience this. The acceptance, genuineness, and understanding need to be *communicated* to the client verbally and nonverbally.

6. *Perception of genuineness.* The client perceives the acceptance and understanding of the counselor. The counselor must be seen as genuine for the client to trust the empathy and caring of the counselor. This type of relationship can facilitate positive change.[5]

The process of change in client-centered therapy is conceptualized as a "combination of consciousness raising and corrective emotional experiencing that occurs within the context of an affirming, and empathic relationship."[5] The counselor listens actively and accurately reflects back the client's thoughts and feelings. This directs the client's attention to become fully conscious of their experiences.

The counselor uses reflection of what the client says by the mirroring back to the client of what he or she is saying to increase awareness. If the client says, for example, "my life is too busy to make food changes," the counselor reflects this back by saying, "So you have a lot of commitments right now." This communicates that the counselor is listening and trying to understand. One should not repeat every phrase as it can have a parrot-like effect. Active listening, reflecting, and paraphrasing are useful. It is important to understand the client and the client's world and determine what the client thinks is important.

If the counselor has these characteristics and attitudes and is able to communicate them to the client, then a relationship develops that is experienced by the client as safe, secure, free from threat, and supportive. The counselor is perceived as dependable, trustworthy, and consistent.

This outcome requires being a good listener, having intuition, providing feedback on both data and feelings, and providing inspiration.[6] It is the type of relationship that supports behavioral change, whether one is working with clients or with staff.

In a client-centered approach, practitioners ask questions and listen carefully to understand the person's viewpoint within the context of their daily lives. It involves supporting the person's ability to self-manage his or her own medical problem or condition emphasizing problem solving, goal setting, and increasing self-efficacy.

Motivational Interviewing

William Miller first described Motivational Interviewing (MI) in 1983 after treating problem drinkers. MI has been described as "Carl Rogers in new clothes" since some of the techniques are rooted in Rogers' approaches.[5] MI has been defined as a "directive, client-centered counseling style for eliciting behavior change by helping clients to explore and resolve ambivalence."[6] It is a person-centered method of guiding to evoke and strengthen a person's motivation and commitment to change.[7]

MI was originally developed from work with addictive behaviors, but the intervention has been used also in a variety of healthcare behaviors.[5] After three decades of research and clinical trials, results have been published for a variety of health problems including diabetes, heart disease, dietary change, and exercise. Studies have shown its effectiveness in weight loss, reducing blood pressure, reducing blood cholesterol, and other medical problems.[8,9] MI is being practiced with a range of cultural groups, and books about MI have been translated into at least 22 languages.[7] Two recent books have applied MI to diabetes care and to MI in nutrition and fitness.[10,11]

Ambivalence

Ambivalence about change is normal and people experience it regularly.[10] Ambivalence is the existence of mutually conflicting feelings about thoughts or ideas, such as "I'd like to lose weight, but I enjoy eating."[9] MI is a counseling style for addressing the ambivalence about change.[7] It has person-centered elements, such as empathy, an egalitarian relationship with a guiding style, and person-centered techniques, such as key questions, reflective listening, shared decision-making, and eliciting change talk.[12]

People may have mixed feelings and an inability to select between two or more actions. There are reasons to change a behavior as well as reasons not to. MI is different in using a collaborative, person-centered communication style and in providing a method and process of moving people toward behavior change and incorporating goals for change. The approach is designed to help people build a commitment and reach a decision to change. The counselor elicits the clients' own motivations for making a change in the interest of their health.

Chances are that clients already know that eating healthier and exercising more promote positive health, but they are enjoying the status quo (a sedentary lifestyle, lack of exercise, and eating the wrong foods) and think of reasons *not* to change. Once people become unstuck from the conflicting motivations of whether or not to change that immobilize them, they can move toward a decision and a commitment to take action. MI helps to resolve the ambivalence and move them toward change.

MI is recognized as an effective approach in Diabetes Self-Management Education.[13] It may be especially useful along with other evidence-based methods when ambivalence or lack of motivation is the main obstacle to behavior change. These would be people in the precontemplation and contemplation Stages of Change discussed in Chapter 5. The approach can be integrated into Prochaska's Stages of Change Model in which people move from being unaware or unwilling to do anything about a health problem, called *precontemplation*, to considering the possibility of change or *contemplation*.[5] In later stages, people prepare to make a change, or determine to finally take action.

CASE ANALYSIS 1

What would you say to Robin to initiate the conversation?

MI seeks to overcome ambivalence and evoke the client's own motivation for change. It promotes the client's readiness to change or to try various courses of action. The client elaborates and the counselor uses reflective listening to mirror back what the client has said. Rollnick and colleagues consider MI a form of guiding rather than giving advice and directing. They suggest that all consultations be based on a guiding style even if full MI is not done.[6]

In a nonthreatening atmosphere, the nutrition and dietetics counselor may explore with clients their ambivalence and have them, not the counselor, voice the reasons for making a change. This approach is also useful in follow-up visits with clients.

Spirit of Motivational Interviewing

As in client-centered therapy, the counselor's style or approach is a central factor in MI. The motivational approach draws on empathic, client-centered counseling that guides rather than directs and does not offer advice. MI has a special character or spirit represented by specific counselor behaviors. The guiding philosophy is not unique to MI and the elements may be found in other approaches. The three components are: (1) partnership, (2) evocation, and (3) honoring client autonomy.[7]

Partnership

MI is a partnership. The relationship is not one in which a passive client is given advice and information by the counselor. It is not something done to a person. MI is done "for" and "with" a person as an active collaboration, recognizing that the client is the expert on his or her environment and life situation although the counselor has specific expertise.

One seeks a collaborative partnership between the counselor and client for conversation to understand the client's situation, points of view, and goals. In the conversation, there is joint discussion of the problems

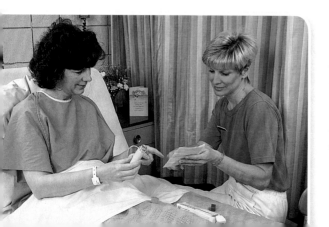

The counselor listens to the client to understand her point of view.

that only the client can solve and change. There should be an empathic understanding and supportive atmosphere in responding to client remarks. This is a way to activate the client's motivation and resources for change.[7]

Evocation

Evocation involves drawing out the client's thoughts, feelings, and situations. One seeks to "evoke" or call forth the clients' own motivations, goals, and aspirations in the interest of their health. Clients know their specific challenges and barriers to change. The counselor's goal is to draw out the client's reasons for change, plans, methods for making changes, and if asked, provide ideas for the client to consider. The role of the counselor is that of a guide who offers assistance along a path to change that the client selects.

Honoring Client Autonomy

Honoring client autonomy means that decisions are left up to the client even though the counselor may have other preferences or opinions. People do not like to be told what to do. Simply giving clients advice to change often is ineffective.[7] The client has the right and freedom to select the path to change. In honoring client autonomy, the counselor recognizes that it is the client who decides and that being told what to do may elicit the "Yes, but . . ." response. For example: "You need to exercise more and eat less." "Yes, but . . ." (See Box 6-1).

The responsibility for change lies with the client: "It's up to you to decide what to do. It's your choice." The goal is to increase the client's motivation, so that change arises from within rather than being imposed from without.[7] The client, not the counselor, needs to develop and speak aloud the arguments for change.

MI can save time by focusing the discussion on changes that make a difference and avoiding unproductive discussion. While the counselor directs the collaborative discussion by guiding it, the focus is on honoring client autonomy in decision making and eliciting the client's own motivation for change.

Spirit of MI	Principles of MI
Partnership	Resist the "Righting" Reflex
Evocation	Understand Your Client's Motivation
Honor Client Autonomy	Listen to Your Client
	Empower Your Client

Box 6-1 ■ Foundations of Motivational Interviewing.

Principles of Motivational Interviewing

In the past, Miller and Rollnick expressed their principles as expressing empathy, supporting self-efficacy, developing discrepancy, and rolling with resistance.[6,14] Recently, they expressed their principles with the acronym RULE.[7,15] These are a guiding framework for selecting approaches and techniques.

1. **R**esist the Righting Reflex.
2. **U**nderstand Your Client's Motivation.
3. **L**isten to Your Client.
4. **E**mpower Your Client.

Resist the Righting Reflex

Resisting the righting reflex refers to the tendency of counselors to give advice to correct or to fix the client's problems in the belief that they have the right answers. This overlooks client ambivalence and does not deal with the need for client change. The problem is that most people tend to resist change and may not view it as possible or necessary if satisfied with their current behaviors. "I know I need to lose weight, but I love good food." The counselor who argues for the benefits of different eating choices, for example, may increase client resistance and decrease the likelihood of change. Instead the client is the one who should be giving reasons and talking about possible changes.

Understand Your Client's Motivation

The client's motivation comes from within the client. We do not instill motivation in people, but instead should try to evoke the client's own motivation and help the person recognize and enhance it. One may explore the client's values, concerns, and perceptions in various situations and have clients tell us what they should change and how they can do it rather than telling and advising them what to do differently. One may ask if the person wants to change and the reasons why it is important to him or her.

Listen to Your Client

Listen rather than giving advice. See the clients' world from their point of view. Communicate empathy and create a collaborative atmosphere where clients can explore the conflicts of making a change in their personal lives. In a collaborative atmosphere, clients can explore suggestions for possible changes while the counselor communicates with empathy.

MI uses the skill of reflective listening with an understanding and accepting attitude of the client's problems, perspectives, and feelings. The reflective listener makes a guess as to what the client means and reflects it back to the client as a statement, not a question.[7] Although counselors have answers to problems, the answer needed for making a change in a behavior comes from the client and requires listening for it as the client talks. The purpose is to have the client continue to explore the problem. Reflective listening is a skill which requires practice.[7]

CASE ANALYSIS **2**

Using reflective listening, how would you comment on Robin's story?

Empower Your Client

Since clients are the ones who have to do the changing, they need to actively engage in the discussion of their healthcare. Some clients may have tried to change in the past and failed. Yet they have personal resources and solutions and can change if they decide to do so. Focusing on past successes rather than failures may increase self-efficacy, the belief that one is capable. The counselor can help clients explore how best to make changes to benefit their health. If the client asks, mentioning another client's successes may offer suggestions (See Box 6-1).

Microskills of Motivational Interviewing

Many counseling approaches also use the same interviewing skills that build rapport, explore concerns, and convey empathy.[5] The MI microskills are expressed by the acronym OARS: (1) Open-ended questions; (2) Affirming; (3) Reflecting; and (4) Summarizing. These help the client explore and resolve ambivalence and any barriers to behavior change.[7,9,10] Training may be needed in developing these skills.

Asking Open-Ended Questions

Open-ended questions are the communication tools to move the conversation along and evoke responses. They are the information gathering backbone of the session in which the counselor discovers what is important to the client. Questions should set a nonjudgmental, collaborative tone that can evoke talk about change. It is helpful to focus first on the person's life, thoughts, and situation before focusing on the problem area and especially to reduce resistance, evoke change talk, and build motivation for change. Later, one can focus on the problem area to develop and implement a plan for change and examine the importance and commitment of the client.[7,8,11]

> **EXAMPLE**   "What concerns do you have about your health?
> "What differences do you think you can try?"
> "What will you do first?"
> "When will you be able to . . ."

In general, MI counselors answer with one or two reflections for every client answer to a question to be sure they understand. For example: "What brings you here today?" "So you're here because of your diabetes," a statement, not a question.

CASE ANALYSIS 3

How would you discuss with Robin her pros and cons of making a change versus continuing her current choices?

In the early stages of the interview, open-ended questions allow individuals to explore the problems and help to establish an atmosphere of trust and acceptance. The counselor may say, for example: "In the time we have together, I want to get an understanding of any issues you have with your choices of foods. I'll be listening so that I can understand your concerns." Or: "I'll also need to get some specific information from you. What do you see as the issues?" Or: "What would you like to discuss first? What concerns you about your food intake?" When responding to change talk by the client, one asks for elaboration to know more about details or examples.

Affirming

Many clients have tried to make changes in the past and ultimately have failed. As a result, it may be necessary to instill hope through affirmations, something positive about the person such as an action, strength, effort, or intention.[7] Examples are statements of appreciation of the personal strengths and internal resources that the client brings. They may include words of understanding of specific positive behaviors, support, or competence in specific situations.[11]

One focuses on the client's strengths and positive attributes. For example, "You must have a lot of strength or resolve to try to lose weight again." Or "You did a really good job keeping food records this week." Center on the word "You." Comment positively on an example of affirming what the person has said. The counselor should not argue for change which may result in the client arguing why it won't work for her. The "Yes, but . . ." response may result.

Reflecting

Reflective listening is a foundational MI skill that counselors use to communicate acceptance, interest, understanding, and empathy, rather than asking questions.[10] It may also be used to strengthen client change talk and ultimately build trust.[7,11,12] Responses should be kept close to what the client said or a similar word to move conversation forward. One may also use it to verbally discuss a thought, encourage more information, or shift away from negativity.[7]

Reflective listening allows the counselor to test a hypothesis of what one has heard and make statements that test understanding of the client's meaning. The purpose is to have the client continue to explore the problem.[7] Simple reflections keep the conversation going. As the conversation progresses, reflections may become more complex.

How the counselor responds to what the client says is an important element of reflective listening. Reflective listening may be one of several types. The counselor may repeat part of what the person said or may rephrase slightly using different words, serving as a mirror to the client.

Paraphrasing is a more major restatement in which the counselor tries to determine the meaning in the statement and reflects back in new words adding to or extending the meaning. Finally, the deepest form of reflection is to reflect feelings in a paraphrase that searches for the client's feelings or emotions behind the statement. The following is NOT an example of reflective listening and is followed by one that is.

> **EXAMPLE**   Client: "I just don't know if I can lose weight, but I need to." (ambivalence)
> Counselor: "Of course you can." (reassuring)
> Client: "But it is so difficult."
> Counselor: "Yes, it is." (sympathizing)
> Client: "I never have eaten breakfast, because I don't have time."
> Counselor: "Just have some cereal and milk." (giving advice)

In the above example, the counselor is not really listening or giving the client a chance to explore the problem. Instead, the reflective listener hears and decodes the message, makes a reasonable guess as to the meaning, and puts the guess into a responding statement. The statement is a declarative one and not phrased as a question, as follows:

> **EXAMPLE**   Client: "I just don't know if I can lose weight, but I need to." (ambivalence)
> Counselor: "It sounds as if you are pulled in two ways. You want to lose weight. At the same time, you wonder if you can do it successfully."
> [Avoid: "You are concerned about losing weight?" as a question.]
> Client: "But it is so difficult."
> Counselor: "You found that your past efforts to change what you eat and lose weight were difficult. I think it's great that you want to try again."
> Client: "I never have eaten breakfast, because I don't have time."
> Counselor: "Your morning schedule must be a busy one."

Reflective listening and responding is a way of checking the meaning rather than assuming that you know exactly what is meant. It is a guess or hypothesis. This allows the client to keep moving in thought. Not every comment is reflected, however. The counselor decides what to emphasize and what to ignore. Standard phrases, for example, are "So you feel . . .," or "It sounds like you . . .," but don't overuse them.

CASE ANALYSIS 4

How would you assess Robin's motivation for change?

A brief reflective listening response, preferable using the client's words, is appropriate. For example: "You work full-time, but think you would have more energy if you lost weight and exercised regularly." This expresses empathy, encourages the client to continue, and is a way to respond to client resistance to change. Reflective listening shows that the counselor is trying to understand, affirms what the client has said, and helps the client to continue expressing thoughts and feelings. Learning reflective listening requires practice and feedback, if it is available. One could try it with a friend or family member.

Summarizing

Summaries by the counselor help to organize the client's thoughts about change, such as client experiences, suggestions, and strengths, or the practitioner may pull together something discussed. Summary reflections should draw together and deliver back to the client any mention of changes that should help the client in moving forward toward a commitment. One gives special weight to client "change talk" in summaries. For example: "Here's what I've heard you tell me so far."[7] Summarizing shows that you are listening and may help clients integrate their thoughts (See Box 6-2). Thus, conversations start with open-ended questions and reflections, affirmations, summaries, recognize change talk, and move the client toward change.[11]

OARS Skills	Communicating
Open-ended Questions Asked	Asking
Affirmations	Listening
Reflective Listening	Informing
Summarizing	

Box 6-2 ■ Motivational Interviewing Skills: OARS Strategy.

Client Change Talk

Many people are uncertain about how they feel about a behavior change. A guiding principle of MI is that behavior change will be more likely if clients verbalize their own arguments and reasons that favor a needed behavior, called client "change talk."[6,7,12] Change talk may be defined as client statements that suggest the target behavior change, such as "I'm going to cook less fried foods to help my weight." Reasons for change, for example, may be discontent with the current situation or seeing the advantages of change. The counselor may ask what the client wants to change and then how he or she plans to do it. This approach requires careful listening.

CASE ANALYSIS 5

How would you evoke "change talk" from Robin?

The client does most of the talking. The MI counselor focuses on the client's concerns and elicits client "change talk" to decrease resistance to change. The counselor listens for statements starting with "I want to . . .," "I could . . .," "I need to . . .," or "I intend to . . ."[7] The counselor may ask what problems concern the person or do a benefit analysis of the possibilities for change. It is important to follow up "change talk" with the reflective listening, reflecting back what the client said to express your interest and invite the client to elaborate.[6]

The emphasis on eliciting certain phrases from the client, or "change talk," is unique to MI. The strength and commitment of the talk is predictive of behavior change. Since many clients are uncertain about making changes and see both the pros and the cons, the counselor's goal is to have the client make several arguments or reasons for change while the counselor avoids the "Righting Reflex." This is an urge to correct the client's ambivalence and set him or her on the correct course, such as recommending exercise to help lose weight. It is the client who should find the reason and make the arguments for change. This is especially important with clients ambivalent about change.

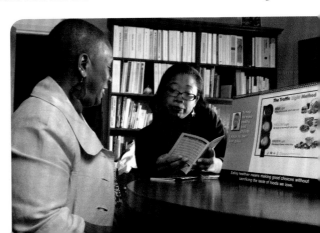

The counselor asks open-ended questions in determining the issues.
Source: Centers for Disease Control and Prevention.

Periodic summaries move the interview along. The professional may summarize the client's statements about the problem, the client's ambivalence, self-motivational statements made by the client, "change talk," and an overall assessment of the situation.[7] Draw together the client's reasons for change. This helps clients make up their minds. It reinforces what they may already know to be true, but may be avoiding. Reflection is especially important after answers to open-ended questions, after self-motivational statements, and after "change talk."

CASE ANALYSIS 6

How would you respond to Robin's "change talk?"

The DARN acronym may be used to generate client statements about change. Change talk may be recognized by statements of *Desires*, *Abilities*, *Reasons*, *Needs* (DARN), taking steps, or commitment to change. Clients who state reasons, desires, or needs for change may exhibit greater intentions and commitments for change although the strength of commitment may vary. The basis for wanting to change may be a health or personal goal.[7] The counselor gathers the examples of change talk and can summarize and reflect them back to the client. The summary should be phrased as a present change in a behavior and not what the person plans to do at a future time.[6]

"I need to get more exercise" is not a commitment to change or the same as saying "I'm going to walk 3 days every week," which is a commitment and action step.[7] A client may acknowledge that change is important, but lack confidence. "I would like to exercise, but never was good at it." One may ask how important this is, and how confident the person is that she could do this if desired. On a scale of 1 to 10 with 10 the highest, how important is this to you?

CASE ANALYSIS 7

If you have other suggestions for Robin, how would you approach her about them?

Counselor Approaches

Traditional nutrition counseling may focus on the assumption that the client has a deficit of information or knowledge which results in the giving of advice and information. Nutrition professionals may talk about the benefits of change and risks of continuing a current behavior in providing information on changes to make.

Instead, the MI counselor asks the client to choose a topic to discuss from several options. One starts with the client's priority while other problems may be examined later. The counselor guides the client to express the reasons for and against change and how current behaviors affect the person's ability to achieve his or her life goals.[7] The guiding style is best suited to counseling about change. The assumption is that a change in behavior is more likely to result from motivation than from giving advice and information. Problem eaters, for example, often already know that they are eating too much or the wrong foods.

One image of the counselor is that of a helper or guide accompanying a person on a journey. The guide "needs the qualities of a companion and the skills of someone who knows the route," but acknowledges the client's freedom of choice and personal responsibility for change.[6] Counselors who conduct MI successfully focus on reflection, including reinforcing positive statements about change, rather than responding with questions and advice. Another factor of importance is the empathic understanding of the counselor in creating an atmosphere of positive regard, acceptance, and safety in which clients feel comfortable discussing the positive and negative aspects of a behavior and exploring the change. A nondirective guiding style uses strategies to elicit the client's own motivation for change.[16]

Communication Skills

Finding and drawing out the client's thoughts involves three communication skills: (1) "asking," (2) "listening," and (3) "informing."[7,17] A guideline is to ask questions that the client can answer with "change talk." Examples are: "What do you want to do differently?" "What small changes could you make?" "What would be some benefits?"[8]

The counselor "asks" open-ended questions for the client to explore the how and why of change in developing an understanding of the problem. For example: "Tell me about how you would go about losing weight and the reasons you want to do it." This is a way to assess the client's choices in considering changes. The counselor may ask the client's thoughts about the options, and how they could affect behavior. For example: "Of the three ways you mentioned, which ones do you think would work best?" (See Box 6-2).

The counselor "listens" to understand the client's frame of reference and experience. The counselor then responds with a brief summary of understanding. The counselor "informs" by first asking permission to provide options and information. One may ask the client's thoughts about the information provided, and how it could affect behavior. For example: "May I have your permission to share some information with you that has helped others. Then I would like to hear your response and thoughts." One tries to find the client's strengths rather than just weaknesses and elicit motivation for change.

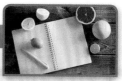

SELF-ASSESSMENT 1

Which of the following client statements represent "change talk?"

1. I guess you will tell me what to do.
2. I want to lose weight to feel better.
3. The doctor says my blood pressure is too high and to eat less salt.
4. I can start eating a small breakfast.

Elicit–Provide–Elicit

MI is described as having an "'elicit–provide–elicit" framework.[6,15] The counselor "elicits" or draws out what the person needs or wants to know or do. One "provides" information in a neutral manner when the client has given permission. One "elicits" what the client thinks about the provided information and what it means to him or her by asking "What does this mean to you?" This emphasizes the client's active involvement and may enhance motivation for change.[6] In this way, the counselor guides the client toward motivation to change by asking open-ended questions and listening to the client. Once the client is motivated to change, behavioral or cognitive counseling strategies discussed in other chapters may be useful.

Eliciting questions may include: "What would you like to know about . . .?" which tells the counselor what is important or of concern to the client.[13] A second approach: "What do you already know about . . .?" has the advantage of saving time and avoids discussing what the person already knows. The counselor learns about the client's experience.

Change

What to change? The client may have mentioned more than one possibility or option for change. If so, one guides the person in examining and determining which alternative to select as it is important for the client to select the one where success is most likely. For example: "With your limited time, which of the two changes do you want to start with?"

Why change? The counselor can expect that the client sees pros and cons of change. It is advisable to ask the client to express both the pros and the cons. If the practitioner has an additional behavioral change goal in mind, one may inquire whether the client would like to hear it. For example: "What do you see as the reasons to change your food intake now as opposed to waiting until you finish the major project at work?" The counselor may summarize the pros and cons in the client's words to see whether this is the best change to try first, but focus especially on the pros.

The concept of the "importance" of the change to the person and of the "confidence" in the ability to make the change are important determinants of readiness to change.[6,17] One may assess readiness for change by asking two questions: How important is the change to you? And how successful do you think you will be regarding the change? Box 6-3 provides a series of questions to use in assessing these two areas with clients.[6]

Useful Questions to Explore Importance

What would have to happen for it to become more important for you to change?

What would have to happen before you seriously considered changing?

How important is this change on a scale of 1 to 10, with 10 the highest?

What would need to happen for your importance score to move up from . . . to . . .?

What stops you moving up from . . . to . . .?

What are the motivators to retain your (current behavior)?

What are some of the concerns you have (or things you dislike) about . . . (current behavior)?

If you were to change, what would it be like?

Where does this leave you now? (When you want to ask about change in a neural way).

Useful Questions to Build Confidence

What would make you more confident about making these changes?

How confident are you about accomplishing this change?

How could you move up higher, so that your score goes from . . . to . . .?

How can I help you succeed?

What have you found helpful in any previous attempts to change?

What have you learned from the last time you tried this type of change?

If you were to decide to change, what might your options be? Are there any ways you know about that have worked for other people?

What are some of the practical issues you would need to address in order to achieve this goal? Do any of them sound achievable?

Is there anything you can think of that would help you feel more confident?

Box 6-3 ■ Assessing Importance and Confidence of the Patient/Client.

Source: Adapted from Rollnick S, Mason P, Butler C. *Health Behavior Change—A Guide for Practitioners.* New York, NY: Churchill Livingston; 1999.

Finally, the counselor can assess the importance, such as on a 10-point scale, as well as assess the client's confidence in the change. For example: "On a scale of 1 to 10 with 10 highest, how important is it to change your food intake and lose 10 lb?" Secondly, one may ask how the client selected a number, such as 5, thus eliciting more "change talk." An alternative is to ask what would have to happen to make the number larger, such as 7 or 8 instead of 5.

Then the counselor may assess the client's confidence. "On a scale of 1 to 10 with 10 highest, how confident are you that you can make the changes you discussed with me?" If the client replies 5, another change or goal should be explored. Or ask what would have to happen to move it up to a 7 or 8. A client whose rating is high in importance, but lower on confidence may need helpful ideas.

Frames

When time is limited, brief interventions have been found to be effective. They include six elements or components, summarized by the acronym FRAMES.[7]

Feedback of personal status

Responsibility (personal) for the change

Advice to change

Menu of options from which to choose

Empathy (counseling style)

Self-efficacy support

After the counselor's initial assessment, *feedback* about relevant health information is given by the counselor to the client. Personal *responsibility* for change is emphasized. "It's up to you to decide. You're the one who has to make changes in your food choices." Choices must be made freely and decisions to change are made only by the client.

The client decides what, if anything, to do with the feedback. Clear *advice* to change or make changes may be given as a *menu* of the variety of alternative ways that changes could be accomplished. Motivation can be enhanced when a person freely makes a decision and feels responsibility for the change. *Empathy* for the client is emphasized and expressed. Finally, attempts are included to strengthen the person's *self-efficacy* for change, to reinforce positive thoughts, and to support the ability to succeed.[1] Note that since advice is given and MI excludes advice, this is not a true MI.

When using MI, the nutrition and dietetics counselor partners with the client to "determine the agenda with empathic, nonjudgmental, supportive, encouraging, and active listening behaviors."[18] For working with clients not in the action Stage of Change, training in MI is recommended. The MI methods have positive effects in many situations, but not all. Null finding have been reported with eating disorders, for example.[6,17]

Applications

A study compared usual care to MI counseling for parents of overweight children ages 2 to 8. At the 2-year follow-up, there was a statistically significant reduction in BMI (body mass index) percentile using MI.[19]

A systematic review and meta-analysis investigated MI's efficacy in 49 studies in medical care settings. The evidence and results suggested that MI provided a moderate advantage to comparison interventions and could be used for a wide range of behavioral issues in healthcare.[20]

A study of parent-involved MI to improve pediatric health behaviors and health outcomes of 5,000 children up to 18 years old was based on building intrinsic motivation to change. Relative to comparison groups, MI was associated with significant improvements in health behavior including diet, physical activity, oral health, and other factors. MI was more successful at improving diets when the intervention included more MI components.[21]

Motivation

The counselor needs to increase the likelihood that the person will move toward change and to note and facilitate any client self-motivational statements.[7] First, the client recognizes that a problem exists. ("I guess my weight is a problem affecting my blood pressure.") Second, the client may express concern about the problem nonverbally, for example, by facial expression, sighing, tone of voice, or verbally. ("I've got to make changes now and eat better for the sake of my health.") Finally, the client may feel positive about the change, thus reflecting self-efficacy. ("I'm sure I can start exercising this week.") Reflecting back these types of statements allows the client to hear the message for the second time and enhances self-motivation. The counselor may question the client to evoke self-motivational statements, for example:

> For problem recognition: "What difficulties have you had in relation to your choices of foods?"
>
> For concern: "In what ways does choosing different foods or eating differently concern you?"
>
> For intention to change: "What are the reasons you see for making a change?"
>
> For optimism: "What encourages you to think that you can make this change?"

When clients reach the action Stage of Change, their questions can still be met with reflections. Here are possible questions to ask:

> "What is the next step?"
>
> "What do you plan to do?"

"Where do we go from here?"

"What good results will occur from this change?"

If the client asks the counselor for information, one approach is to offer several alternatives rather than only one. For example: "I can give you several alternatives. Then you can tell me what you think will work for you." When the client selects an alternative, he or she is more likely to try it and adhere to it than if the counselor provides only one option. The client takes responsibility for a personal choice. In the case of only one alternative, the client may say: "That sounds good, but it won't work for me," thus rejecting the solution.[7] The counselor may ask: "On a scale of 1 to 10 with 10 the highest, how confident are you that you can do this?" "How important is this to you on a scale of 1 to 10 with 10 the highest?"

Thus, there is a relationship between the counselor's interpersonal style and client outcomes. A counselor's collaborative, rather than authoritarian style, may evoke the client's motivation and better outcomes. If motivations and confidence are present, setting goals and plans for change may follow.

Reading this chapter is not sufficient to fully acquire skills in MI and be able to use them. Further reading, training, and practice are needed. The website of the Motivational Interviewing Network of Trainers (MINT) is www.motivationalinterviewing.net. It provides information such as books, videos, and other resources.

Goal Setting

Once the ambivalence is resolved and the patient is motivated to make a change, the practitioner must decide when to transition to goal setting and an action-oriented planning phase of counseling.[10] Reaching a final plan requires setting clear goals, since having goals can facilitate change.

Goals have been found to motivate change because they set a standard against which the client can compare a current behavior with a new one. Allowing the client to select a goal believed to be achievable supports client autonomy. They should be clearly stated, reasonable, and attainable. Selecting goals enhances personal choice and control, making it more likely that the person will succeed. The goal-setting process is discussed in Chapter 5.

Effective counseling helps clients to identify and overcome any barriers to change and acknowledges that lapses and relapses are a normal part of the change process. Barriers may include, for example, lack of time, cost, family environment, lack of social support, nonsupportive friends, fear of adverse psychological or physiologic consequences, and the like.

Clients need feedback about the change to enhance motivation. It can be provided in many ways, such as self-monitoring records; results of improved medical laboratory tests; positive comments from friends, family, and the counselor; and the client's own positive self-talk ("I'm doing better").

Health Belief Model

One of the first public health theories to try to influence health behaviors was the Health Belief Model (HBM) that was designed to understand people's use of preventive health services.[22–24] The theory assumes that health behaviors are motivated in relation to a degree of fear or perceived threat of illness. The HBM uses four constructs to explain people's readiness to act: perceived susceptibility; perceived severity; perceived benefits; and perceived barriers.

If a person imagines being susceptible and it would be a serious illness, such as cancer or stroke, one may be more likely to reduce the threat of illness by making changes in health behaviors. These concepts might account for a person's "readiness to act" and make changes.[23–25]

Perceived *susceptibility* may be defined as a person's opinion of how at risk or vulnerable he or she is to getting an illness or an adverse medical condition.

Perceived *severity* is the opinion of how serious the adverse condition is. The threat may be influenced by other factors, such as knowledge, education, age, socioeconomic status, and cultural group.[1]

Perceived *benefits* are the opinions of whether or not a behavior change, as a preventive action, is needed to reduce the risk or threat of disease and that positive results may be expected. Perceived *barriers* are the opinions of the personal costs, time, challenges, or problems of taking action to change a behavior.[1,23,24]

Later, additions were made to the HBM to better explain behavior. Environmental *cues to action*, such as giving the person how-to information or media reports, could direct motivation promoting readiness to act and make changes. *Self-efficacy*, one's belief that one is capable of taking a necessary action or making a change that will lead to an outcome one desires was recognized to fit the more complex behavior challenges.[23] The HBM suggests that people will engage in healthy behaviors if they value the outcomes. Ways to enhance a person's self-efficacy are discussed in Chapter 8.

To illustrate the six constructs, an overweight person with a family history of diabetes mellitus may perceive a *threat* or risk of diabetes due to the

Pregnancy motivates new health behaviors.
Source: Centers for Disease Control and Prevention.

family history. She may understand that she is *susceptible* and that there could be *serious* consequences. She perceives that weight loss and more exercise are actions or behaviors that are *benefits* in reducing the threat. She may question whether or not the *barriers* of lack of motivation, time, and others can be overcome.

A *cue to action* may be that the relative's condition has worsened. Benefits need to outweigh barriers to action. As people weigh the pros and cons of a health behavior change, they make a decision as to whether or not to take action. People with a high degree of confidence or *self-efficacy* will be more likely to be successful in changing and improving health behaviors than those with a low level of confidence.[23]

The HBM may be helpful in analyzing people's framework of thoughts about health actions especially when they have no symptoms as well as examining their understanding of health behavior changes. A client's inaction or lack of adherence to recommended changes may be explained by examining the person's thoughts and perceptions when it comes to choosing and carrying out health behaviors. It has been suggested that perceptions of severity could be more important to those already diagnosed with a disease and less important to those considering only prevention behaviors.[24]

Directive Counseling

This section focuses on the general applications of directive counseling strategies as they may be used in the supervisor/manager–employee relationship. Directive counseling tends to be most appropriate when the manager is aware of a problem or is concerned about the behavior of the employee, but the employee is unaware of the problem or is unwilling to address it. Counseling may also involve discussions of superior performance or promotion counseling.

In directive counseling, the professional initiates the discussion or approaches the staff member based on a direct referral from another manager or recognizing an employee problem situation. Staff may exhibit anxiety or become defensive and resist problem solving under the conditions. They are more likely to become hostile and defensive because they are "called in" rather than doing the "calling," and they may be more concerned with exonerating themselves of any blame than with collaborating to solve the problem. For this reason, counselors need to be especially sensitive to all verbal and nonverbal behaviors and to be supportive while attempting to explore the issue at hand.

Employee Counseling

Employee counseling includes the discussion of a work-related problem to address employee performance that needs improving. Counseling of staff should be limited to job-related concerns and should not include probing into personal problems. For such personal problems, the manager should provide referral to employee assistance programs. When employee counseling loses its problem–performance orientation, it runs the risk of being interpreted as an invasion of privacy.

Managers have an obligation to conduct work-related counseling sessions with employ-

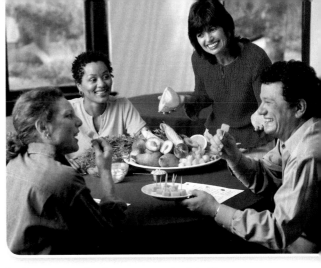

Employee counseling focuses on work-related issues.
Source: *US Department of Agriculture.*

ees. These should be held as often as necessary, assisting the staff in their professional development as well as dealing with career problems as they occur. The manager should not postpone employee counseling until the annual or semiannual performance appraisal interviews. Allowing problems to accumulate and handling them all at one time is generally ineffective. Employee counseling should occur as close to the incident as possible.

Applications of Directive Counseling

Managers have a skill set that is different. Often, individuals who are extraordinary in their professional expertise or ability to perform a professional task are selected to manage others. Although nutrition and dietetics practitioners have a strong foundation regarding the competencies for being a supervisor or manager, additional experience or continuing professional education in directive counseling or conflict resolution may be desirable.

An example of the use of directive counseling is for discussing unsatisfactory job performance. Counseling occurs after the manager has assessed that the employee knows his or her job description, has been trained for the position, and knows the performance expectations. Directive counseling of employees can be a form of discipline. The root of the word "discipline" comes from Latin and means "to train" or "to mold." Rather than the role of a judge, the attitude of the counselor needs to be that of a caring coach who wishes to assist the other in improving. The objective of employee counseling is to change behaviors and develop productive members of the team.[26]

Guidelines for Directive Counseling

Managers prepare for the counseling session in advance, selecting a suitable time and private place free of interruptions. One gathers specific instances of superior, average, and/or substandard performance, such as attendance records or customer service, and organizes the information prior to notifying the employee. Written performance standards should be based on job-related requirements from the job description.[26] There are several stages in the counseling interview. They include involving, exploring, resolving, and concluding stages.

Involving Stage

After a manager has assembled information on quality and quantity of employee job performance, reviewed the company written policy, and consulted with human resources if the problem is serious, facts must be shared and discussed with the employee on a timely basis. To begin, the manager needs to establish an appropriate atmosphere. In opening the discussion with the staff member, the counselor must be explicit in the desire to solve a problem rather than to punish. The aim is to improve the staff member's performance.[26]

One way of keeping the conversation appropriate is to keep remarks performance-centered rather than to make judgments about the person. It is more supportive and factual to say, "You have been late six times in the past 2 weeks," than to say, for example, "Lately you don't seem to care about your job; your attitude is poor." Inferences are not facts. The manager could not possibly know the quality of the employee's "caring" for his job or the condition of his "attitude," but does know the objective facts—that the employee has been late six times in the past 2 weeks.

Exploring Stage

In the exploring stage, the issues are discussed. Preferably the manager has documented job-related problems and examples from personal observation. Throughout the interview, the counselor focuses on company policy, objective facts, being specific about what has been seen, and about what behaviors need to be improved. If the complaint is from others, and the supervisor or manager is unable to document the examples from personal observation, discuss the effects of the situation with the individual with an emphasis on clarifying the issues and hearing from the staff member's vantage point. The manager proactively makes an effort to improve the employee in fixing the problem at hand.[27]

Resolving Stage

Next, the manager should discuss employee options on how to correct the behavior and the consequences of failing to improve. The resolving stage should result in specific goals and a plan of action. As in nondirective counseling, the counselor should provide adequate opportunity for employees to tell their side of the story, and their remarks should be paraphrased. Not only do people not know what they do not know, but they easily fall into traps of seeing, hearing, and selectively perceiving what they expect to see and hear.

Giving employees an opportunity to tell their side of the story and then paraphrasing it and empathizing with what the employee is feeling usually leads to collaboration in the resolution process. There may be extenuating circumstances that no one on the staff is aware of, which account for the behavior of the employee. Perhaps the employee is late to work because of a family member with a terminal illness or a car pooling problem, for example. Having employees explain the problem from their own perspective may add significant insight and understanding. Employees are held responsible for their actions and the responsibility for improvement belongs to the employee. The manager makes responsible efforts for helping.

Concluding Stage

After an agreement on a solution has been reached, the manager should describe as specifically as possible what the consequences will be if the agreed-upon changes in the employee's behavior are not actualized in the defined time limit. One might say, for example, "If you are absent without notice again, I am going to file a warning notice with human resources." The manager needs to remember at this point not to exaggerate the consequences or to mention consequences that will not be carried out. If the employee does continue the problem behavior, the manager must go to the next level of the disciplinary process. The manager closes the session and documents the goals and plan of action.[26]

Although verifying understanding is important in nondirective counseling, it is equally important in directive counseling. The tendency for employees to experience physiologic stress symptoms from the threat of being called in by the manager heightens the possibility of their misunderstanding some of the communication. Both the manager and the staff member need to paraphrase one another to verify that each has understood the other and that they agree on the final solution.

An expression of confidence and support by the manager can help ensure successful implementation of an action plan that both parties have agreed on. Rather than saying, "Well, let's see what will happen," the manager provides more motivation by saying, "I think these are the kinds of ideas that can make a difference." Employees should be reminded that they are an important part of the team and that their contributions to the team are valued. If the action plan includes a multistep process for improvement, it would be wise to set follow-up meeting dates. Doing so not only confirms commitment, but adds incentive to begin the performance changes.

As in nondirective counseling, managers must attend to the supporting nonverbal behavior throughout the interview. The spatial dynamics of the location should allow the two people to feel close, since feelings are being shared and help is being given to solve the problem. The manager needs to act, talk, look, and gesture in a manner that allows the subordinate to infer that the purpose of the counseling session is to change a problem behavior, not to reject or punish. Finally, the manager has to remember to allow adequate time for full expression of thoughts and schedule multiple sessions when appropriate.

Measuring the Outcomes of Counseling

The outcome of successful counseling is attaining the desired goals or changes in behavior. These goals may be those of the employer, counselor and, most important, the clients or employees. The measurement may be short-term or long-term. Beyond individual client or staff outcomes, practitioners systematically need to assess the results of their counseling to determine effectiveness. Questions, such as the number of counseling sessions generally needed to create change, are essential to determine recommendations for care and confirm outcomes. Self- and periodic evaluation of one's counseling skills will assist in your professional counseling skill development.

Summary

Communication effectiveness is enhanced when the nutrition professional uses appropriate evidence-based theories and strategies that promote behavioral change. This chapter examined several theories and models used in counseling. These include directive and nondirective counseling, Motivational Interviewing, and the Health Belief Model. Further information on counseling is found in the chapters that follow.

Review and Discussion Questions

1. Identify three differences between nondirective and directive counseling.
2. What are the key points in the Health Belief Model?
3. Discuss the four principles of motivational interviewing.
4. What counselor style or approaches are recommended in motivational interviewing?
5. Define and give two examples of reflective listening.
6. Why is it better to give clients more than one suggestion when they ask for advice?
7. Explain the four-stage process of counseling used in the directive counseling section. Provide an example of how this would work with an employee absenteeism issue.

Suggested Activities

1. To practice reflective listening statements, form groups of two, one playing the role of a client and one a counselor. Each client should think of two or three things about himself or herself that he or she would like to change (e.g., get more sleep, eat better, lose weight, get more organized and use time better, overcome procrastination, be happier, watch less television, make more friends). This can be stated as: "One thing I would like to change about myself is . . ." The counselor develops one or two hypotheses of what the person means and puts one of them into a reflective statement rather than a question. A reflection may be started with the following: "You are feeling . . ." "It sounds like you . . ." "You are saying that . . ." "So you think . . ."
2. During the next week, practice paraphrasing what others say. What reactions do you get? Does your paraphrasing tend to cause the other to go on talking?
3. Write both a paraphrase and an emphatic comment to the following comments made by a counselee:
   A. "I feel awkward discussing my eating habits. I feel embarrassed about my diet."

B. "With working all day and a hungry family when I get home, I don't have time to cook."

C. "I am at a point now where I don't believe I will ever lose the weight."

4. Form triads consisting of a counselor, counselee, and observer. Each individual should take a turn in each of the roles for 5 to 7 minutes to try the motivational interview approach to counseling. The counselee should play the role of a client interested in healthy eating or one who wants to lose weight. After each round, the observer should share reactions to the counselor's approach and encourage feedback from the counselee to the counselor. From the counselee's perspective, what did the counselor do that helped their interaction; what did the counselor do that hindered it? At the end, discuss how the approach helped you.

5. Repeat the activity in number 4. The counselee is a staff member who is not completing his work in a timely manner. Which approach was most helpful here and why?

6. During the next week, make arrangements to view a nutritionist's counseling session, noting particularly what occurs during each stage of the process. What behavior on the part of the counselor facilitates the building of rapport and trust? What techniques did you see that were reflected in the chapter? Discuss which characteristics of a successful counselor were expressed.

7. After each of the statements below, use the FRAME acronym approach to consider the comment.

A. "My work situation is impossible. It seems that I'm the scapegoat for everybody. I'm beginning to wonder if I should consider looking for another job."

B. "It doesn't seem fair to me that I should have to work weekends when the staff members who have been here only 2 years longer don't have to."

C. "It seems easy every morning to promise myself that today I will stick to the program we designed. By noon, however, I begin thinking that I'll never be able to comply with the dietary changes for the rest of my life, so why bother?"

8. To practice developing understanding and using reflective listening, divide into pairs. Ask each person to prepare to discuss a personal experience that would be difficult for someone else to understand. The counselor can use open-ended questions but primarily reflections. The task is to use verbal and nonverbal skills to seek to understand the experience being described by the other. After 10 to 15 minutes, the pair may switch roles. At the conclusion, the instructor may wish to answer questions and ask for reactions to the activity.

9. Count the Fs in the following statement:

FASCINATING FAIRYTALES ARE THE RESULT OF YEARS OF SCIENTIFIC STUDY COMBINED WITH THE EXPERIENCE OF CREATIVE MINDS.

Compare answers with several people. Why did you get different answers? How does this relate to issues as a counselor?

CHAPTER 7

Counseling for Behavior Modification

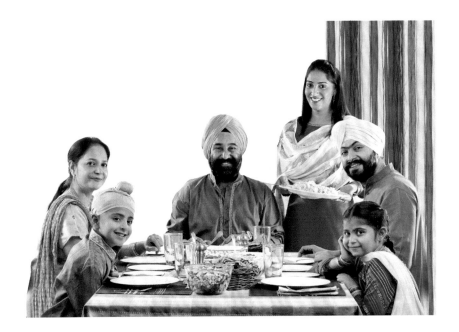

Objectives

- Define and distinguish learning styles of classical conditioning, operant conditioning, and modeling.
- Apply behavior modification principles in clinical situations such as

weight management, diabetes mellitus, and cardiovascular disease and in human resource management.
- Analyze eating behaviors according to the "ABC" framework.
- Compare self-monitoring and self-management techniques.

Martha M. was recently diagnosed with type 2 diabetes mellitus. She is 50 years old, 5'6", and 180 lb. A homemaker, she is married to an electrician, and their only child is away at college. She is finding it increasingly difficult to motivate herself to get involved in outside activities now that the house is empty.

Martha describes her typical daily eating pattern as follows: She wakes up in the morning at the same time as her husband, makes coffee for both of them, and prepares a warm breakfast for him before he leaves for work. She continues to drink her coffee but does not eat. She gathers her "to do" list and completes it around 11:00 AM. Then she rewards herself after a busy morning with a pastry and makes another pot of coffee. For the rest of the afternoon, she will clean the house or work on crafts until about 5:30 PM. She does not engage in regular physical activity. She will then begin making dinner so that it will be prepared by about 7:00 PM, when her husband arrives home. Standard dinners may include sausage lasagna and a small side salad; or fried chicken, mashed potatoes and gravy, and canned corn; or spaghetti and meatballs with toasted garlic bread and milk. Usually, they will have dessert and share a bowl of ice cream or a brownie when they watch a movie at home.

> *Treat a man as he is and he will become who he is; treat a man as he can and should be and he will become as he can and should be.*
>
> —Goethe

Introduction

Lose weight! Quit smoking! Control your blood sugar! This advice is easily uttered but requires a process to implement and maintain. This process is referred to as behavior modification. Changing behaviors is one of the most difficult tasks for people because human behavior is quite complex. Complex behaviors usually are based on a combination of inherited and acquired characteristics. The inherited characteristics cannot be changed, just as it is impossible to alter any genetic attribute. However, the acquired characteristics, those shaped by a person's environment and experience, can be altered. Behaviors that are learned or acquired can be changed or modified, but this usually requires the right approach at the appropriate time.

Consequences drive behavior. Most undesirable behavior is acquired and maintained by the same principles as optimal behavior, and in some cases the unhealthy behaviors will naturally change.[1] However, the role of a counselor in behavior change is warranted in some situations to highlight for the patient the cost–benefit trade-off or reveal how the "pros" outweigh the "cons" of change.

In behavior modification, the counselor attempts to alter previously learned behavior or to encourage the development of new behaviors.[2] For example, it is often difficult to influence patients who may not see the health danger in their current habits. Food preferences and eating behaviors have deep roots within the individual and may be highly resistant to change. In addition, behaviors may define individuals in terms of what they think and feel and how they react to certain situations.[1] Reluctance to make changes may occur when a good rationale and a stepwise process to change are not identified. Counseling for behavior change can help reduce the resistance to change.

Simply furnishing information about what to eat is often insufficient to promote alterations in eating behaviors or adherence to medical nutrition therapy. In these instances, it may help to differentiate between diet instruction and behavior modification. In fact, the standardized language of the Nutrition Care Process (NCP) distinctly separates nutrition knowledge from client behaviors that influence nutrition-related goals.[3]

Contrary to traditional diet instructions, nutrition counseling for behavior modification steers the client into assuming responsibility for change.[4] The transfer of decision-making power from the professional to the client reduces the risk of relapse and failure. Over time, even individuals in the best designed, short-term intervention can relapse after the formal program ends. If the responsibility for decisions is transferred to clients, they are much more likely to modify eating choices. As difficult as this seems, it is even more challenging to effectively implement this approach in acute care nutrition intervention settings. Along with information on nutrition, behavior modification principles may be used because they offer the nutrition and dietetics professional an additional dimension to counseling—that of combining the sciences of psychology and physiology with the art of therapy.[4]

Behavior modification principles are applied in various aspects of medical nutrition therapy. One of the earliest and the most frequently used applications was in the treatment of obesity. Therapy for undesirable eating behaviors related to diabetes mellitus, cardiovascular disease (CVD), and other chronic diseases are other potential uses of behavior modification. In prevention, behavior modification can be applied in wellness and disease risk reduction. If unhealthy eating behaviors are modified in favor of healthy alternatives, the incidence of nutrition-related diseases could decrease.

CASE ANALYSIS **1**

In preparation for your initial counseling session with Martha, compile a list of initial behavioral modification ideas and strategies that may be appropriate.

In human resource management, supervisors may be interested in altering the behavior of employees and encouraging the development of new behaviors. More effective interaction between peers and supervisors may also be a goal. Although the term *behavior modification* in the context of human resource management may sound manipulative, an honest and understanding supervisor may use the principles by sharing with employees the goals of the process. Modeling is a technique that is used frequently in employee training programs. Likewise, people in leadership positions may use techniques to help employees assess situations and make adjustments, or behavior changes, as needed to obtain the desired results.[5]

This chapter reviews the principles of learning and the process of behavior modification that have evolved from research. Included are classical conditioning, operant or instrumental conditioning based on positive reinforcement or rewards, and observational learning or modeling after others. The behavioral modification principles are discussed within the context of selected practice applications and human resource management. The role of cognition—the individual's mental perceptions of events and their effect on behavior—is covered in more detail in Chapter 8.

Classical Conditioning

The methods of behavior modification are based on principles of learning that have been discovered mostly in the experimental laboratory. Perhaps the best-known animals in the history of psychology were the dogs housed in the laboratory of Ivan Pavlov, the Russian physiologist, who was conducting research on digestive processes.[6] Serendipitously, Pavlov noted that his laboratory animals salivated not only when food was presented but also when the laboratory assistant who regularly fed them came into the room; at times, they even salivated at the sound of the laboratory door opening. Pavlov spent the rest of his life investigating a type of learning based on association, now known as classical conditioning.

Pavlov realized immediately that the response of salivation to laboratory assistants and noisy doors was not a part of the physiologic makeup of the dog. The dogs were salivating when events occurred that had regularly and repeatedly come before the presentation of their food. An association was apparently formed between some event and the future appearance of food.

Pavlov noted that certain environmental events or stimuli would reliably trigger or elicit a particular behavioral response. For example, food in a dog's mouth would reliably produce saliva. The triggering event, food in the mouth, became known as the *unconditioned stimulus*, whereas the response that was triggered salivation was called the *unconditioned response.* This relationship was built into the organism and hence unconditioned.

Conditioning occurs when a neutral stimulus—one that originally does not trigger a particular response (e.g., salivation)—eventually comes to produce that response. This occurs by pairing the originally neutral stimulus with the unconditioned stimulus. When conditioning has occurred, the *conditioned stimulus* (CS), which was originally neutral, produces the same response as the unconditioned stimulus, or one that is very similar. In the example, the CS was the presence of the laboratory assistant. Pavlov showed that bells, tones, lights, and many other stimuli could serve as the CS and could come to elicit the response of salivation, which is labeled a *conditioned response* because it is triggered by or produced by a CS.[6]

Many types of responses have been found to react to classical conditioning principles. Not only reflexive responses, such as salivation and eye blink, but also complex emotional responses can be classically conditioned. The heart pounds and beads of perspiration appear on the forehead as one hears the siren of an ambulance approaching a neighbor's home. The same phenomenon may occur when the teacher passes out examination questions. Try to construct a scenario to account for this response in terms of classical conditioning principles or think of situations in nutrition and dietetics in which classical conditioning might play a part in human behavior or emotional responses.

Operant Conditioning

At about the same time that Pavlov was delineating the principles of classical conditioning, a young American scientist, Edward Thorndike, was pursuing the investigation of learning principles from another perspective. Thorndike used many types of animals in his research and designed and constructed "puzzle boxes" for cats. A hungry cat was placed inside the box with food located outside. To have access to the food, the cat had to solve the puzzle of how to escape from the box. Thorndike observed that the cats made trial-and-error responses until escape was achieved and the food consumed. Gradually, the time required to complete the puzzle decreased. Furthermore, the behavior that achieved success in solving the puzzle became dominant, and unsuccessful behaviors were eliminated.[6]

Thorndike proposed an explanation for this phenomenon based on a principle he called the Law of Effect. This law stated that behaviors could be changed by their consequences. Responses that were followed by satisfying consequences would be strengthened. Behaviors not followed by satisfying consequences, or behaviors followed by annoying consequences, would be weakened and less likely to occur in the future. Thorndike's Law of Effect was applied to principles of learning and formed the foundation for the study of operant or instrumental conditioning, which is learning based on reinforcement or reward.

The focal point of research on the Law of Effect is the relationship between responses, or behaviors, and the consequences of those behaviors. Four types of response–consequence outcomes have been characterized.[6] First, responses or behaviors may produce positive outcomes, a consequence known as *positive reinforcement.* An example of reinforcement would be the praise and attention an overweight person may receive after losing a noticeable amount of weight. Second, responses may produce negative outcomes; this consequence is known as *punishment.* Punishment decreases the future likelihood of a response. Examples of punishment include the receipt of a traffic ticket for an improper left turn or the inability to fit into a favorite outfit after gaining weight.

Third, responses may result in the removal of adverse stimuli that are already present. This consequence is known as *negative reinforcement* or escape and is similar to positive reinforcement in that it increases the future likelihood or probability of a response. Examples of negative reinforcement include escaping devastating cold by going into a heated building, escaping a boring television show by changing channels, or eliminating or reducing hypoglycemic agents in type 2 diabetes by losing weight and following a sound meal plan.

Finally, responses may prevent an unpleasant event from occurring. Examples include avoiding the cold by staying indoors or engaging in regular physical activity to prevent weight gain. The avoidance of adverse events increases the likelihood of the response, as does positive reinforcement. Behaviors that are neither positively nor negatively reinforced should typically decrease in strength.

Later behaviorists continued where Thorndike concluded. B.F. Skinner is best known for championing a set of methods and terms to explain behavior on the basis of the principles of operant conditioning. Skinner developed a situation in which behavior could be observed in discrete units and subsequently recorded. This situation was an operant chamber, which has been dubbed a "Skinner box." The lever presses of rats and key

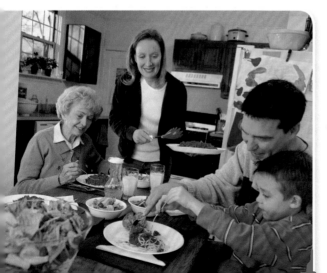

Parents and caregivers shape children's eating habits.
Source: US Department of Agriculture.

pecks of pigeons have been the most frequently studied responses. Skinner's enthusiasm for the behavioral approach was not limited to lower animals, however, as he proposed wider application for the principles that were established. In fact, the behavioral approach has become an important practical technique in many settings, such as classrooms, mental health interventions, prisons, offices, and self-management situations.[1,5]

Modeling

In addition to classical and operant conditioning as modes of behavior change, a third form of learning is known as observational learning or modeling. Learning by modeling involves the observation of some behavior or pattern of behaving, which is followed by the performance of either the same or a similar behavior. Albert Bandura is associated with this method of learning by modeling.[7] In behavior modification for weight reduction, for example, a person could "eat like a thin person" to model after the appropriate food choices, portion sizes, and duration of meals of someone who demonstrates the skill.

The effectiveness of learning by modeling appears to be directly related to certain characteristics of the model. The two characteristics found to be most relevant are the observer's similarity to the model and the status of the model. The more similar the characteristics of the model are to those of the observer, the higher is the probability that learning by modeling will occur. Movie and television stars and other well-known persons capitalize on modeling by producing books and videotapes of their fitness and nutrition programs. Many people model after the behavior of a person with "status," even though equally effective or superior programs could be developed by relatively unknown but professionally trained nutritionists and exercise physiologists.

Shaping behavior begins at an early age. Parents and caregivers of children serve as role models in forming eating habits and behaviors. Both good and poor eating habits and healthy or restricted behaviors can be modeled and thus communicated to children and adolescents who are shaping eating behaviors that will likely remain with them through adulthood.[8] Long-term food choices of children can stem from the dietary patterns of parental figures. Nutrition counseling may be geared toward parents for their benefit and for the health of their children.[8,9]

To take advantage of modeling, nutrition professionals may try sharing success stories of people who have made permanent dietary modifications for the benefit of their health. In group therapy, clients who have succeeded in changing eating practices may serve as models for others. Keep in mind that the client often views the counselor as a model, and to this end, nutrition professionals should be following the healthy nutrition recommendations given to others.

Behavior modeling is used in employee training programs to teach basic supervisory techniques, selling skills, and a variety of other verbal skills through observation of films and videotapes. New employees may be assigned to work with current employees who serve as models of desirable behaviors. Managers should make sure that their own behaviors exemplify what they expect of employees.[5] If the supervisor adds an extra 10 minutes to the allowed time for a coffee break, for example, employees may model after the example set.

A great deal of human learning and behavior undoubtedly is a result of modeling, even though traditionally emphasis has been placed on the stimulus–response or behavior approach to explaining changes in behavior, or the acquisition and extinction of responses.[6] These three approaches—conditioning, operant conditioning, and modeling—form the basis of behavior modification. The behavioristic position is that many behaviors are learned or alterable through use of these three learning principles.

Note, however, that individuals might be more or less resistant to behavior change depending on where they are on the continuum of Stages of Change (see Chapter 5 for an in-depth discussion of the Stages of Change model). One barrier to effective communication is that a counseling approach may be implemented erroneously in a particular stage, but may be effective in a different stage. Consequently, counseling for behavior change may employ various approaches to counseling at particular stages.[4,5]

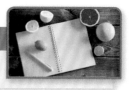

SELF-ASSESSMENT 1

Describe examples of modeling you may have experienced.

Changing Eating Behaviors

As the principles that govern behavior and behavior change became more clearly defined, it became increasingly apparent that nutritionists and behavioral scientists should work together to provide methods of using these principles in applied settings where changes in dietary habits are the primary goal. The American Heart Association has been one of the leaders in encouraging this type of collaboration and has developed a clinical practice guideline on lifestyle interventions.[10] The most common application has been the behavioral management of obesity, but cooperative programs have led to application in such diverse areas of concern as CVDs, eating disorders, and diabetes mellitus.

Dietary behaviors should be studied in terms of the client's total environment, which includes the physical, social, cultural, psychological, physiologic, and environmental factors compounded by all conditions and events that precede and follow eating. Behavioral scientists have referred to this as the "ABC" framework, derived from an analysis of the *Antecedents* stimuli or cues, the *Behavior* response itself or eating, and the *Consequences* reinforcement or reward of the behavior.[11]

For an example of the ABC framework, consider the following scenario: a man at home alone notices a package of cookies left on the kitchen counter; this may be considered the antecedent or cue. Next, the man eats some or all cookies in the kitchen; this is considered the behavior. After eating the cookies, the man may experience the consequence, that of satisfaction from the taste of the cookies, with reduced feelings of hunger or frustration to reinforce the behavior. The nutrition counselor and the client must find ways to decrease unhealthy eating behaviors and increase new desirable ones.

Antecedents

Behavior modification techniques work by regulating the antecedents, the behavior of eating itself, and the consequences or rewards. Analysis of antecedents of behavior seeks to control or limit the stimuli or cues to eating. For example, a cue may be seeing or smelling food, watching television, arriving home from work or school, attending a social event, or noticing the presence of extra food on the table at mealtime. Behavior may be influenced by both internal and external factors. There may be internal cues, such as physiologic feelings of hunger or psychological feelings of loneliness or boredom. Other external variables may cue eating, such as noting the time of day or passing an ice cream shop in the street. Both internal and external factors may be mediated by cognitive factors, such as not caring about current weight levels or not wishing to dull one's appetite for the next meal.[12]

Once the antecedents are identified, the mediating variable theory calls for identifying the variable most strongly associated with the behavior.[13] The premise is that if one alters the mediating variable, one would expect to influence the behavior associated with that variable. Conversely, if the behavior is only weakly associated with a variable, changes to the mediating variable are not expected to manifest in successful behavior change.

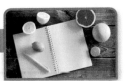

SELF-ASSESSMENT 2

1. What are your cues for eating?
2. What are strong mediating variables to your eating behaviors?
3. The introductory paragraph included the example of a man eating cookies in the kitchen. How could the cues in this situation be modified?

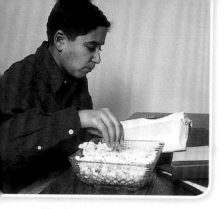

Studying may be a cue to eating.

Source: Copyright Wolters Kluwer.

The behavior-modifying strategy involves decreasing the exposures to situations in which food is used as a reward or as a focal point of an activity. A list of suggestions for changing behavior that have been recommended by various authors for persons desiring to lose weight is found in Box 7-1.[5,11,12] To modify antecedents, the nutrition counselor may suggest removing negative cues (not buying inappropriate foods); introducing new, more positive cues (exercising instead of eating); restricting behavior to one set of cues (eating only at designated times); cognitive restructuring (discussed in Chapter 8); and role-playing (new responses to old antecedents telling a friend you would rather go to a movie than out for pizza). Breaking response chains and preplanning behavior are other strategies.[2,4]

Preplanning meals and snacks and having only appropriate foods in the house are preferable to expecting self-control when hungry. Preplanning social occasions and exercise are helpful. Small portions of favorite foods may need to be included in the diet to avoid feelings of total deprivation and potential abandonment of dietary changes. Doing the right thing is enhanced by stimulus control. The goal of preplanning to control antecedents is to decrease the number of times the person is exposed to tempting situations so that the client's behavior is tested as seldom as possible.[14]

I. Provide Incentives to Aid Patients in Maintaining Commitment

    A. Determine ways to focus attention on successful experiences. A positive comment by the counselor is helpful, and you can always find something positive to say.

    B. Encourage people to tell others about dietary goals. This public commitment often will aid in maintaining a course of action.

    C. Have the person anticipate problems that might come up and consider possible solutions before a problem arises. Having a plan ready will make focusing on the goal easier.

    D. Concentrate on allowed foods and portions rather than the disallowed. Be positive.

Box 7-1 ■ Techniques for Behavior Modification

Source: From Farmer RF, Chapman AL, American Psychological Association. Behavioral Interventions in Cognitive Behavior Therapy: Practical Guidance for Putting Theory into Action. 2nd ed. Washington, DC: American Psychological Association; 2016; Wadden T, Butryn M, Hong P, et al. Behavioral treatment of obesity in patients encountered in primary care settings. JAMA. 2013;1217:1779–1791; and Lin JS, O'Connor E, Whitlock EP, et al. Behavioral counseling to promote physical activity and a healthful diet to prevent cardiovascular disease in adults: a systematic review for the U.S. Preventive Services Task Force. Ann Intern Med. 2010;153:736–750.

E. Keep reminding the person that dietary change is a gradual process. Dietary habits were not developed in a brief period of time and probably will not be significantly changed in a short time. Set realistic goals for immediate and long-term change. Encourage successive approximations to the desired behavior.

II. Learn Eating Habits and Exercise Habits by Record-Keeping

A person cannot change a habit until he or she knows what it is. Self-monitoring with accurate records of the foods consumed is necessary for behavioral control of eating. This record-keeping exercise can identify the person's patterns of food intake and those cues that are associated with food consumption as well as the emotional outcome of eating. The person will become more aware of the environmental stimuli that are associated with eating behavior. Information to consider recording would be

A. What food was eaten
B. Quantity of each food
C. What the person was doing just before eating to help identify cues
D. Place of eating cue providing
E. With whom eating occurs, or alone cue providing
F. How the person felt cue providing
G. Time of eating cue providing

III. Control the Stimuli Cues and Restructure the Environment

A. Physical environment

1. Based on the records kept, have the person identify physical stimuli in the environment that are associated with, and therefore are cues to, inappropriate eating behaviors. Different stimuli become associated with the act of eating and can become signals for appropriate or inappropriate food consumption.

2. Ask the person to identify physical stimuli that could remind him or her to eat properly. Examples of these would be charts or graphs, cartoons, signs, and the like. The presence of appropriate foods in the home is probably the best cue to appropriate eating, supplemented by the elimination of inappropriate foods.

3. Have the person specify a special place where food should be consumed, such as at the dining table and not in front of the television set or kitchen sink.

4. Make those foods that are acceptable in the nutrition plan as attractive as possible. Use good dishes, crystal, and so forth to make dining a pleasant event.

5. Set up shopping trips based on the following suggestions:

a. Shop for food only after eating.
b. Use a shopping list.

Box 7-1 ■ (continued)

   c. Avoid ready-to-eat foods.

   d. Do not carry more money than needed for shopping list.

6. Set up specific plans and activities:

   a. Substitute exercise for snacking.

   b. Eat meals and snacks at scheduled times.

   c. Do not accept food offered by others.

   d. Store food out of sight.

   e. Remove food from inappropriate storage areas in the house.

   f. Use smaller dishes.

   g. Avoid being the food server.

   h. Leave the table immediately after eating.

   i. Discard leftovers.

7. Regarding special events and holidays:

   a. Drink fewer alcoholic beverages.

   b. Plan eating before parties.

   c. Eat a low-calorie snack before parties.

   d. Practice polite ways to decline food.

   e. Do not get discouraged by occasional setbacks.

B. Social environment

   1. Have the person identify the types of social situations that con-
      tribute to poor eating habits. Examples of stimuli in the social
      environment that might contribute to difficulty for the person would
      be negative statements from family members or friends and social
      situations in which there are expectations for eating inappropriate
      or disallowed foods.

   2. Have the person identify the kinds of social interactions that
      would support good eating habits and following the nutrition plan.
      Role-playing, in which the person practices how he or she will ask
      others to help change his or her eating habits, can be useful.

C. Cognitive or mental environment

   1. Have the person identify the thoughts and feelings that are likely
      to make attempts to change eating habits unsuccessful.

   2. After the person has identified possible negative thoughts that
      could lead to discouragement, help him or her develop some posi-
      tive thoughts that can be used to counteract the negative ones.

   3. Avoid setting unreasonable goals.

IV. Change Actual Eating Behavior

A. Slow down.

   1. Take one small bite at a time.

Box 7-1 ■ (continued)

    2. Put the fork down between mouthfuls.

    3. Chew thoroughly before swallowing.

    4. Take a break during the meal. Stop eating completely for a short period.

  B. Leave some food on the plate.

  C. Make eating of inappropriate foods as difficult as possible.

  D. Control snacks.

    1. Save allowable foods from meals for snacks.

    2. Establish behaviors incompatible with eating.

    3. Prepare snacks the way one prepares meals—on a plate.

    4. Keep on hand a quantity of low-calorie foods such as raw vegetables; have them ready to eat and easy to get.

  E. Instruct the person that when eating, he or she should not be performing any other act. The cues associated with eating should be restricted to that act, so the person should not eat while reading, sewing, watching television, and so on.

  F. Have the person continue self-monitoring.

V. Change Exercise Behavior

  A. Routine activity

    1. Increase routine activity.

    2. Increase use of stairs.

    3. Keep records of distance walked daily.

  B. Exercise

    1. Begin a supervised exercise program under a specialist's direction.

    2. Keep records of daily exercise.

    3. Increase exercise gradually.

VI. Set Up a Reward-and-Reinforcement System

  A. Have family and friends provide this help in the form of praise and material rewards.

  B. Clearly define behaviors to be reinforced.

  C. Use self-monitoring records as a basis for rewards.

  D. Plan specific rewards for specific behaviors. Use written contracts.

  E. Gradually make rewards more difficult to earn.

  F. Use creative reinforcers, such as dropping quarters in a bank, putting money away for each goal reached and earmarked for something desirable. Take money back as a punishment if the goal is not reached.

Box 7-1 ■ *(continued)*

In some instances, responses occur in chains in which each response produces the stimulus for the next response. An example of a chain is watching television, going to the kitchen at commercial breaks, getting a snack, eating the snack, and feeling satisfied or less bored reinforcer. The components of the chain should be identified, and then a break in the chain should be planned, such as doing stretching exercises or laundry at commercials.

CASE ANALYSIS 2

What are Martha's possible antecedents or cues to eating? Can you identify any response chains?

Behavior

After identifying antecedents, the nutrition professional and client can explore the eating behavior itself by investigating the speed of eating, the reasons for eating, the presence of others, and activities carried on during meals or snacks, such as watching television. The chain of eating too rapidly, for example, can be broken by introducing delays in eating, such as resting the utensils after a bite of food or pausing for conversation. Also, eating behaviors can be modified by encouraging the person to focus on eating as a single event in which he or she concentrates on the act of eating and enjoying the flavors of the foods.

CASE ANALYSIS 3

Identify two specific behavior changes that Martha may want to try.

Consequences

Consequences of eating are described as reinforcements or rewards. Because behavior may be maintained by its consequences, efforts are made to arrange consequences that will maintain desirable behaviors. The consequences of eating may be positive, negative, or neutral. In general, positive consequences are more effective in promoting change than negative or punishing consequences. Reinforcers may be earned over a long period of time or they may be of short term. For example, a long-term reinforcer may be fitting into smaller size clothes after a weight loss program. A short-term reinforcer may be avoiding purchasing "empty calories" from the snack machine, setting the money that would have been spent on the snack aside, and then purchasing a book at the end of the week with the money saved. Alternatives to eating may be included, such as walking or exercising, calling a friend, gardening, or working on a hobby.

If the client's current eating habits are pleasurable and if food is considered its own reward, then new and different rewards must be established. Eating is a powerfully motivated behavior, the occurrence of which is necessary to maintain life, a positive reinforcement. The nutrition professional can help to identify new reinforcers with clients and introduce healthier food choices.

Acquired taste can be developed for a broader selection of foods and can steer choices to healthier selections. In some cases, a client may be aware of foods prepared only one way, which were not pleasing to eat. If a new preparation method is described, the client may be receptive to trying the food. For example, a client may dislike asparagus because he or she knows it only as the long skinny vegetable that is boiled and covered with Hollandaise sauce. If the client is told that asparagus can be grilled for a delicious flavor, he or she may be open-minded enough to try it again and perhaps develop a taste for this low-fat vegetable. Changes in eating patterns that are pleasurable are self-reinforcing. If new patterns are a chore and are disliked, they will fail to provide self-reinforcement.

The counselor can work with the client to establish reinforcers. Asking "What do you like to do with your leisure time?" may identify activity reinforcers. Reinforcers may be walking; attending movies, plays, or sporting events; taking a bath; gardening; knitting; playing cards; or reading. Social reinforcers may be found by asking "Whom do you like to be with?" Reinforcers may include visiting or calling family or friends. Other questions are "What do you find enjoyable?" and "What do you like to buy when you have extra money?" other than unhealthy foods, of course.[4] Box 7-2 summarizes the identification of reinforcers.

1. Make a list of leisure-time activities and hobbies that you enjoy.
2. Make a list of people you like to be with.
3. Make a list of things you would like to purchase with small amounts of extra money.
4. What do you find relaxing?
5. What do you do for fun?
6. What are your favorite possessions?

Box 7-2 ■ Identifying Reinforcers

A very important point here is to recognize that the counselor is also part of the reinforcement. Rather than focusing on failures, the counselor should emphasize what the person has done right with verbal reward and praise. Remind clients to reward themselves cognitively by telling themselves they are making progress and have done something right. For the obese, the ability to fit into smaller-sized clothes hanging in the closet and the weight loss itself are reinforcing. New reinforcers need to be established and introduced for weight maintenance, such as engaging in enjoyable activities, joining a gym for physical activity, engaging in social events not centered on eating, or walking laps around shopping malls. The reinforcement provided by significant others and self-monitoring are discussed later in this chapter.

SELF-ASSESSMENT 3

1. What rewards do you get from eating?
2. What rewards do you think others receive from eating?
3. Identify one or two reinforcers that may help you change an eating behavior.

After one or two eating changes or goals are identified, a schedule of reinforcement needs to be discussed and established. The schedule specifies which behaviors, if any, will be reinforced and how frequently reinforcement will be provided. Continual reinforcement is the simplest method, but this may lose its effectiveness if the reinforcer is used excessively. An alternative is intermittent reinforcement, such as reinforcement three times a day or once a day. Eventually, the time may be lengthened between reinforcements. The schedule should be appropriate to the behavior one is trying to strengthen, convenient for the person to apply, and applied immediately for the greatest effect. Never reinforcing a behavior leads to its extinction.[2,5,11]

In some cases, contracts may be desirable. Contracts are clear statements of target behaviors of the individual; they specify the type of reinforcers to be used, the person who will deliver the reinforcers, and the frequency of reinforcement. They are signed and dated by the counselor and the client. Contracts ensure that all parties agree on the goals and procedures and provide a measurement of how close the client is to reaching the goals. The signatures help to ensure that the contract will be followed, since signing is a commitment and may provide added motivation to change.[4] Figure 7-1 is an example of a contract.

Patient/Client Name _____

Date _____

Goals:

   Example: Increase physical activity 3 times a week.

   1.

   2.

Strategy to Modify Goal:

Time Frame:

   Example: Get up a half-hour earlier than usual for a brisk walk in the neighborhood Tuesdays, Thursdays, and Saturdays.

   Use the stairs instead of the elevator, especially if only one floor.

   1.

   2.

_____   _____
Patient/Client Signature   Dietitian's Signature

Figure 7-1 ■ Example of a behavioral contract for change.

An alternative to a formal contract is encouraging the client to write out a list of behaviors to change and a few strategies to implement the change. Also, a simple list of pros and cons of modifying food choices can become a key eye-opener to some.

CASE ANALYSIS **4**

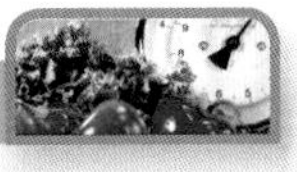

What would be some eating changes or goals that might be created with Martha's input? Identify one or two reinforcers that may help change Martha's eating habits.

Completion of behavioral assessment, including a consideration of the Stage of Change, is needed before counseling begins. Examination of the ABC framework antecedents, behaviors, and consequences by the nutrition counselor and the client assists both parties in understanding current eating behaviors and allows discussion of what can be changed. Maintaining new behaviors when under pressure or stress is especially difficult. The counselor may consider assessing client self-confidence and the ability to cope with stress or anxiety. This evaluation may help identify clients who will need additional support at particularly stressful times.

Goal setting and problem solving in a supportive environment are key factors of behavior modification.[15] Goals must be set realistically yet high enough to provide significant change. The role of the counselor is to help the client develop his own integrated plan geared toward defined and measurable goals. The nutrition counselor serves as a guide or facilitator of change rather than a director or controller of change by suggesting behavioral techniques appropriate to the situation. The counselor should assist the client in assessing the triggers to eating problems and should suggest possible goals, strategies, and techniques to deal with them.[5]

Ultimately, the client must determine which suggestions seem manageable at that time and must be willing to implement them. It is also a good idea to ask the client to give an example of the specific behavior change rather than the concept by stating, for example, "The next time I am out of milk I will buy low-fat milk instead of whole milk." This is a concrete action plan compared with merely stating "I'll try to follow a low-fat diet."

Since clients are not routinely in daily contact with the counselor, they must be ready to assume personal responsibility for sound dietary changes and eventually become independent. They must learn to analyze and solve their own eating behavior problems. Have the client start with small, easy changes, which are most likely to be successful, and progress incrementally to more difficult ones in later sessions.

To be self-reinforcing, the eating changes should be pleasurable ones. If clients enjoy potato chips, ice cream, pizza, and beer, they have to find substitutes they enjoy, such as baked chips, fresh grapes, unbuttered popcorn, and calorie-free beverages or light beer. It may be sufficient to start by reducing the quantity of favorite foods consumed. However, some people may elect to avoid a food item entirely to reduce the temptation of having more. Needless to say, strategies must be highly individualized, and what is appropriate for one client may be inappropriate for another.

Nutrition counselors have the opportunity to share the experiences of others. By having counseled patients and clients on various issues and using customized approaches, counselors learn to assist patients at every point of change. The process of counseling can be compared with making bread. Every baker knows that particular ingredients, kneading, and rising time are essential to making a loaf of bread, but he or she also introduces artistic expression and ingredient variation to make a unique loaf of bread that meets the distinct tastes of loyal customers. When preparing a new recipe, it is often helpful to see pictures of the finished product; however, the baker or chef must sometimes adjust the recipe for cooking at different altitudes or with varying ingredients. Similarly as counselors, we need to be cognizant of the right things to convey at the right time and be able to customize along the way.

The counselor should discuss with the client the possibility of deviations from the planned behavior, especially when under physical or emotional stress. Expecting

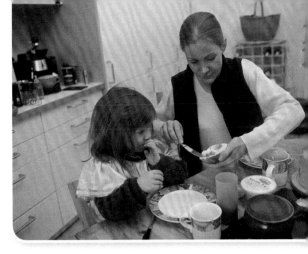

The mother influences the child's cues for eating.

Source: Copyright Wolters Kluwer.

immediate, total control over change is unrealistic and may lead to diminished self-esteem in clients who have problems following diets, with eventual abandonment of the dietary changes. Learning any new skill requires practice over a period of time. Repetition of the same new behaviors gradually becomes reinforcing and habitual. Support and forgiveness should be provided during any lapses.

Enthusiasm for change may be expected to drop rapidly after the initial period, especially if frustration and disappointments arise. Weekly appointments, or alternative methods of communication phone or e-mail, with the counselor may be needed and are desirable in the beginning, tapering to bimonthly and monthly. However, preestablished rules and limits should be set forth in advance of embarking on alternative communication.[16]

Self-Monitoring

Self-monitoring, or keeping records of eating behaviors to be controlled, was intended originally as a means of supplying the counselor and client with data for analysis. Clients record what, where, when, and how much they eat; the circumstances, for example, eating while watching television or while feeling bored; and the persons present (Table 7-1). The exercise of keeping records has additional value of its own; it increases client awareness and understanding of current eating behaviors and the influences on them and leads to such realizations as "I'm eating too much during evening hours while I watch television." Data provide a basis for setting goals for change "I'll eat a low-calorie snack instead." and finding ways to reinforce new behaviors "I'll tell myself how well I'm doing."

Keeping records serves as a measure of the person's commitment to change. In addition, by having to write down the foods and beverages

183

Time	Food/Amount/ Prep Method	Room/ Place	Others Present	How You Felt Before Eating	Activities at the Same Time
Example:					
9:30 PM	8 cookies, 10 oz milk	Family room	Husband	Bored, tired	Watching television

Table 7-1 ■ Self-Monitoring Food Record

consumed, the client may think twice about actually consuming an item rather than eating it out of habit or while distracted. Patterns of weight change, physical exercise, blood sugar, and blood pressure are other self-monitoring techniques. In a systematic review of the literature on self-monitoring for weight loss, Burke and colleagues [17] determined that an association between self-monitoring and weight loss was consistently reported despite weaknesses in study design. Self-monitoring may be conducted by traditional paper and pencil diaries or more advanced use of technology such as a digital recorder or online tools.

Self-Management

In most behavior modification programs for weight control, the client and counselor are together only for a brief duration at specified intervals. Consequently, the counselor cannot be continually in control of dispensing rewards and punishments or withholding them for appropriate and inappropriate behavior, which is the basis of behavior modification. Therefore, self-regulation or self-management techniques are taught to clients so that they can regulate and control their own behavior. In this way, progress may be achieved in the interval between meetings of the client and counselor.

Research has shown the importance of developing behavioral self-management techniques. Skinner[18] explained that self-management or "self-control" occurs when the individual manipulates the variables on which the behavior rests. Self-management programs have been designed to help persons become aware of and modify antecedents of eating and to self-administer rewarding consequences for eating differently. As self-management programs have evolved, more emphasis has been placed on cognitive change. People have been helped to modify thoughts and beliefs that interfered with adherence to specific dietary regimens and to make use of self-reinforcing thoughts when appropriate behaviors occur. Becoming aware of one's inner state can assist in achieving the desired self-management. For example, referring to a diet has connotations of an ephemeral event, whereas adapting a lifestyle change leads to a more permanent behavior modification.

What self-management and/or self-monitoring techniques might be successful for Martha?

Social Support

Clients' social environments consist of people they are in contact with daily. It is important to include the person's family and significant others when planning lifestyle and dietary changes. The nutrition professional should include family members in counseling for change whenever possible, since the changes in food plans at home may affect them as well. Cultural and social factors may be contributing factors to obesity. If the family system supports an obese lifestyle with high-calorie foods and little physical activity, change will be difficult for the client unless the whole family participates in the challenge.[4,19] The involvement and support of spouse and family play an important role in weight loss.[19]

Ideally, family and friends are supportive of the client's efforts to change eating behaviors. The counselor may need to discuss with clients the important role of support in achieving permanent change. The professional may suggest that clients request help from family and friends by seeking their agreement not to eat inappropriate foods in front of them and not to purchase or prepare the unhealthy foods. In addition, clients might ask their spouses, families, and friends to offer positive reinforcement for their efforts. Role-playing some of these situations with clients may be helpful.

When family members are present at the counseling session, they should be asked to discuss ways in which they can contribute to the client's lifestyle change. Reinforcing proper behavior by the use of praise is an example. Controlling antecedents by having proper foods available is of great assistance. Family and friends should avoid acting the role of judge. "You shouldn't eat that," "It's bad for you," and "I told you so" are not helpful remarks. Jealous and envious reactions may also be expected. "You've lost enough weight," "Just this once won't hurt your diet," and "Your skin is getting to look awful" are remarks that the client may need to tolerate or confront.

Applications

Weight Management

The most common application of behavioral principles and methods to the treatment of nutritional problems has been in the management of body weight. Although there has been much success using behavior modification in weight loss regimens, weight regain is common and is a result of the failure to impose weight maintenance behaviors.[20] Research into the characteristics among people who successfully maintain weight loss reveals that weight regain is due in part to not fully adhering to behavior change strategies.[21] Successful patterns of behavior and strategies to implement on a routine basis include maintaining consistent eating behaviors on all days of the week, self-monitoring weight, eating breakfast regularly, and choosing a diet without excess calories.[22]

Overweight and obesity are complex and not easily treated. While excess weight may manifest from a variety of reasons, only one of which may be related to inappropriate eating behaviors,[19] strategies to control weight should be targeted to the etiology of the weight gain. The Academy of Nutrition and Dietetics position on weight management emphasizes a lifelong approach to healthful lifestyle behaviors including sustainable and enjoyable eating practices and daily physical activity.[19]

The American College of Sports Medicine, in a position statement, stressed that lifelong weight control requires commitment, an understanding of your eating habits, and a willingness to change them.[23] Realistic goal setting, combined with a reduction of caloric intake plus a sound exercise program, is recommended. Tailoring practical applications to a client's lifestyle achieves the greatest success. Physical activity may have an additive role in weight management as it can attenuate emotional overeating and improve dietary control.[24]

Motivation and readiness must be present for behavior change. This is particularly true of eating behaviors and physical activity. Several factors are relevant to the prediction of success in weight control, one of which is motivation to reduce weight. After the Stages of Change model is applied to assess the readiness to change behavior, realistic and individual goal setting is critical.[25,26]

Explaining realistic weight loss achievements is essential. Clients may see improvements in comorbidities associated with overweight/obesity when there is an initial reduction of about 10% of their body weight over a 6- to 12-month period.[26] To expect more than that initially would be a setup for disappointment; however, weight goals can be reevaluated after successful weight loss. Another motivator may be a deposit-refund system in which patients are asked to deposit money that is later returned if the patient attends meetings faithfully, or achieves a previously determined weight loss, or both.[4] However, a financial reward system may not be effective for long-term behavior change.[27]

An added benefit of significant weight reduction based on cognitive-behavioral treatment in a long-term therapeutic setting has been the reduction in psychosomatic symptoms, anxiety, and depression in treated clients. More adaptive behavioral alternatives in longer goal-oriented programs seem effective in promoting continued weight loss.[25] Taken together, these results emphasize the fact that there is no quick fix in weight reduction and that the outlook must be long term.

Diabetes Mellitus

Behavior modification methods have proved to be a useful component in the management of diabetes mellitus. Patient adherence to appropriate dietary regimens to control glucose is challenging. Behavioral interventions such as cueing, self-monitoring, and reinforcement for appropriate behavior can be successfully implemented to improve glycemic control and reduce risks of complications in patients with diabetes. As previously noted, though, the problem of control of overweight and obesity from the standpoint of any particular treatment is complex.

Behavioral management techniques may be used to prevent progression to diabetes in people with prediabetes and to reduce the burden of diabetes complications in those with diagnosed disease.[28] The American Association of Diabetes Educators advocates seven self-care behaviors that should be emphasized in patient care, including healthy eating, physical activity, glucose monitoring, medication adherence, problem solving, reducing risks by seeking preventative services, and coping.[29] Additionally, clinicians should help patients identify factors that help self-management and burdens, and factors that hinder behavior change.[29] Implementation of structure and use of technology to increase counselor and social support are important and effective strategies to achieve optimal behaviors.[30] Proactive management by care providers and self-management by patients is warranted and has demonstrated positive outcomes.[26,29]

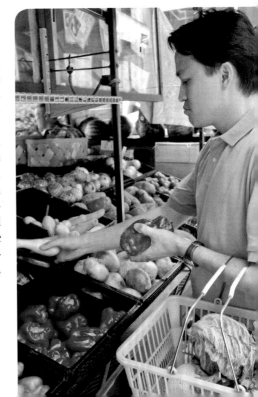

The National Diabetes Education Program supports the work of the other organizations in diabetes management and sets forth initiatives for comprehensive care. These initiatives and additional resources can be viewed on its web site at http://ndep.nih.gov. Behavioral interventions, when used in the management of diabetes mellitus, should be geared to the developmental stage of the individual in treatment.[31] An understanding of life span changes,

The goal of counseling is self-management.
Source: CDC/Amanda Mills.

that is, preadolescence, adolescence, and adulthood in relation to life role, peer conformity pressure, eating disorders, and hormonal changes needs to be taken into account. A strategy that is effective for an adolescent with diabetes struggling with peer conformity pressures may differ markedly from the one that will be of assistance to a pregnant woman with diabetes. There is a definite need to individualize interventions directed toward behavior change.

Cardiovascular Diseases

The American Heart Association (AHA) has established a definition of ideal cardiovascular health to include health behaviors and clinical factors that should be met to reduce the risk of cardiovascular disease CVD.[32] To be successful, the AHA advocates for lifestyle habits to include good dietary behaviors, physical activity, and avoidance of tobacco. It is recognized that reduction in morbidity and mortality from CVD can be significantly reduced by modest, sustained changes in lifestyle behaviors. Additionally, these positive effects accrue over time so that long-term success at behavior modification is warranted for CVD reduction.[33]

Evidence supports goal setting, self-monitoring, reinforcement, and modeling as effective in modifying behaviors related to diet and physical activity.[33] Other important elements of long-term success in behavior change include frequent and prolonged contact of patients with their healthcare providers who advocate positive behaviors, as well as enabling the client to problem-solve, especially during times of relapse, which may be a normal part of behavior change.

A policy statement from several European and American organizations calls for a model to combat noncommunicable diseases using healthy lifestyle interventions on a global perspective.[34] Since it is generally recognized that CVD may result from self-selected behaviors such as smoking, inappropriate eating behaviors, lack of physical activity, and the pursuit of stress-prone lifestyles, it is encouraging that the initiation of the behavior is by choice and that modification of these self-defeating behaviors is possible. Because the risk factors are behavioral in nature, it is particularly appropriate to attempt to alter them using psychological methods based on behavior modification. The degree of difficulty with such behavior modification partially depends on how long the undesirable behavior has been in place.

Human Resource Management

The behavior of employees is of major concern to supervisors interested in productivity and good human relations. Setting observable, measurable goals and noting the discrepancy between actual and desired performance may help in actualizing desired behaviors. Supervisors need to convert ambiguous affective goal statements into a format that is useful for producing improved performance. In this way, employees are encouraged to periodically assess their own performance and adjust behavior as needed for improved results. Rather than attempting to catch employees doing things wrong or inefficiently, managers are encouraged to positively reinforce when employees are doing something right or approximately right and then gradually move them toward the desired behavior. Positive reinforcers include the following:

- Praise
- Positive feedback
- Recognition employee of the week, month
- Added responsibility
- Compliments
- Special assignments
- Social events
- Knowledge of results
- Thank-you letter
- Salary increase
- Bonus
- Promotion

Praise is used immediately to reinforce proper behavior. Eventually, some employees begin to praise themselves for the proper behavior, which provides additional reinforcement. A gentle reprimand may also be used, concentrating on the improper behavior and not on the person.

An important aspect of job satisfaction and performance is the employee's sense of personal control; therefore, it is imperative that supervisors refrain from using behavior modification in ways that are seen as manipulative and degrading to employees. Intrinsic motivation should be encouraged to emphasize the importance of a self-reinforcing loop.[5]

Summary

There are numerous applications and major advantages of behavior therapy. Programs integrating behavioral approaches appear to hold the most promise for effecting lasting changes. In particular, comprehensive programs that consider the psychological, cultural, environmental, and behavioral factors are more apt to be successful.

Eating patterns are not altered easily, but behavior modification therapy offers promising techniques that may be helpful to both the client and the counselor. Analysis of the ABCs—the antecedents of eating, the eating behavior itself, and the consequences of eating—by the counselor and client leads to understanding of the problems, the setting of goals, and the development of strategies for change. Efforts should be made to arrange consequences that reinforce and maintain desirable changes, with an ultimate goal being independent client self-management. Behavior modification may be used in conjunction with other counseling and education strategies.

Review and Discussion Questions

1. Describe the similarities and differences in learning styles of classical conditioning, operant conditioning, and modeling. Are there situations or cases in which you would prefer using one style over another?
2. Give two examples of a chain of events using the ABC framework.
3. Describe two methods of self-control discussed in the chapter and discuss how each aids in successful behavior modification.
4. List one important behavior modification strategy for each of the applications discussed: obesity, diabetes, CVD, and human resource management.
5. Apply the nutrition care process and nutrition care process terminology to the case challenge of Martha using the steps of nutrition assessment, nutrition diagnosis, nutrition intervention, nutrition monitoring, and evaluation.

Suggested Activities

1. Complete a food diary for 3 days using written or digital format. Identify your cues for eating. Identify your reinforcers. Set one goal for change with identified reinforcers.
2. Record and identify your own ABCs related to an activity other than eating, such as studying, exercising, and smoking. How can these

behaviors be made to occur more or less often by rearranging the antecedents, consequences, or both?

3. Role-play and record a counseling session. How often did you reinforce positive behaviors?

4. Arrange to watch an adult interact with a child or children for half an hour. Tally the number of times the adult attends to desirable behaviors, which reinforces them, versus the number of times desirable behaviors are ignored, which may lead to their extinction. Note whether the adult responds to undesirable behaviors, which reinforces them.

5. Identify your own reinforcers by making a list of leisure-time activities that you enjoy, people you like to be with, and things you would purchase with extra money. Select an appropriate reinforcer for yourself for the next time you have a book to read or a paper to write. Identify a time schedule for dispensing the reinforcer.

6. Select an undesirable behavior of your own that you would like to diminish. Record the situations in which the stimulus or the behavior occurs for 3 days. Identify the controlling stimulus conditions just before the behavior and the reinforcement.

7. Identify three situations in which modeling occurs.

8. Discuss your personal experiences at work and compare them with those of others. Does your supervisor praise or punish? What are the consequences of the supervisor's actions on your behavior and that of other employees?

CHAPTER 8

Counseling for Cognitive Change

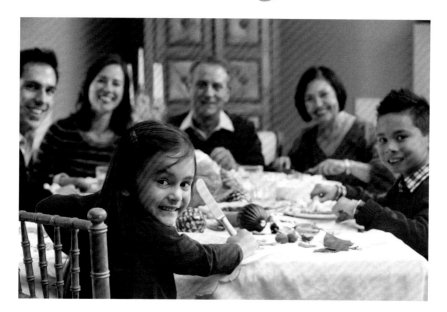

Objectives

- Explain how cognitions affect people's behaviors.
- Discuss the types of cognitive distortions and the effects they have on people's behaviors.
- Explain the three phases of cognitive restructuring.
- Discuss self-efficacy's role in the initiation and maintenance of health behavior changes and in a person's choice of activities.

- List the advantages and disadvantages of the four sources of efficacy information.
- Explain the use and advantages of self-monitoring of cognitions.
- Explain high-risk situations and the cognitive–behavioral model of the relapse process.
- List determinants and predictors of lapse and relapse and how to assess them.
- Identify treatment strategies to prevent lapses and relapse.

Carol Jones is a 50-year-old woman recently diagnosed with type 2 diabetes mellitus. Her maternal grandmother had diabetes. Mrs. Jones was an overweight child and is now an overweight adult at 5'4" and 180 lb. She is married and works part-time at a retail clothing store in a local mall.

Dr. Smith referred her for counseling to lose weight. Joan Stivers, the nutritionist, notes in her assessment that Mrs. Jones seems to have a problem with low self-image and negative cognitions and that her overweight is related to cognitive distortions. As a result, the current priority is cognitive restructuring.

If you think you can or you think you can't, you're right.

—*Henry Ford*

Introduction

The prevention and treatment of health problems and chronic diseases require theory- and evidence-based interventions. Changing behaviors is a challenge for most people, many of whom are coping with a serious health problem. The Stages of Change discussed in Chapter 5 examines people's readiness to change. The professional then decides which theory to consider in counseling for behavior change.

Cognitive Behavior Theory integrates two theoretical approaches—the behavioral approach described in Chapter 7 and a cognitive approach. The behavioral approach focuses on observable, measurable behaviors, such as overeating, and concentrates on the interaction of the person's external environment and behavior.

The cognitive approach focuses on the role of the mind, specifically on cognitions or one's thoughts, as determinates of behaviors and feelings. Behavioral explanations require knowing what people are thinking and feeling internally. It is one's thinking that causes people to feel and act the way they do. How we think (cognition), feel (emotion), and act (behavior) all interact. Cognitive behavior theory seeks to modify a person's thinking and belief system to bring about changes in behaviors.[1] As indicated in the above quote by Henry Ford, your thoughts influence what you believe you can or cannot do. An advantage is that we can change the way we think in order to feel and act better.

There are a number of evidence-based theories of behavioral change that may be appropriate in a nutrition counseling intervention. This chapter explores cognitive-behavioral therapy, self-monitoring client's cognitions and emotions, identifying maladaptive and negative thoughts related to food and eating as the basis for cognitive restructuring, and relapse prevention. Enhancing client self-efficacy (SE) and the influence of observational learning, or modeling, are components of social cognitive theory. These are factors within the person's internal thoughts that affect eating and health behaviors.

Validated behavior change theories are integral to the Nutrition Care Process guiding nutrition assessment, interventions, and outcome evaluation.[2] There is growing evidence that interventions developed with theoretical foundations are more effective than those lacking one and that combining multiple theories, models, and approaches leads to better results. These methods are important in client-centered disease prevention and management.[3]

Cognitive–Behavioral Therapy

Cognitions may be defined as one's thoughts or perceptions at a particular moment in time. These thinking patterns can profoundly influence people's behaviors, actions, and feelings. Many emotions we feel are preceded and caused by a thought.[4] When strategies for dealing with a client's cognitions are incorporated into behavioral programs, the term "cognitive–behavioral therapy" (CBT) is used.

Eating disorders, for example, are essentially cognitive disorders. For bulimia nervosa, CBT is an effective treatment and leading evidence-based treatment for eating disorders.[5,6] In adults with eating disorders, CBT was found to be a "potent treatment." Evidence-based forms of CBT had strong outcomes in routine clinical settings.[7]

There are three fundamental propositions in CBT: (1) Cognitions are learned and can affect one's behaviors, thoughts, and feelings; (2) A person's cognitive activity can be monitored and changed using evidence-based intervention strategies; and (3) Cognitive change may effect a desired behavior change. The major aim is to produce changes in the automatic thoughts that maintain a person's behavior that needs to be changed. There is a difference between thinking "I can't do it." and "I can try."[4,8]

CASE ANALYSIS 1

Mrs. Jones: "I have always been heavy. I don't think that I can ever lose weight."
YOUR RESPONSE:

NOTE: In each Case Analysis for this chapter, "Your Response" indicates an opportunity for you to practice cognitive counseling. Rather than giving advice, seek further information with a paraphrase or a thought or a feeling Mrs. Jones expresses or a reflective summary of what she said.

It is evident that "multiple interventions at multiple levels are often needed to initiate and sustain behavior change."[9] Evidence exists to support the use of a combination in facilitating modification of targeted dietary habits, weight, and cardiovascular and diabetes risk factors.[9] Weight control programs, for example, may include assessing readiness to change, motivational interviewing, stimulus control, cue reduction, self-monitoring, cognitive restructuring, self-efficacy, outcome evaluations, realistic goal setting, physical activity, stress management, relapse prevention, contracting, social support, and dietary change.[3,10]

People who are overweight can benefit from cognitive-behavioral strategies to reduce weight, especially when combined with exercise and dietary strategies, at least in the short term. The practitioner needs to individualize a nutrition counseling intervention that is directed toward resolving the nutrition diagnosis. The assumption that a person's knowledge will lead to improved food choices is only partially correct as other factors are influential.

CBT applies interventions and techniques to modify dysfunctional and negative thoughts and beliefs that may underlie a problem. It focuses on what people think or thinking errors rather than what they do. Introduced by Aaron T. Beck in the 1960s, it explores the relationship between cognitive processes or thoughts and the lifestyle problem in question, such as the need for changes in food, exercise, and health behaviors.[1] These types of thinking affect one's feelings, moods, and how one acts.

The key is to realize that it is not events by themselves that may affect behavior, but how we perceive the events mentally. Feeling tired and somewhat unhappy after a long day of work, for example, may be perceived in different ways. Some may feel happy to be home while others may think of a food or drink reward or treat. What goes through your mind at the end of a tiring day? How does it affect your choice of behaviors? Over time, these thoughts become automatic so that they are repeated when one finds oneself in the same situation again.

The approach in working with clients is problem-oriented in helping them identify their thoughts about food and eating in specific daily situations. Distorted thinking and unrealistic cognitive appraisals of events can negatively affect one's feelings and behaviors.[8] While the client may consider the thoughts as "truths," counselors use the tool of cognitive restructuring to help clients identify, evaluate, and respond to negative thoughts about diet or a health problem.

Cognitions

Cognitions are thoughts that occur in one's stream of consciousness. Beck refers to them as "automatic thoughts," since they run through the mind automatically. Others refer to them ongoing "internal dialogue" or as "self-talk."[1,4] Since our thoughts are subconscious and seldom noticed, we are barely aware of them even though they can create powerful feelings.[4] They may be positive, negative, or neutral and are usually believed to be true.

Negative thoughts, such as "It's not worth the effort to eat less" or "I'm too tired to exercise" are obstacles to behavioral change, affect people's feelings, and may decrease self-efficacy or people's beliefs about their ability to perform specific behaviors. ("I can't do it"). This can lead to lapses or relapse in the behavior change process. ("I'll eat whatever I want."). Individuals with positive cognitions, such as "losing weight is worth the effort," and perceived SE ("I can do it") tend to call upon their coping skills and regulate their behaviors better.

CASE ANALYSIS 2

Mrs. Jones: "I lost 10 lb once before. But it was just a fluke. I couldn't do it again."
YOUR RESPONSE:

Times when individuals are more likely to engage in self-talk include when they are integrating new thoughts and actions, such as making lifestyle and dietary changes, performing a new job, or experiencing intense emotions. According to Albert Bandura, cognitive processes play a major role in the acquisition and retention of new behavior patterns.[11] See Box 8-1 for examples of self-talk.

Counseling is based on the hypothesis that people's feelings and behaviors are influenced not by events, but by their perception of events or situations.[1] The perception is often expressed in an internal dialogue or self-talk that influences subsequent feelings, behaviors, and even physiologic responses. For example, someone who has lost 5 lb on a new eating plan (event) may be thinking that dieting is difficult (thought), is not worth the effort (thought), and is feeling deprived and hungry (feelings). Having successfully lost the weight is not as influential

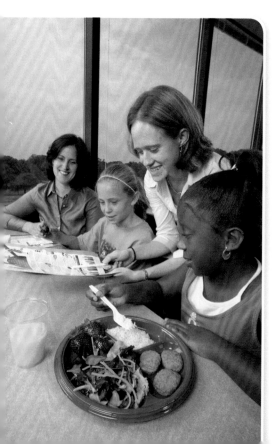

This tastes good is a positive cognition.
Source: US Department of Agriculture.

"I'm going to get a college degree so I'll have a successful career."

"I need to get up earlier tomorrow so I'll arrive on time."

"It's the holidays so I'm going to eat whatever I want."

"My New Year's resolution is to get more exercise."

"I'd be in better health if I lost some weight, but it's hard to do."

"I look fat."

"I hate to exercise because it makes me sweat."

"I have no will power."

Box 8-1 ■ Examples of Self-talk

as the perceptions that it is difficult or not worth the effort, resulting in psychological feelings of deprivation and physiologic feelings of hunger. As a result, the individual may abandon plans for further weight loss even though successful at losing weight.

SELF-ASSESSMENT 1

What is the result of each of the following cognitions?

1. "I don't feel like studying tonight."
2. "I might as well do my homework now and get it over with."
3. "I don't have time to exercise today."
4. "I'll feel better if I take a break and walk for 20 minutes."

Your understanding of cognitive restructuring will improve if you start applying it to yourself when you identify negative and dysfunctional thoughts.

Cognitive Distortions

Since negative and dysfunctional thoughts inhibit behavioral change, it is necessary for individuals to first become aware of distortions in their thought patterns. Faulty thinking almost always contains gross distortions, often has little to do with actual reality, and may be self-defeating and destructive. Twelve common cognitive distortions have been identified[1,4] (See Box 8-2). The counselor can assist clients in reevaluating these.

Cognitive distortions are thinking traps that have been learned over time. These negative thoughts create adverse feelings that may lead to a negative self-image or sense of worthlessness. In addition, they can become a self-fulfilling prophecy. Because they are learned, they can be changed or relearned with practice. Since some people have had these thoughts for years, however, change may require extended effort and counseling.

1. All-or-Nothing Thinking: The tendency to evaluate oneself, one's experiences, people, and things in either black or white, good or bad, without seeing a middle ground, and is the basis of perfectionism. For example, "I ate this piece of pie and I shouldn't have. I'm a failure."

2. Overgeneralization: An isolated negative event is generalized to other situations. For example: "I ate too much. I will never be able to lose weight."

3. Mental Filter: A single negative detail is dwelt upon, causing the whole to be perceived as negative. For example: "If I can't eat whatever I want at the restaurant, it won't be any fun."

4. Discounting the Positive: For example: "I am following the diet now, but I probably won't be able to do it tomorrow."

5. Jumping to Conclusions: People assume the worst. "I don't think I can follow the diet." or "I'll feel less lonely if I eat this bag of cookies."

6. Magnification and Minimization: "Everyone will hear I goofed up. I'm ruined." Or "I lost a tiny bit of weight today, but hardly any"

7. Emotional Reasoning: Negative feelings are considered true. "I feel inadequate so it must be."

8. Should Statements: To try to motivate oneself: "I should eat fruit and I shouldn't eat cake."

9. Labeling and Mislabeling: For example: "I'm a pig." or "I'm a failure.

10. Personalization: Seeing oneself as the cause of a negative event. For example: "What happened was my fault because I am inadequate."

11. Tunnel Vision: One sees the negative in situations. For example: "She can't do anything right."

12. Mind Reading: People think that they know what others think and feel: For example: "She is not interested in being my friend."

Box 8-2 ■ Cognitive Distortions

Cognitive Restructuring

Cognitive restructuring techniques refer to a variety of approaches the counselor may use to assist in modifying the client's thinking and the assumptions and attitudes underlying them. Based on learning theory, it involves unlearning maladaptive associations between stimuli and our responses as we learn new ones. While much self-talk is harmless, the focus is on the false thoughts, inferences, and premises. Thus the counselor attempts to become familiar with the client's thought content, feelings, and behaviors in various situations or events and helps the client identify specific misconceptions and distortions and to test their validity and reasonableness. Changing the thoughts to positive ones can modify and improve one's feelings and behaviors.

"When I go out to a restaurant, I won't get my money's worth if I don't eat the food they serve."
YOUR RESPONSE:

Phases of Cognitive Behavior Modification

Cognitive modification consists of three phases, not necessarily in progression. They include (1) recognizing the problem, (2) exploring it, and (3) making changes. The aim is to produce changes in the thought processes maintaining a behavior that needs to change.

Recognizing the Problem

The first step involves helping the client recognize and understand the nature of the problem. A basic principle is that people cannot change a behavior without increasing their awareness, raising their consciousness, or noticing a pattern in how they think, feel, and behave, and the impact of the behavior in various situations.

Rarely does a person recognize that thinking processes are a source of the eating problems which is the reason why homework is necessary. This is true in eating disorders, overweight, and other dietary changes. The counselor can enlist clients in a collaborative, investigative effort to learn and understand. Clients self-monitor by keeping a written log of self-observations to become aware of the relationship between negative and self-defeating thoughts, feelings, and eating choices as in Table 8-1.

Daily record of _____		Date: _____
False Thought or Belief	**Type of Distortion**	**Self-Defense, Coping Thought**
"I shouldn't have eaten those cookies. I'm a failure."	All-or-none thinking	"Eating 3 cookies does not make me a failure. I can improve."
"I ate the pie. I'm a pig."	Mislabeling	"Pigs are animals and I am human. I don't have to be perfect."
"I don't have time to eat right or exercise."	Fortune-teller error	"I have just as much time as anyone else. I can make time."

Table 8-1 ■ Assessing and Altering False Thoughts

Date & Time	Place	People	Situation	Thoughts/ Feelings Before Eating	Food Eaten	Thoughts/ Feelings After Eating
1/10 & 2:15 PM	Home	Family	Snacking	"I'm hungry and upset."	6 cookies, cola	"I feel better."

Table 8.2 ■ Daily Record of Thoughts and Feelings

The log is a source of material to discuss in counseling sessions. Avoiding the terms "maladaptive" and "dysfunctional" thoughts with clients is advisable. Examples of maladaptive thoughts are: "Everyone at the party is sampling the foods, so I will too (thought)." "Just this once won't hurt."

Self-monitoring records are useful in lifestyle intervention programs.[12] They may include a false thought or self-criticism, the type of thinking error it represents, and a self-defense response or the substitution of a more objective, coping, self-enhancing thought. Others suggest records that include the situation or event with thoughts and feelings before and during eating as well as after eating as in Table 8-2.

Self-monitoring is a learning experience. The homework gives the person a central role in solving the problems as well as providing the counselor with information about them.[13] Since negative and self-critical self-talk may be at a subconscious level, self-monitoring can bring it to a level of awareness. Records of thoughts, emotions, dietary behaviors, physical activity, and other measures may be recorded. Evidence substantiates the effectiveness of self-monitoring and self-management.[13]

CASE ANALYSIS 4

Mrs. Jones: "My husband likes me the way I am. He does not complain about my weight"
YOUR RESPONSE:

The client may be asked to (1) discover negative thoughts by writing them down; (2) recognize the relationship among events, thoughts, feelings, and one's behavior; (3) test the validity of the automatic thoughts; (4) substitute more realistic thoughts for distorted ones; and (5) identify and alter underlying beliefs and assumptions that predispose him or her to engage in faulty thinking patterns.[8] This homework is important to help the client understand and overcome eating problems, recognize lack of coping, and avoid lapses and relapse. The counselor reviews the homework records with the client at the next appointment, reinforcing any positive and coping thoughts while helping clients recognize and reevaluate negative ones.

The client's learned internal dialogue or self-talk may be positive and supportive, negative, or neutral. Positive cognitions support behaviors, as for example, "These dietary changes are not so bad." Negative cognitions inhibit people's ability to change, such as, "These dietary changes look difficult to follow". Thoughts can be self-critical, such as "I'm fat," or self-indulgent, such as "I deserve a treat."

In eating disorders, such as anorexia nervosa and bulimia nervosa, dysfunctional thoughts and beliefs about "fattening" foods, fear of weight gain, body image distortion, and feelings of low self-worth require identification, challenging, and restructuring.[6] In managing subordinates, an employee may be thinking, "I like my job," or "This job is boring." Thoughts affect one's feelings and behavior.

Because cognitions are learned responses, the counselor views the client's cognitions as behaviors that can be modified or changed. Many people cannot improve their eating habits until they recognize and change their thoughts about food, eating, drinking, and exercise. Overeating and drinking can be an individual's way of coping with stress, depression, and other emotions. The approach is to help the client get rid of unproductive, debilitating thoughts or beliefs and adopt more positive, constructive ones. In the Women's Intervention Nutrition Study (WINS), for example, dietitians applied behavioral, cognitive, and motivational counseling techniques including identifying negative thoughts about diet change and cognitive restructuring to turn negative thoughts into positive ones.[14]

Exploring the Problem

During the second phase, the counselor helps the client to explore and consolidate the cognitive problem found in self-monitoring records. As the client reports negative, self-defeating, and self-fulfilling prophecy aspects of thoughts, the counselor can ask how these affect actual behavior and how they can be modified into more positive, coping thoughts. For example:

> "What happens when you are thinking you are bored and want to eat something?"
>
> "What happens when you think you are too tired after working all day to do any cooking?"
>
> "What happens when you think the food isn't as good tasting or satisfying as before?"

Note that the counselor does not provide advice or solutions to the problem and must resist this temptation. While the counselor may be tempted to give advice, it is not helpful. Rather than providing answers, asking clients questions about their thoughts promotes self-discovery, thus helping people learn to solve their own problems. Clients need to recognize that negative thoughts sabotage lifestyle change and decrease motivation.

What good does it do to focus on negative thoughts? Is there another way to look at the situation or a different explanation?

What is the worst that could happen versus the likeliest outcome? What if it happens?

What is the factual evidence supporting or challenging this negative thought? Is it really true?

How helpful or hurtful is this to my goals?

Do I benefit from thinking this way? What would happen if I change my thinking?

What can I say about myself in self-defense?

Am I exaggerating a negative situation? Is there an alternative explanation?

Is it as bad as it seems? What is more realistic?

Box 8.3 ■ Questions to Ask Oneself

The client learns to interrupt the automatic nature of negative self-talk and appraise and challenge the situation. The negative cognitions or thoughts are viewed not as facts, but as hypotheses worthy of testing. The client can be encouraged to ask the questions in Box 8-3.

In addition to client records of food, exercise, and thoughts, the counselor can discuss with clients the range of eating situations, past and present, during which they have had false thoughts, such as hopeless thoughts about previous attempts to lose weight or follow specific dietary changes.

Using the Socratic method and a collaborative approach, the counselor asks open-ended questions so that clients verbalize their thoughts and feelings concerning food, eating, and the dietary goal or change. One may ask: "How do you feel about . . .?" and "What do you think about . . .?" to determine what individuals are thinking to themselves about the eating behavior to be changed, about their ability and desire to change it, and at follow-up appointments, about their progress.

EXAMPLE "How do you feel about eating more fruits and vegetables instead of cookies?"

"How do you feel about cutting down on the amount of fried foods you eat?"

"What do you think about your ability to make these changes starting tomorrow?"

"On a scale of 1 to 10 with 10 being the highest, how important is this to you?"

In group counseling, cognitions can be discussed such as the negative self-talk of obese people. Clients need to realize the self-defeating and self-fulfilling aspects of their thoughts.

Making Changes

In the third phase, actual change takes place. The counselor helps clients modify their internal self-talk to produce new, more adaptive thoughts and behaviors. Clients are encouraged to control negative, self-destructive thoughts, to talk back with positive self-statements as a coping strategy, and to reinforce themselves for having coped. The goal is for clients to start noticing and interrupting negative thoughts as they occur.

An obese woman who is eating differently, for example, can tell herself how well she is doing and to keep it up. The "power of positive thinking" greatly enhances motivation and results. As clients learn to respond in new ways and eat differently, the counselor can note the results of the intervention and document it.

For a future desired behavior, cognitive rehearsal with visual imagery permits attention to the important details. A client may rehearse, for example, his or her food order at a restaurant or the amount of food and beverages to consume at a party. If individuals think about or imagine themselves overcoming barriers and performing adequately, actual performance is likely to improve.

One's motivation is partly influenced by cognitions or thoughts. People form beliefs about what they can or cannot do, set goals for themselves, and plan actions to achieve results they value. The ability to represent future consequences or outcomes in positive thoughts provides a source of motivation.[11] For example, positive thoughts that one will feel better, look better, or be in better health may contribute to motivation.

CASE ANALYSIS 5

Mrs. Jones: "When the holidays come, my friends bring me candy and treats. My husband and I eat them. We can't waste food."
YOUR RESPONSE:

Self-Efficacy

An "efficacy" expectation is the belief about how capable a person is of performing the change in behavior required to lead to the desired health outcome. SE refers to the person's confidence in the ability to perform a health behavior or dietary change and to persist over time. It affects how much effort a person gives, what level of performance is attained, and whether or not healthful behavior changes are maintained. A male client may or may not believe, for example, that he can reduce his dietary sodium intake continuously (SE) to attain the "outcome" of lower blood

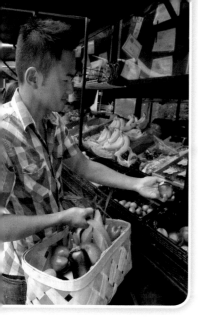

Positive thoughts about fruits and vegetables affect one's choices.
Source: CDC/Amanda Mills.

pressure. Among staff, an employee may believe that performing work optimally will lead to the desired "outcome" of a promotion, but may or may not believe that he or she is capable (SE) of optimum performance on a continuous basis.

Given a choice, would you be more likely to take on a task if you believed you might NOT be successful or would you select a task where you were confident of success? SE may determine whether or not a person will attempt a task and how long the person will continue. Ways to increase a person's SE include setting reasonable goals for change, enjoying rewards for accomplished changes, keeping self-monitoring records, and reinforcing successes. An increase in a person's SE may improve motivation. SE is a central concept of Social Cognitive Theory in predicting and promoting lifestyle behavior change.

SE is a situation-specific judgment of one's ability to perform specific behaviors or tasks without relapsing, as for example, eating differently, exercising more, or coping in high-risk situations.[15] These perceptions about performing and overcoming barriers, not necessarily one's true capabilities, influence whether people consider changing, whether they mobilize the perseverance and motivation to succeed, whether they have the ability to recover from setbacks, and whether they can maintain behavior changes.[16]

A client on a weight reduction or diabetic regimen, for example, may have a strong degree of SE when eating at home, but a weaker one when eating in a restaurant, thus affecting motivation and performance. There are many things people do not pursue because they think they are not capable or harbor self-doubts about their abilities.

Does will power have anything to do with behavior change? Albert Bandura does not believe that appropriate behavior, such as healthful eating and regular exercise, is achieved by a feat of will power. He recognized that learning and behavior change are influenced not only by external cues and rewards that are discussed in Chapter 7, but also by the interaction of demands on one's coping capabilities.

In Bandura's view, successful therapies work by increasing an individual's skills and confidence in the ability to engage in or practice a specific behavior.[11] This allows individuals to exercise greater self-control over their behavior, motivation, and environment. Participants in an online intervention of nutrition and physical activity found success depended on users developing SE for behavior change, the extent for setting personal goals, and tracking and receiving positive feedback on targeted behaviors.[17]

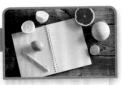

Bandura distinguishes between "efficacy" expectations ("Can I do it?")
and "outcome" expectations ("What I expect will happen if I perform the
behavior").[18-20] An "outcome" expectancy is a person's estimate or belief
that a given change or behavior will or will not lead to an outcome the
person values.[21] For example, the behavior of reducing dietary sodium will
result in an outcome of lower blood pressure and better health; following a dietary regimen will lead to an outcome of weight loss and better
physical appearance and health; or successfully completing a project for
one's superior will result in a salary increase or promotion. Besides cost
and benefit outcomes, people weight the outcomes of social approval or
disapproval, pleasurable or aversive expectations, and personal standards
against which one evaluates oneself.[20]

SE and outcomes are differentiated because people may believe that
certain actions can produce an outcome, but they may have serious doubts
about whether or not they can cope with the necessary changes and overcome barriers to reach the outcome. These perceptions and evaluations,
not necessarily the person's true capabilities, may apply to performing a
desired behavior, such as eating less, as well as abstaining from a problem
one, such as overeating.

Choice of Behaviors and Activities

Efficacy expectations are a major determinant of people's choice of activities.[11]
Clients involved in a change of behavior, such as eating or exercising, must
make decisions about whether or not to attempt different food choices,
how long to continue, how much effort to make, and in the face of difficulties, whether or not to persist. Bandura believes that these decisions are
partly governed by judgments of SE. People tend to avoid situations that
they believe exceed their coping capabilities, but are willing to undertake

activities they judge themselves capable of executing.[21] The stronger the perceived SE, or sense of personal mastery, the more persistent are the efforts, even in the presence of obstacles. When difficulties arise, those with lower perceptions of SE make less effort or may give up entirely.[20]

A study of levels of exercise among adults with type 2 diabetes found variables in moderate intensity exercise included task SE, self-monitoring, overcoming barriers, making time to exercise, self-reward, social support from family and friends, and self-evaluative outcome expectations.[22] Increasing SE was associated with physical activity in healthy nonobese adults who did self-monitoring.[23] Interventions with cancer survivors found meaningful changes in nutrition behavior and physical activity.[24]

A person's SE is generally a good predictor of how that individual is likely to behave on specific tasks.[11] SE affects whether or not people consider changing a health habit, whether they mobilize the motivation and perseverance to succeed, whether they are able to recover from setbacks and relapses, and whether they are able to maintain the changes made.[20] The evidence is overwhelming that there is a close association between SE and nutrition and health behavior change, and that SE is a powerful predictor of change.

In addition, personal goals enhance performance.[20] Motivation to perform a task can improve in part through one's self-evaluation of performance, such as having lost 2 lb, when compared with an adopted goal of losing weight. A person with strong SE increases effort and persistence in achieving subgoals and that results in higher performance. For clients, the counselor needs to break down tasks into easily mastered steps that are within the person's capabilities while requiring some degree of effort. Behavioral contracting and self-monitoring discussed in other chapters may be helpful also.

Dimensions of Efficacy Expectations

The counselor needs to assess clients' thoughts and confidence concerning their abilities to make changes in eating and exercise behaviors. Different dimensions of thoughts may be examined, such as level of difficulty of the task, strength of SE to succeed at the task, and generalization to other situations. When tasks have different levels of difficulty, efficacy expectations may limit some people to the simple tasks, while others may feel comfortable with more difficult ones. Weak self-beliefs are easily extinguished by disconfirming experiences, whereas those with strong efficacy expectations will persevere in their efforts even through difficulties.[20]

Measuring Self-Efficacy

A two-step approach to measuring SE is suggested. First, given a group of tasks of varying levels of difficulty, ask clients which dietary goals or changes they can undertake. It is preferable to start off with the simpler ones in order to guarantee success as that will increase SE. Then the client can work up slowly to more difficult ones.

Second, for each designated change in the behavior, ask clients to rate the strength of their confidence of success in making a specific change on a 5-point scale, with 5 being very confident to 1 being not at all confident. If not confident, a different task or goal should be found. Self-appraisals are reasonably accurate, because people successfully execute tasks within their perceived capabilities, but shun those that exceed them.

Efficacy expectations and performance should be assessed periodically during the dietary change process, because the stronger the perceived efficacy, the more likely people are to persist. In the Transtheoretical Model or Stages of Change, discussed in Chapter 5, SE scores were generally found to increase in the later stages of change and were significantly higher for those in action and maintenance stages. They are low in the precontemplation and contemplation stages, where people may have little confidence in their ability to change.

Sources of Efficacy Information

When planning food and exercise interventions, it is important to consider the four major sources of efficacy information. Beliefs about SE are based on (1) actual performance accomplishments, (2) vicarious experiences (modeling) by observing the performance of others, (3) verbal persuasion, and (4) physiologic and emotional states.[11,18,20] All four have been used in food and exercise interventions.

Actual Performance

The most influential and effective way to increase SE is actual performance accomplishments. The counselor needs to divide changes into many small, easily managed steps, let the client select the ones to try first, and be sure the person has the confidence to succeed. Setting personal goals and self-rewards may be beneficial in enhancing performance and increasing SE. An increase in SE and motivation results from successfully performing the behavior and attaining subgoals.[16] For example, attaining the subgoal of following the dietary change today is an immediate commitment rather than a future goal of never eating desserts again. With employees, a goal of improving performance today is preferable to a more distant goal of improving during the month.

Personal successes raise mastery expectations while failures lower them, especially early in the course of a health behavior change. Repeated success in overcoming obstacles through perseverance strengthens SE. People also perfect their coping skills. Success begets success; failure begets failure.

Modeling

A second source of efficacy information comes from modeling or observational learning followed by guided performance. Bandura believed that people learn by watching or observing the actions of others.[16] Clients can learn how to handle situations by observing a model demonstrating the appropriate behavior, such as ordering healthful food from a restaurant menu or saying "no thank you" to dessert offerings. The vicarious experience of seeing another perform can generate expectations that if another person can do it, "so can I."

To enhance imitation, the model should be perceived as similar to oneself or possessing competencies to which one aspires. Clients should then be given an opportunity to perform the modeled behavior successfully. In group counseling sessions, negative role models are a problem and should be avoided. Employees also learn by observing and modeling after other employees. Stronger efficacy expectations, however, are produced by personal accomplishments than by only observing another.

Verbal Persuasion

A third approach, verbal persuasion, is widely used by counselors in attempts to influence behavior, but is among the least effective approaches. Telling people what to do, that they possess the ability to do it, and informing them of the benefits, is not as helpful, especially if the individual has failed to follow dietary changes. The encouragement of the counselor, or support from others, may vary greatly depending on their perceived credibility, their prestige, trustworthiness, and other factors. The counselor saying: "I know you can do it" isn't effective and the client may not mobilize efforts to change.[11,16]

Physiologic and Emotional States

Finally, people partly judge their capabilities from physiologic states and emotions. Situations in which an individual has to cope with lifestyle changes may produce anxiety, stress, hunger, fatigue, and tension. Those who regain the weight, for example, may have lowered self-esteem and SE. Those susceptible to anxiety may become self-preoccupied with their perceived inadequacies rather than with the task at hand. Stress-reducing activities and discussion of correct interpretation of body signals may be of help.

In summary, an effective intervention program should increase SE as well as increase the value of the outcome. Personal mastery of a dietary change or accomplishment of a goal is the most compelling. Small "wins" build confidence for additional changes. Good role models, such as former clients, may be enlisted to explain how they overcame difficulties. Anxiety, hunger, and stress, should be explained to make sure that the individual does not misread body signals and abandon efforts.

With employees, personal accomplishments give better efficacy information than telling people that they are capable of performing a job.

Modeling after the performance of others, such as seeing that hard work leads to a promotion, is another source of efficacy information. Behaviors, both good and bad, may be adopted from seeing what others are doing.

Cognitive Appraisal of Efficacy Information

The extent to which success raises SE depends partly on the amount of effort expended. Laborious effort suggests less SE than success achieved through minimal effort. One's performance suggests higher SE if attained through continuous progress rather than through discouraging reversals. In addition, various factors enter into personal appraisals. People with high SE set higher goals with a firmer commitment, attribute failure to lack of effort, and may increase effort and persistence in achieving a goal.

If people are not fully convinced of their personal efficacy, they abandon the skills they have learned when they fail to get quick results. Those with low SE may attribute it to low ability and those with negative self-beliefs do not discard them readily.[16] Even when actual performance attainments are beyond their previous levels, they may discount their importance or credit their achievements to factors other than to their own capabilities.

Thus, in their daily lives, people approach, explore, and try to deal with health situations within their capabilities, while avoiding situations they perceive as exceeding their ability. People weigh various sources of information in deciding their choices of behaviors, how much effort they put forth, and how long they will persist in the face of difficulties.[11,16] SE expectations are presumed to influence one's level of performance by enhancing intensity and persistence of effort.

Relapse Prevention

I ate the whole thing!

G. Alan Marlatt and others developed a model of the relapse process originally for addictive behaviors.[25,26] A relapse can be defined as a complex, multi-determined process that may be considered as an individual's response to a series of lapses, a loss of control over food and health choices, and a return to a previous problem eating behaviors.[25] Relapse is high in obesity interventions involving weight and behavior change.[27] The major goal in counseling is to provide the skills to prevent a complete relapse, regardless of the situation or impending risk factors.[25] Relapse prevention (RP) includes both behavioral and cognitive components.[28]

Behaviors may be seen as overlearned habits that can be analyzed and modified. The eating behavior of individuals with anorexia nervosa, bulimia, and obesity, for example, may be viewed as maladaptive habit patterns with maladaptive coping mechanisms.[29] These behaviors are generally followed by some sort of immediate gratification, such as feelings of pleasure or the reduction of anxiety, tension, boredom, or loneliness. When eating takes place prior to or during stressful or unpleasant situations, it represents a maladaptive coping mechanism.

A Relapse Model

The model of relapse is based on the assumption that relapse events are preceded by a high-risk situations.[28] An individual's control continues until the person encounters high-risk situations, or "those that challenge the individual's ability to cope."[29] When faced with some situations, people tend to use maladaptive responses they are familiar and comfortable with, such as excessive eating. See Figure 8-1 for a modification of Marlatt's Model of Relapse adapted for food.[25]

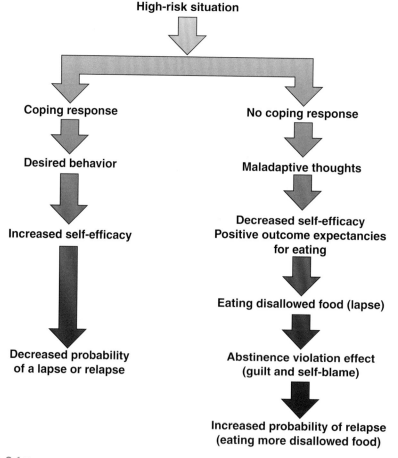

Figure 8-1 ■ Cognitive-behavioral model of the relapse process.

Source: Modified from Marlatt GA, Gordon JR, eds. Relapse Prevention. New York, NY: Guilford Press; 2005.

High-Risk Situations

The problem of giving in to temptation is a challenge for clients engaging in dietary and other health behavior changes. Most people making lifestyle changes experience temporary setbacks. If they don't know how to cope and recover, they may give up all efforts and relapse permanently.

RP is based on a group of cognitive–behavioral strategies for assisting people who are changing a behavior. The self-management program is designed to help individuals identify, anticipate, and cope with cravings and setbacks, thus maintaining adherence to the targeted changed habits.[30]

A distinction exists between a "lapse" and a "relapse." A lapse, such as one overeating episode at a restaurant, is a slight error, or one instance of return to a previously discontinued food behavior. A lapse should not be viewed as a personal failure leading to feelings of guilt, but as a learning experience as one examines the immediate precipitating circumstances and ways to correct them in the future.

The goal is to assess with clients their high-risk situations associated with relapse.[31] For a person on a restricted diet, common tempting situations are emotional distress, negative emotions, moods, feelings, cravings, social situations, and negative physiologic states.[26] These include clients' exposure to events, places, persons, thoughts, and other cues to eating ranging in different intensities.

Negative emotional moods and feelings, such as depression, anxiety, stress, frustration, anger, boredom, loneliness, and feelings of deprivation prior to or at the time of the lapse are related to relapse.[29] Uncontrolled eating is a common response when a person is alone. The emotional reactions increase the chance that one lapse will occur and increase to a relapse. Negative cognitions, self-defeating thoughts, and low SE ratings are of concern because they are predictive of relapse. Individuals with positive cognitions and perceived SE tend to call upon their coping skills and regulate their behaviors better. Bandura does not believe that appropriate behavior, such as choosing appropriate foods and avoiding others, is achieved by a feat of willpower. When people do not behave optimally even though they know what they should do, thoughts or cognitions may be mediating the relationship between what one knows and what one does.[11,16]

Positive emotional states in which one desires to increase feelings of pleasure or celebrate an event are also a problem. A study of dieters found that negative emotional states occurring when the individual was alone and positive emotional states involving other people, such as at social gatherings, were both difficult high-risk situations to handle, suggesting that managing these situations should be incorporated into nutrition counseling.[29]

Besides individual factors, situational or environmental factors also play a role in relapse. The support of family, friends, or self-help groups is

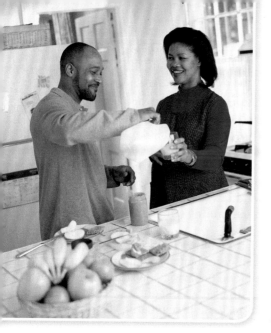

When happy and hungry, foods may present a high-risk situation.

Source: US Department of Agriculture.

associated with better success, while interpersonal conflicts, such as disagreements or hassles in relationships with family, friends, or an employer, may signal the possibility of relapse.

Eating cues in the environment, for example, may include holidays, restaurants, and social gatherings where overeating is socially acceptable. In the Women's Intervention Nutrition Study (WINS), examples of high-risk situations included holidays, restaurant dining, special occasions, and emotional cues.[14] Social pressures from others occur when individuals tempt or coax ("Eat it. Just this once won't hurt you.") and when a person sees others consuming foods not on his or her dietary regimen. ("Everyone else is eating it. Why shouldn't I?")

Finally, negative physiologic factors may contribute to relapse. Urges and cravings for foods, feeling of hunger, fatigue, or headache, may increase the chance of relapse. See Box 8-4 for examples of high-risk situations.

SELF-ASSESSMENT 3

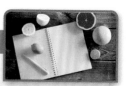

Using the examples of high-risk situations in Box 8-4, identify those that are high-risk situations for your own eating.

Physiologic feelings of hunger, fatigue, food cravings, tension, stress
Attending social affairs, parties, eating in restaurants, holidays
Low self-efficacy or inadequate motivation
Negative self-talk
Lack of social support from family, friends, or coworkers
Interpersonal conflicts
Positive emotional states (i.e., fun and celebration of an event)
Negative emotional states or moods (i.e., depression, anxiety, frustration, anger, boredom, loneliness, feeling deprived, upset, sad, or worried)

Box 8.4 ■ Examples of High-Risk Situations

Identification and Assessment of High-Risk Situations

Assessment of high-risk situations may be viewed as a two-stage process. In the first stage, an attempt is made to identify specific situations that may pose a problem for a client in terms of a lapse or relapse. Self-monitoring food records are helpful in identifying these situations as well as in raising the individual's awareness of food choices made. Self-monitoring is an intervention in itself that may reduce some of the behaviors.

Eating may be an automatic response that cannot be dealt with until there is a conscious awareness that one is eating without any conscious decision to do so. SE ratings can be assessed by giving clients descriptions of specific situations and asking them to rate how difficult it would be to cope. Situations with the lowest SE ratings are the highest risk situations for a lapse.[32] The counselor may ask the client to identify the difficulty of coping on a 5-point scale, with 5 being the most difficulty. Descriptions of past relapses may be informative. People who coped successfully may have relied on avoidance of events or on cognitive strategies, such as thinking positively about goals for change or the negative consequences of a lapse.

Coping versus Failure to Cope in High-Risk Situations

There are two possibilities when a person is in a high-risk situation—a coping response or lack of one. If the individual copes, SE is increased and there is less probability of a lapse or relapse. For example, the client thinks coping thoughts: "I'm not hungry so I won't eat," "I'll take a walk instead of eating," or "I'll phone my friend instead of eating."

After identifying high-risk situations, the second stage is an assessment of the client's coping skills or capacity to respond involving both thoughts and actions. One can evaluate these in simulated situations with role-playing or in written form. An individual can role-play responses to high-risk situations with the counselor or fellow group members.

Abstinence from less preferable foods is frequently viewed by individuals from an all-or-nothing perspective. Marlatt postulates a cognitive and affective "abstinence violation effect" (AVE) when a person violates the commitment to change food choices and consumes a food that he or she should not eat.[25] The cognitive component examines whether the lapse is considered internal and uncontrollable or external and controllable. The affective component is related to feelings of guilt, shame, and hopelessness. Possible responses to giving in to temptation are the following:

- One feels guilty, has lowered self-esteem, and blames oneself for the loss of control or indulgence in food. ("I shouldn't have eaten it, but I did. I'm guilty.")
- An obese individual may continue to eat to relieve the guilt ("I ate one cookie and I blew it. I might as well eat the whole bag.")
- A person may alter his or her cognition from being a restrainer to an indulger. ("I lack willpower and never could follow the diet anyway.")

- The person may rationalize. ("I deserve a break today. I owe myself this food.")
- The person may change his or her commitment to save face. ("I changed my mind about following this dietary regimen and decided to eat whatever I want.")

Lapses affect both people's thoughts and their feelings. If there is no coping response and the person feels unable to exert control, he or she experiences a decrease in SE, sometimes coupled with a sense of helplessness or a passive giving in to the situation. ("It's no use. I can't stop myself.") In this all-or-nothing perspective, a single lapse leads to giving up. If the person has positive outcome expectancies of immediate gratification from eating ("It will taste delicious. I will feel better if I eat this.") and ignores the negative health consequences, the probability of lapse or relapse is enhanced. The individual experiences a conflict of motives between a desire to maintain control and the temptation to give in. The person consumes less desirable foods, a lapse has occurred, and there can be a problem in reestablishing control. After a lapse, the person either copes and gets back on track or may proceed to relapse.[32]

It is important to educate clients about the relapse process since it is unlikely that people will recognize the range of situations that may trigger eating. When the individual's unique high-risk situations (thoughts, feelings, people, and situations) are identified, counselors can teach the person to look for cues, such as an upcoming party, vacation, holidays, or stressful time at work. The client can take preventive action and make advance decisions about how to cope. The goal of treatment is to help the client learn to anticipate and prevent the occurrence of lapses and relapse or help the individual recover from a lapse before it escalates into a full-blown relapse.

Lapses are inevitable. The counselor needs to advise clients to expect this and prepare them to handle it. Failure to do so deprives the client of the opportunity for developing skills to cope with a lapse or relapse or minimize damage. Using the term "lapse" avoids the value judgment associated with a term like "cheating" on the diet. Everyone will, on occasion, overeat or eat tempting foods. Each mistake is viewed as a learning opportunity, not a personal failure. The goal is to teach the individual how to identify situations with a high risk for lapse and relapse, to use problem-solving and coping strategies when confronted, and to deal with the negative thoughts (guilt) that accompany a lapse.

The most dangerous time is that immediately following a lapse.[32] The reward of instant gratification may far outweigh negative health effects in a distant future. Thus, a single lapse, or series of lapses, may snowball into a full-blown relapse from which it is more difficult to recover. Figure 8-2 is an example of failing to cope at the grocery store and at home in the presence of the external cue of potato chips. The loss of control and dysfunctional self-talk results in binge eating and relapse.

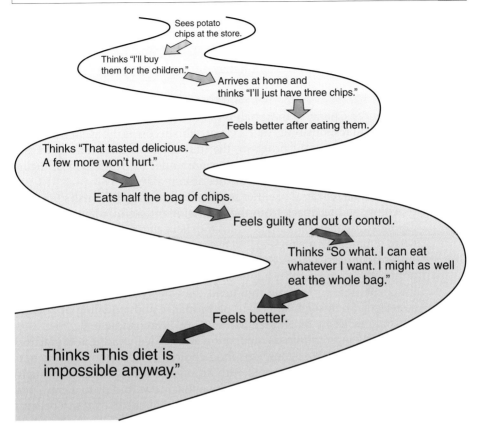

Figure 8-2 ■ When failing to cope, one's thoughts affect eating.

Other Treatment Strategies

Coping skills include cognitive responses, such as positive self-talk ("I can do it."), behavioral responses, such as calling a friend instead of eating, and beliefs about SE, or judgments concerning whether or not one can respond effectively. Coping skill training implies the actual acquisition of a new behavior through essential practice and rehearsal of coping skills. "Practice makes perfect," as an old saying goes.

Cognitive restructuring may be used also to counter the cognitive and affective components of the abstinence violation effect (AVE).[25] Instead of seeing the first lapse as a sign of failure characterized by conflict, guilt, shame, and personal attribution, the client can be taught to view it as a single event or small mistake rather than a total disaster, to renew the commitment to lifestyle change right away, and to learn from mistakes by reviewing the environmental and psychological factors in the lapse situation.

Clients initiate dietary changes with varying degrees of motivation and commitment. In addition, some who appear to be highly motivated initially may discover that long-term change is more difficult than first imagined. Patients who lose some weight, for example, and those who struggle but adhere to their dietary regimens, may be able to cope with temporary setbacks. Motivation may differ among people from collective cultures where people interact in the group.[26]

Food habits or eating behaviors are assumed to be shaped by prior experiences. Changing these habits or behaviors involves the active participation and responsibility of the client, who becomes the agent of change. In a self-management program, the individual acquires new skills and cognitive strategies so that behaviors are under the regulation of higher mental processes and responsible decision-making.

Behavioral rehearsal of either actual or hypothetical high-risk situations, coaching, and feedback from the counselor are useful. Mental rehearsal through imagined scenarios in which the client engages in coping responses when temptations are present and feels good about it, may be used to cope with reactions to a lapse. Role reversal with the client teaching the practitioner how to cope with a high-risk situation and handle a lapse will give the client more convincing arguments than any counselor could provide. Increasing SE through successful performance and modeling of positive self-statements are recommended, such as "I can handle it.[25]

Training in mindfulness meditation and guided mindfulness practices may enhance making conscious food choices and developing awareness of eating cues.[33] If confronted with an urge to binge, clients are taught to imagine their urge as an ocean wave that grows, builds to a crest, and gradually subsides. Not acting on the urge strengthens SE. Wansick believes that the answer to mindless eating is not to eat mindfully, but to set up our environments to control external cues so that we mindlessly eat less.[34]

As an antidote to stress, relaxation training; positive self-talk; meditation; exercise instead of eating; visualization of relaxing, pleasant scenes or of carrying out coping behaviors when tempted; and stress management procedures may be needed.[29] In visualization, clients are asked to close their eyes and think of a stressful or tempting situation. The counselor can ask questions that create a visual picture of the situation and the accompanying emotions. If imagining a party, for example, the counselor may ask: "What do the surroundings look like?" "What are you doing?" "What are other people doing?" "Where are the foods and beverages?" "What will you choose?" "Who can you turn to for support?" "What will you say?" "How do you feel?"

Relapse rates for clients with obesity are high. Patients can make written plans for lapses and relapses, identifying early warning signs of a slip, and strategies to stay on track. Adopting a problem-solving orientation to stressful situations or modeling problem solving by thinking out loud with clients is helpful. The counselor and client can review the events and emotions in past lapses and relapses since patterns may repeat themselves.

When lapses are discussed, it is preferable to discuss how the individual might have succeeded in preference to focusing on the failures.[35]

Models and Theories of Change

In Chapter 5, Procheska noted that people recycle through the Stages of Change as people do not maintain gains the first time. He changed his Transtheoretical model from a linear to a spiral pattern.[30] In the model, recycling to a previous stage is expected as people go through the six stages of precontemplation, contemplation, preparation, action, maintenance, and termination. RP strategies are important, especially in the action and maintenance stages. Patients with eating issues and challenges can be expected to progress through all stages with frequent backsliding.

People in the action stage will encounter high-risk situations, stresses, and temptations that tax coping efforts. They may slip or lapse in one situation and resist in another. The majority are not successful at the first attempt at change. Relapse commences with recycling to an earlier stage and can be viewed as a learning opportunity. Just as Rome was not built in a day, neither is successful dietary change accomplished in a short period of time.

Clients need to learn self-monitoring and self-management skills to cope with the normal urge to lapse into old habits. They should be more successful when they keep in contact with a counselor, at least by phone, for a year or more. The model of life-long treatment is used by several groups, such as Alcoholics Anonymous, Overeaters Anonymous, and the lifetime membership offered in Weight Watchers.

One would hope that our models and theories of health behavior change would explain and predict change. Social cognitive theories, the Health Behavior Model, the Transtheoretical Model, and other theories have limited success in explaining dietary change. Food practices are the result of a number of interacting variables.

Interventions do not change behaviors directly, but can be designed to change mediating variables. A change in strongly related mediating variables (psychosocial, behavioral, environmental, and biologic) can result in behavioral change. Changes in family food practices, for example, may be a strongly related mediating variable resulting in change.

Summary

While all theories and models are valuable, additional scientific research is needed as a basis for planning more effective, evidence-based interventions that are appropriate for the individual client. The nutrition professional may combine a number of counseling approaches with clients. This chapter describes the use of cognitive restructuring of negative and dysfunctional thoughts, and outlines methods that increase the client's self-efficacy or self-confidence to change a behavior. The problems of lapse and relapse that require coping skills and relapse prevention approaches are included.

Counselors should give clients a summary or overview of the relapse process. With an increased level of awareness in high-risk situations, clients are better prepared to utilize their coping skills and take remedial action to avoid a lapse or relapse. People need to see themselves as capable agents of control rather than as helpless victims in situations beyond their control.

Review and Discussion Questions

1. What is cognitive therapy?
2. What effect do negative cognitions have on behavioral change?
3. What types of cognitive distortions do people have?
4. Explain the three phases of cognitive restructuring.
5. What is the relationship between an outcome expectancy and an efficacy expectancy?
6. How do self-perceptions of efficacy affect a person's choice of activities?
7. Explain an individual's four sources of efficacy information. How does each affect behavior?
8. Explain the relapse model.
9. What are examples of high-risk situations?
10. What strategies can help to prevent relapse?

Suggested Activities

1. Keep a record of what you eat during one day noting your thoughts about food before eating, during eating, and after eating. What percent are positive? Negative? How did this increase your awareness?
2. Identify your own high-risk situations for eating and how you respond. What happens if you cope with the situation? What happens if you are unable to cope with the situation? How do you feel?

3. For each of the following client cognitions, forecast how the client will behave. Then develop a more positive, coping thought.

   A. "I've never been able to stick to any low-calorie diet for more than a week."

   B. "The food doesn't taste any good without salt."

   C. "There are chocolate chip cookies in the cupboard, and I sure could use a few after the day I've had. I deserve a treat."

   D. "Here is a commercial break on my television show. Guess I'll check the refrigerator."

   E. "That leftover pie looks good, but I don't need it."

   F. "I've blown my whole diet eating that apple pie with ice cream. What's the use?"

   G. "I don't have time to prepare all of that special food today."

4. For 2 days, keep a tally of the number of times people use the terms "should," "shouldn't," "must," "have to," or "ought to" in statements about themselves. Or keep a tally of the number of times you use these terms.

5. For 2 or more days, consume a modified diet (low fat, low calorie, restricted sodium, high fiber, etc.). Keep a log of your thoughts. Identify any high-risk situations.

6. Each evening for 2 days, make a written list of all of your successes or things you accomplished. Give yourself a verbal pat on the back with a positive cognition.

CHAPTER 9

Counseling Through the Life Span

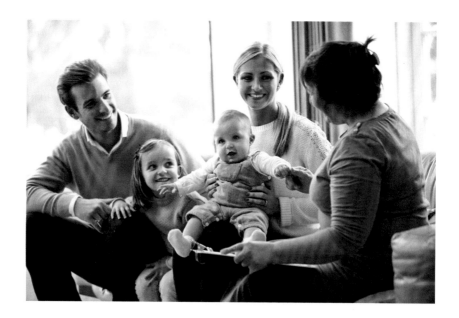

Objectives

- Identify life span age groups.
- Recognize strategies for effective counseling through the life span.
- Evaluate the preventive health nutrition focus for each life span group.
- Define self-management concepts in chronic diet-related disease.

Mrs. Smith, a widow, is 76 years old. She is 5'3" tall and weighs 150 lb. She has arthritis in her knees and hands which limits her mobility. She does not drive, and there is no grocery store within walking distance of her home. She takes aspirin or over-the-counter anti-inflammatory agents. She lives on a small pension and Social Security. Last month, her granddaughter Sarah (age 35, 12-weeks pregnant) moved in with children Charles (age 15) and Chelsea (age 4) while Sarah's husband is on overseas military duty. The family will be coming to your office for nutrition counseling.

The journey through life is a process of growth and change.

—Anonymous

Introduction

National nutrition objectives, including Healthy People 2020 and Choose MyPlate, address all age groups across the life span.[1,2] It has been reported that adults make more than 225 diet-related decisions each day.[3] As medical research and technology increase the longevity of our population, new emphasis on the quality of life is emerging. Public awareness of the role of nutrition in preventive health is increasing. Nutrition professionals have a wide array of opportunities to disseminate accurate information and deliver innovative educational strategies to accomplish key goals such as maintaining a healthy body weight through the life span.[4] The purpose of this chapter is to discuss key counseling strategies that are most effective by individual life span groups, by family groupings, and within the context of chronic diet-related diseases.

Prenatal and Pregnant Women

Nutrition education should ideally begin in the prenatal phase of child-bearing years when women are at risk or when they are planning to become pregnant. This is an excellent opportunity to assess current food habits and align to healthy intake goals. This also provides a sound nutrition beginning for the earliest weeks of gestation when women typically have not confirmed their pregnancy. Women often do not have access to a nutrition professional at this point. Innovative ways to reach this audience might

221

include partnering with gynecologists, primary care providers, physician assistants, or nurse practitioners to offer coordinated preventive health conversations. Community outreach to educate existing mothers prior to their next pregnancy is also another potential way to reach this audience.

Life span counseling continues with pregnancy. The quality of the diet of the pregnant mother has been clearly linked to better outcomes for both mother and fetus.[5] Long-term effects of nutrient deficits during gestation are also well known. Nutrition education should focus on the pattern of weight gain and selection of foods to meet fetal growth goals. Nutrition counseling addressed to these issues can also reduce the incidence of excessive weight gain during pregnancy that may evolve into gestational diabetes.

Group classes for expectant mothers are common but often are only implemented in later trimesters. Involvement of husbands and partners in individual and group counseling can help create a healthy environment setting that can be sustained after the baby is born. Postpartum activity to return to prepregnancy weight is an important counseling strategy to reduce risk of obesity.[6]

CASE ANALYSIS ● 1

Sarah comes to your office for nutrition counseling. She admits she was not very aware of her diet during her other pregnancies and wants to be more informed during this pregnancy. What are some key nutrition education and counseling strategies you may want to incorporate in your first session?

Infants up to 2 Years of Age

Parents or caregivers are the primary decision makers in the feeding of infants during the first year of life. Full-term infants may only require minor adaptations to their food intake to achieve nutrition goals such as changing from a milk-based to a soy-based formula. Preterm infants may require extensive stepwise interventions to address both growth and food tolerance issues.[7] For example, the feeding may need to be adapted for nutrient density when the feeding volume is changed. Breast-feeding or commercial infant formulas are recommended to be the single source of nutrition during the first 4 to 6 months of life. Breast-feeding has been shown to have positive nutrition outcomes for both mother and infant, particularly during the first 3 months of life. Breast-feeding for the first full year of life may also reduce the incidence of toddler obesity.[8] Mothers can continue to express milk even when returning to work but need to be instructed on collection procedures and safe milk storage. Most mothers, especially first-time mothers, need lots of support in order to be successful. Resources for lactation support include lactation consultants, professional organizations such as the La Leche League International, and peer mother networks.

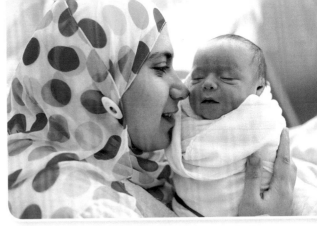

A mother influences the earliest feeding decisions for her newborn.

Counseling Strategies

Individual counseling may be most effective when addressing unique issues or providing specific individualized strategies. Observing actual breast-feeding practices may help in solving problems. Group support may be more appropriate when both mothers and infants gather to interact. The nutrition professional can act as a facilitator for discussion and guide the conversation to pertinent topics. Family members and child-care partners can also be involved to replicate feeding environments and larger cultural conversations.[9]

The nutrition professional should be objective when providing feeding information and respecting parental attitudes toward breast-feeding. It is important to be up-to-date on all commercial formulas and their nutrient composition. This information is necessary to deliver accurate and sound data upon which to make feeding assessments for growth and tolerance.

Nutrition education is most critical when counseling about the choice and amount of complementary foods introduced at 4 to 6 months of age. The American Academy of Pediatrics and other professional organizations have published recommendations for the introduction of solid foods.[10,11] Using recommendations from recognized authorities derived from evidence-based analysis provides validity to education sessions. Many of the first foods served to infants are higher in sodium than recommended, a direct result of parent choices in feeding the foods they preferred or had available rather than more nutritious first choices.[12] The risk of childhood obesity is less when infants are breast-fed during the first year of life along with low intake of sugar-sweetened beverages during the toddler years.[8] Educational efforts can help parents make better choices for their children.

Preschool Children, Age 2 to 5 Years

Nutrition counselors should work with parents and caregivers to influence the eating behaviors of preschool children. The primary goal of health and nutrition education for this life span group is to promote healthy growth and development. This is an opportunity to set the stage for future food choices and to prevent chronic diseases of adulthood, such as obesity. Children's food habits are learned through family food settings, personal experiences, and education. Children of this age are just beginning to make food choices within the controlled environment and choices of their caregivers.[13]

Influences on Eating Habits

Many children of this age attend day care settings that provide at least one meal per day. The content of foods served in a day care center is a direct influence of the caregivers' expectations. A higher level of involvement by parents may result in a higher nutrient level of foods served. Therefore, caregivers must work together with teachers to mutually reinforce learning about nutrition and making proper eating choices. Parents may also want to provide their child's teacher with information about specific dietary restrictions they impose to ensure that the child's diet consists of similar foods both at home and in school.[14]

In the preschool years, family and cultural practices are a major influence on what children eat. Young children are unable to make informed decisions, but can vocalize their likes or dislikes. Most young children tend to eat the same food as their parents or the types of food their parents believe are healthy. For example, if parents routinely eat fruits and vegetables, it is more likely that their children will eat them; whereas if parents routinely eat cake and cookies for dessert, it is more likely that their children will eat these sweets.[15]

The attitudes and practices of caregivers themselves also have a direct influence. For example, if a mother believes that oatmeal is a good source of soluble fiber then her child will more likely eat oatmeal for breakfast. On the other hand, if a mother thinks that two eggs are a healthy breakfast because they are full of protein, then her child will more likely grow up expecting eggs for breakfast. Thus, parents, siblings, and caregivers must explore their own nutritional beliefs and try to model and choose appropriate eating behaviors and choices.[14,15]

Another characteristic of preschool children is their reliance on the physical and visual concept of the food. Familiarity with a food is a strong concept.

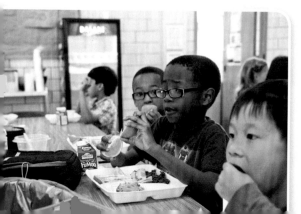

Young children often will not try new foods unless provided in an innovative and positive environment. Also, children of this age have been shown to judge satiation and satisfaction

Preschool children explore visual and physical concepts of food.
Source: CDC.

by the familiarity of the foods served. Thus, they may continue to look for more food and large portions if they feel they did not "eat" food, but rather an unfamiliar alternative.[16] Exposures to televised food commercials could influence preschool children's food preferences, leading them to pressure parents to buy particular food items at the grocery store.[15,17]

Counseling Strategies

Nutrition professionals are often faced with challenges when counseling preschool-age children. One challenge is to assess the food pattern of the child. This involves collecting accurate information from the caregiver, who may not be present at all the meals consumed by the child. Food records directed at this life span age group have been adapted with reasonable accuracy for children 9 to 36 months of age.[13] Another issue they may face is the changing diet pattern of the child. Young children tend to change their behaviors rather quickly; for example, a child who is a good eater as an infant may be a fair to poor eater as a toddler. Children may also neglect to eat a particular food for weeks to months without any explanation. A child who is entering a phase of growth spurt may increase intake and variety for a short time, only to revert to a different food pattern the next month.[13]

In addressing these challenges, nutrition professionals should provide the child and caregivers with suggested food patterns that offer a variety of food choices. Food patterns can be found from various professional sources. The ChooseMyPlate education initiative from the United States Department of Agriculture offers specific resources for children. Nutrition counselors should also recommend that the child should be exposed to a wide variety of foods rather than offering the same type of food repeatedly. Emphasis should focus on nutrient density and appropriate portion size. For example, the counselor could advise caregivers of preschool-age children to control the quantity of juice drink boxes consumed daily by alternating beverage consumption among 100% juice, water, and milk.

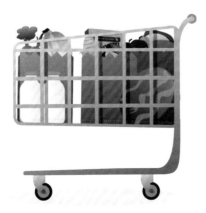

Figure 9-1 ■ Shopping drives food choices.

Another strategy to address a fickle preschool-aged eater is to let the child determine the quantity and frequency of his or her eating patterns. Nutrition professionals may want to encourage young children to be accountable for their dietary habits and allow them to decide how much and how often they should eat. However, this method must be approached with caution because children may be unable to make informed or logical decisions. Counselors should also provide nutrition learning activities for the child. Recommended strategies for teaching nutrition to young children include action stories, songs, videotapes, tasting parties, visiting vegetable and fruit gardens, puzzles, art projects, and field trips.

Nutrition assessment with a diet history, when needed, may take longer to accomplish at these ages. As preschool-age children tend to be fickle, it may be difficult to determine the quantity or frequency of particular food consumption. To address this challenge, nutrition professionals may recommend a consecutive daily food record or journal that lists the type and amount of food consumed by the child. To make this activity fun for the child, you may suggest that older preschool-age children draw pictures of what they eat or caregivers can take pictures of meals on their mobile phones to share at subsequent counseling visits.

CASE ANALYSIS 2

Which education and counseling strategies would you consider using when working with Chelsea and her family?

School-Age Children, Age 6 to 12 Years

School-age children, defined as ages 6 to 12 years, begin to have increasing control over their food choices. These new lifestyle choices can affect later development and behaviors, particularly body weight and image foundations. It is essential that children be provided with guidance and advice to assist them in establishing healthy dietary and exercise habits. Partnerships of children, schools, and families can promote health and well-being and influence these necessary lifetime food habits.

During this stage of the life span, nutrition education seeks to provide children with the knowledge needed to select healthy foods. Age-specific guidelines are available to assist nutrition professionals to plan education content. Nutrition counselors seek to facilitate the development of children's analytical and evaluative skills so that they may be better able to understand food and nutrition information. Because risk factors for some chronic diseases begin in youth, behavioral-focused nutrition education is appropriate. This type of education encompasses cognitive learning, in which children learn how to select a healthful diet; affective teaching, in which children and counselors address motivation for dietary change; and behavioral components, such as selecting new food choices and lifestyle behaviors. Studies show that these types of interventions, which focus on specific behavior changes, result in more effective changes than a general nutrition education approach.[13,15,18]

Influences on Eating Habits

During the school years, family, culture, and the body's physical composition greatly influence what children eat. What children eat is also affected by food insecurity and poverty status.[15,18] Therefore, nutrition professionals need to assess the child's social, physical, and psychological environment as well as his or her overall health when counseling children and their caregivers on the types of dietary changes that they should make to ensure a well-balanced diet and a healthy lifestyle. Since a 6 year-old is very different from a 9-year-old, an evaluation of the developmental stage of the child according to theories of child psychology and of the child's cognitive level must also be done before a healthcare professional can plan any nutrition intervention. In addition, a nutrition counselor should be familiar with scientific studies that specifically focus on the behaviors within this age cohort. For example, studies have shown that involvement in an active gardening program helped influence vegetable consumption in young children.[19] Dietary modeling, or replacement of familiar low-nutrient-density food choices with higher-nutrient-dense options, has been shown to be effective in increasing nutrient density.[13,15] This concept can be further reinforced by involving the child in the process of helping to prepare bran muffins for breakfast to share with the family rather than choosing a packaged donut. Caregivers with higher nutrition knowledge, particularly with food labeling, have also been shown to be able to make better choices more readily for their children.

The dietary behaviors of many school-age children, like those of preschool-age children, are often formed away from the home, particularly in school or at after-school programs. The position of the Academy of Nutrition and Dietetics is to support the nutrition integrity of the entire school environment, not just formal feeding lunch opportunities.[20] Nutrition professionals should collaborate with members of the school faculty, school lunch program, athletic department, and local community so that together they can teach children about nutrition and assess children's dietary trends. It is also important to address the content of home-packed meals brought to school. Children and caregivers need guidelines such as the ChooseMyPlate.[2] Counselors can also assist teachers to incorporate nutrition principles into academic coursework, such as using portion sizes and weights in math classes.

Nutrition professionals should assess and note the child activity patterns, including number of hours spent exercising, participating in athletic events, watching television, or playing video games. During the school-age years, children tend to be heavily influenced by peers and classmates. In addition, they are more exposed to the various forms of technology, such as television and social media. In particular, there appears to be a strong relationship between obesity or weight gain and sedentary status and snacking patterns.[15,21]

Counseling Strategies

As with preschool-age children, nutrition professionals must address various challenges when counseling school-age children and their caregivers about healthy nutrition plans. One challenge that the counselor will encounter is a child's busy, and often unpredictable schedule. Many adults and their children do not eat breakfast. Another option is that they may pick up a fast-food breakfast from a drive-through location and eat it on the way to school. Children who eat a healthy breakfast are more likely to have lower cholesterol levels, maintain a healthy weight, and exhibit a higher level of awareness and concentration in school.[13,15,21] Nutrition counselors should recommend to school-age children and their parents or guardians the value of eating breakfast.[13,15] They can reinforce this concept by providing examples of quick nutritious breakfast options. In addition, traditional breakfast foods (i.e., scrambled eggs, toast, and cereal) can be interchanged with nontraditional foods (i.e., peanut butter, bean burrito, and pizza) to keep continuing interest and involvement in food choices.

After-school snacks are often required to meet the child's energy needs. Children who become involved in competitive sports or after-school vigorous activities may need additional nutrients or have an increased appetite. Conversely, children who are sedentary after school may require snacks that are more appropriate to their lower energy needs than active counterparts. Many children consume a significant percentage of their calories after school when they have more time to eat and/or a wider array of foods may be available as in the home setting. The nutrition counselor should provide caregivers and coaches proactively with healthy snack ideas appropriate to the child's needs.

Counselors should be aware of the nutritional trends and patterns among school-age children. The number of school-age children who are overweight is of concern because it has more than doubled in the past decade. Physical inactivity, parental overweight and obesity trends, and skipping meals may contribute to overweight in children.[21] Globally and as well as within the United States, a significant number of children are estimated to experience food insecurity defined as an unstable access to food. Although this differs from chronic malnutrition, professionals should be vigilant in identifying children and families at risk.[22]

School-age children also have many concerns about their body image and appearance. It is during these years that many children become preoccupied with their weight and may start dieting. About one-third of children think they weigh too much. Many children also believe that their weight is above average cultural and societal standards. As a result, nearly half of all children have attempted to lose weight or have engaged in a diet plan within the previous year.[13,15]

Health educators should create nutrition activity programs that seek to educate children about appropriate and healthy food choices and nutrition behaviors. Children want learning to be fun.

Active learning activities for children area recommended. For example, nutrition professionals can have children actively measure quantities or amounts of food by providing them with actual ingredients, scales, and measuring cups. Specifically, if they are trying to demonstrate to children how much sugar is in a can of soda, they may provide the children with a measuring cup and a bag of sugar. Allow them to measure the amount of sugar as indicated on the nutrition label. Older children can compare how much sugar is in two different types of cereal, one high-sugar type and one low-sugar and high-fiber option. They can read the nutrition label, measure the amount of sugar, and record and chart the amount of sugar in each cereal. Children can discuss what they discovered in small groups such as which cereal is the better nutritional choice. For homework, children can bring food labels from home or search online for product information under supervision.

Nutrition counselors should also use visual aids and materials to appeal to conceptual learners. Experiments with new foods and methods of preparing them are appropriate activities for children. For example, children can play nutrition-focused games or participate in scavenger hunts where they must locate specific foods. When discussing the basic food groups, they may use the ChooseMyPlate concept with portion size models to teach the importance of understanding serving size on different dishes and plates.[2] Nutrition professionals may also engage students in oral activities such as describing their favorite foods or written activities such as keeping a food diary or meal journal.

Educators could also use technology and social media under supervision to provide students with self-directed activities. For example, they can connect students from another culture and country using video media or use web-based sites to search for nutrition programming.

The nutrition counselor should try to choose words that children understand. Consider presenting complicated terms, such as "glucose," in conjunction

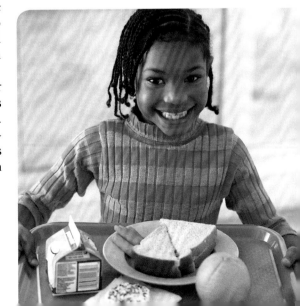

Food served at school lunch programs contributes to total nutrition.

with visual models (i.e., food models ranked by glucose content) and the use of simpler terms such as "sugar." Define difficult-to-understand words and pair with recognition connections such as flash cards. Choose words that have a positive connotation, rather than a negative one. For example, many children and adults consider the word "diet" to be negatively associated with weight and being fat. Therefore, use words such as "food plan," "food choices," "meal plan," or "menu" to indicate the type of foods the child should eat.

Professionals who counsel children in an office can create a warm, welcoming feeling by using color and visual images to create an inviting space. The office environment can be made attractive with colorful food models, magazine pictures, posters, food packages of commonly eaten foods, and beverage glasses of various sizes and shapes.

Adolescents, Age 13 to 19 Years

Adolescence is a period of cognitive, physical, and psychosocial change. As teenagers experience these rapid and unknown changes, they need to adjust their nutritional behaviors by increasing their healthy dietary habits and decreasing those that are unhealthy.

Before a nutrition counselor can plan an educational session, the adolescent's overall health must first be assessed. This includes, but is not limited to, assessing the following: current body weight, weight fluctuation, physical growth, timing of growth spurt, physiologic maturation, and activity level. Teenagers vary in rates of physical growth, in the timing of the growth spurt, and in physical activity patterns. The growth spurt of most adolescent girls occurs between 10 and 12 years of age. Adolescent boys, however, experience a growth spurt typically 2 years later at ages 14 to 16. Rates of growth may vary among either gender because of external influences such as poor diet, prenatal health conditions, or chronic illnesses. Physical activity patterns may also vary. For example, teenagers who participate in sports engage in high levels of physical activity, whereas those who frequently watch television or play video games are considered to engage in minimal to moderate activity.

The nutrition counselor must be familiar with the characteristics and external pressures that are associated with the teenage years. Adolescence is a time of awkwardness, self-awareness, and experimentation. Take a moment to recall your teenage years: suddenly, you are given more accountability and responsibility, yet you are unable to fully exercise your new freedoms because you are still under the jurisdiction of your parents and teachers. As you try to exert your independence and search for your identity, you are faced with the challenge of balancing freedom with responsibility and personal preferences with authority. Do these thoughts sound familiar? Many teens that nutrition professionals treat will be experiencing these internal conflicts and emotions. In addition, they will be balancing the demands of their quasi-adult, yet quasi-child, environment that includes school, friends, family, and even work. One of the most demanding issues is the hectic schedule that many teens follow. Such schedules provide challenges to eating right as well as even having time to plan when to eat. As a healthcare professional, it is imperative to keep these factors in mind when counseling adolescents.

Influences on Eating Habits

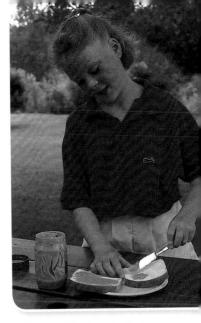

Adolescents like to make their own food choices.

Why do adolescents make the food choices they do? A study of adolescents assessed their perceptions of factors influencing their food choices. These factors included hunger and food cravings, appeal of the food, taste of the food, time considerations, convenience of the food, food availability, parental influences on eating behaviors (such as culture or religion), health benefits of foods, situation-specific factors, mood, body image, habit, cost, media influences, and vegetarian beliefs. However, the most influential factor was the adolescent's desire to fit the social norms of the peer group, that is, teenagers' food choices were most likely influenced by what their best friend was eating.[15,23]

Food is often a social experience and eating often occurs when one is surrounded by one's friends or peers. Because adolescents are uncomfortable with anything that makes them seem different from their peer group, they may tend to eat whatever snacks or meals their friends are eating. Sometimes, this may be a positive experience, as when adolescents mimic the healthy eating habits of their friends. But it may have a negative effect if adolescents choose to mimic the unhealthy dietary choices of their peers. Peer interaction can also affect food choices at parties and sporting events, entice after-school snacking, and induce consumption of alcohol. Thus, the challenge for the counselor is to help individual adolescents incorporate healthful eating habits into their lifestyle, rather than mimic the unhealthy eating habits of their peers.[15]

Although almost all public schools participate in the school lunch programs, many high schools have competitive vending machines on site that may sell low-nutrient-dense foods such as soft drinks, candy, chips, and high-fat foods. Currently, initiatives are being made by local governments and school boards to ban or reduce the number of unhealthy snacks and sodas available from school cafeterias and vending machines, yet the fact remains that adolescents will continue to seek out these food items.[24] Thus, effective dietary interventions and counseling require that nutrition professionals explore the external factors influencing food choices so that healthy changes can be made.

Adolescents are also eating out more with their families or consuming take-out foods within their own home more than once a week. A recent study found an increased healthy eating index score if youth were encouraged to learn how to prepare some of their own foods.[25]

One particular trend, dieting, is a common practice among teenagers. Dissatisfied with their weight and body, many adolescents reduce their caloric and fat intake through intermittent elimination of food quantity and quality. By cutting calories without thought to the nutritional value of foods, adolescents may eliminate important nutrients from their diet, leading eventually to marginal nutritional status. This sustained practice can evolve into eating disorders in both girls and boys.[26]

Adolescents are more prone to poor body image issues. Professionals have to be aware of how an adolescent's negative body image can affect his or her nutritional habits. For example, girls may go through puberty and suddenly see their hips begin to widen and their breasts begin to develop. Uncomfortable with these changing features, young girls may develop a poor body image because they do not realize that this change is "natural" and will balance out as they get older.

The depiction of extremely slim actresses and models by the media tends to enforce unrealistic, idealized standards of weight; yet many adolescents strive to look like them and resort to drastic dieting, refuse to eat food, take diet pills, or overexercise. Nutrition professionals must realize that they cannot treat these serious eating disorders alone. Although they must provide nutrition counseling, they must also provide a nutrition intervention for the adolescents who are suffering from these disorders. Often, eating disorders occur because of one's dissatisfaction with his or her personal life or because weight appears to be the one area of life that he or she can control. Thus, effective treatment requires an interdisciplinary team approach in which psychologists and medical specialists collaborate to assess and treat patients across a continuum of care.[26]

Becoming a vegetarian or a vegan is another common trend among this age group. Those who become vegetarians may be vulnerable to nutritional deficiencies if their food intake is not balanced properly. Vegan practices are even more restrictive on protein sources. Adolescents who adopt these practices need to be assessed for essential nutritional deficiencies as well as signs of potential eating disorders. Nutrition professionals particularly need to watch their vegetarian and vegan clients and ensure that they are not abusing their bodies or becoming preoccupied with weight loss or body image.[15,26]

In treating adolescents, nutrition counselors must be knowledgeable about the importance of exercise and sports. Many teens are involved in competitive sports activities. Athletic participation can have both a positive and a negative impact on healthy adolescents. Positively, in some sports, such as wrestling, adolescent boys may be highly motivated to learn about nutrition to improve their athletic performance. On the other hand, boys may be trying to lose weight by inappropriate means so that they may wrestle within a lower-weight class. Nutrition professionals should be proactive in recognizing nutrition misinformation and fads with this group by providing interesting and accurate education materials and programs.[27]

Counseling Strategies

Cognitive-behavioral therapy intervention strategies should target the affective domain, or feelings and attitudes, and not just give information to increase knowledge. Adolescent attitudes and patterns related to food choices and physical activity should be explored, since they may persist into adulthood.

Nutrition professionals and adolescents may engage in either one-on-one counseling or group counseling sessions. In one-on-one counseling, personal decisions related to self-care can be explored privately between the counselor and the adolescent. Group efforts can use the power of peer support to discuss and share how adolescents can handle challenging food situations when among peers.

Counseling adolescents that are also pregnant requires enhanced focus. These pregnancies are at greater risk than adult pregnancies because many teenage girls have poor nutritional intakes and/or have not yet completed their growth spurt. Pregnant teens are at a greater risk of having premature or low-birth-weight babies and developing concurrent health conditions such as anemia and hypertensive disorders. They may be reluctant to change their food patterns compared with their peers. Pregnant teens require significant caloric intake in order to support the growth and development of the fetus, as well as to support their own personal growth needs.[5]

Collecting information on dietary patterns of adolescents can be challenging. The use of digital photography to aid in dietary assessment or to record food intake prospectively using an adolescent's smartphone if available may add validity and interest to the process.[28] Because food is so closely linked with what the adolescent is doing, meal patterns should be assessed with an activity time line to be most effective. In this way, the counselor can understand what is triggering the eating pattern and how to integrate recommendations within that environment. Adolescent snacking patterns are often connected with social media use and traditional television viewing. By understanding the setting, positive information on alternate food choices can be presented, rather than assuming an adolescent would avoid the environment or choose not to eat.[15]

Another effective counseling approach is to address the food environment directly. School, home, and popular food service settings can be encouraged to present a wider array of interesting healthy foods in general. Healthier foods can be priced more attractively. Individual refined-grain products can also be substituted with higher fiber whole-grain alternatives.

CASE ANALYSIS 3

What specific education and counseling strategies would you consider using when working with Charles?

Family Counseling

Family is the most prominent influence on children's eating patterns from preschool through adolescence. Nutrition professionals must include parents, family members, or guardians in nutrition counseling sessions. The goal of effective family nutrition counseling is to use the shared environment to influence positive nutrition and health patterns and to foster healthy food consumption practices.

To provide effective nutrition guidance, counselors must be aware of the client's family composition and family roles and responsibilities as they relate to food procurement. Family nutrition counseling involves providing guidance and advice to people who live in the same household. In many households, families are composed of "nuclear" relatives, such as parents and siblings, as well as "extended" relatives, such as grandparents, aunts, uncles, or cousins. In others, children may be raised by only one parent. Many children of divorced parents share time between households, which may have different food challenges.

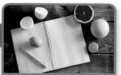

SELF-ASSESSMENT 1

1. Describe your own family household.
2. Who is responsible in your family for food purchasing and menu planning decisions?
3. Can you identify the origins of your own food preferences?

Because changes in family food buying and food preparation influence the child's adherence to the regimen, it is essential that the nutrition professional know which family member primarily engages in these activities. Historically, in many typical households, a child's mother was the person responsible for food shopping and food preparation. In today's society, this is no longer true of all households. Many women work outside the home, and other members of the family (fathers, grandparents, and older siblings) may have the primary responsibility for menu planning, purchasing food, and preparation of food. In some households, none of the family members has time for these responsibilities or for menu planning. In other circumstances, older children may be responsible for preparing their own breakfasts, bag lunches, and after-school snacks. When only nutritious food is brought into or made within the home, children are given environmental cues that enhance their healthy dietary regimen and reduce their intake of high-fat, high-calorie foods.

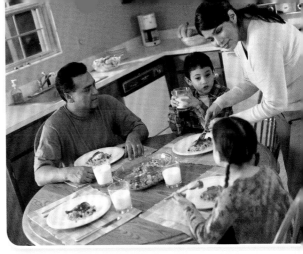

Parents may be motivated by concerns about child nutrition.

Source: US Department of Agriculture.

Members of a household share common biologic, social, cultural, psychological, or environmental spheres, and it is the task of the dietetics professional to provide a food program that addresses each of these spheres. When family members cooperate and provide the child with social, psychological, and environmental support, they greatly assist in fostering the child's dietary changes and help other family members improve their diet habits as well. Dietary changes often benefit everyone in the family.[29]

Preschool-age and school-age children, and even adolescents, are highly influenced by their parents or guardians' eating behaviors. Family members can serve as good role models by eating healthy food and rewarding healthy habits in the child. Children frequently mimic their parents' food habits. For example, if a boy sees that his father refuses to eat broccoli, he will be more likely to refuse broccoli. Thus, parents need to set a good example. The counselor must help parents and guardians to be the role models by helping them negotiate changes in what is purchased, prepared, and eaten by members of the family.[13,15]

Nutrition professionals may face some challenges while providing counseling to families. Some clients do not wish to involve certain family members; stepparents may refuse to participate; spouses and parents may be overly controlling and negative in dealing with the child; and mutually acceptable times for appointments may be difficult to arrange for several people. In these cases, other sources of social support may have to be located and collaborative relationships will need to be formed.

Other concerns may be present. Parents may not be good role models or supportive of their children. They may use sweets and desserts as a reward or bribe: "Eat this and you can have dessert," for example. Siblings may tempt and tease a brother or sister who is not supposed to eat certain foods. Parents who take a food plan too literally may create a stressful environment in the family, leading to food battles and conflicts. Nagging, criticism, and policing about food and weight issues should be replaced with positive reinforcement and praise when correct dietary behaviors are observed.[13,15]

CASE ANALYSIS ◉ **4**

Make a list of potential challenges and opportunities in providing nutrition counseling to Mrs. Smith and her extended family.

Adults, Age 20 to 64 Years

Healthy adults are the target group for the majority of the chapters in this book. Nutrition counselors should encourage preventive health by providing education using ChooseMyPlate and other simple messages for everyday food intake.[2] The 2015 Dietary Guidelines provide five broad guidelines that encourage healthy eating patterns as shown in Table 9-1.[30] Many online resources are available to download with colorful brochures that highlight the aspects of a wide range of common topics such as bone health and prevention of osteoporosis in adult women and men.

The nutrition professional should keep abreast of the ongoing research in dietary patterns. The Women's Health Initiative (WHI), for example, is an observational cohort study of women age 50 to 79 years that continues to follow women for dietary and lifestyle risks of cardiovascular disease. Counseling of postmenopausal women on a healthy diet with adequate calcium content to promote strong bones is another area of high interest in preventive adult nutrition.[31]

The nutrition professional must keep current on existing and evolving research in the area of nutrition. Food patterns, such as the Mediterranean diet and low glycemic index, are more extensively studied. Novel food patterns and complementary medicine health practices will require evaluation by the nutrition professional prior to conversations with clients.

1. Follow a healthy eating pattern across the lifespan.

2. Focus on variety, nutrient density, and amount.

3. Limit calories from added sugars and saturated fats and reduce sodium intake.

4. Shift to healthier food and beverage choices.

5. Support healthy eating patterns for all.

Table 9-1 ■ 2015 to 2020 Dietary Guidelines

Adults, Age 65 Years and Older

The aging of the global and US population presents challenges to families, policy makers, and healthcare providers. Many older adults enjoy a standard of living and increased life span unknown a century ago. These older adults also have more concurrent medical conditions requiring nutrition counseling to remain healthy or to lower the risk of complications.

Today's older Americans are generally better educated than previous generations. This factor can influence socioeconomic status, health, and quality of life. Many continue to live independently. A large majority enjoy social contacts with friends and relatives, including activities such as going to restaurants for meals. Although economic resources are sufficient for many, there are significant disparities in income and wealth that may create food insecurity. A new trend for older adults is choosing to live within healthcare communities such as assisted living where some meals are provided each day. Others will spend a decade or more in long-term care communities where all meals and medications may be provided.

In general, older Americans need to be assessed by functional status rather than age alone. Independent and active older adults may still be working part-time, with few health issues. Others may be living with limited independence, serious health problems, or disabilities. The evaluation focus of each older adult needs to be individualized to their unique needs.

Counseling Strategies

A comprehensive nutrition assessment of any older adult should be performed that considers the economic, psychosocial, cultural, health, physiologic, and lifestyle factors influencing food intake before planning a nutrition intervention. Primary goals are not as strong on prevention as on maintaining adequate nutrition status. Many older individuals eat smaller meals and have lower activity levels, but may not achieve minimal nutrition requirements. Poor dentures may affect chewing and digestion. Preference for lower-nutrient-density food choices such as apple pie compared with a fresh

Older adults dine together at a community site.
Source: Punchsock.

apple may decrease some nutrients such as fiber. Smaller portions need higher-nutrient-density focus, but may not be the choice of the client.[32]

Nutrition professionals need to stay current on published literature. Evidence-based systematic reviews, practice and position papers, and other critical analysis formats can aid in developing education content. Controversy is often present in many areas of practice such as the relationship between nutrient intake and cognitive changes,[33] calcium supplementation,[31] or optimum weight status. For example, fragility of bones in osteoporosis may not benefit from more body weight but rather from selected weight-bearing exercises in conjunction with bone health nutrition awareness. There is ongoing debate if obesity should be actively addressed after the seventh decade of life or emphasis placed on lean body mass.[4]

CASE ANALYSIS 5

What socioeconomic, physiologic, and lifestyle factors influence Mrs. Smith's food intake? What are two key nutrition issues you might discuss with Mrs. Smith during your first session?

People aged 85 years and older are the most likely individuals to live in nursing homes. Those in nursing homes tend to be more impaired functionally and may need assistance with eating. Malnutrition affects about two of every five elderly nursing home residents. Several assessment tools are available to perform nutritional and dysphagia screening.[29,34]

A primary nutrition focus in long-term care facilities is the risk reduction of pressure ulcers and other wound healing issues by providing adequate calories and nutrients under the direction of a registered dietitian.[35] The Academy of Nutrition and Dietetics has an active practice group of specialized members that focus on this area of geriatric expertise and have published standards of practice for their field.[32]

Achieving and maintaining optimal nutritional status of the older population is the primary goal for nutrition counselors. A few counseling recommendations are found in Table 9-2. Nutrition counselors should be aware of local and government community programs to access for older adults. Food assistance programs and food pantry systems are often available. Government programs may provide meals at little or no cost in a social setting such as community or recreational centers, senior citizen centers, and churches. Home-delivered meals are another common resource in many communities.

Changes in resting energy expenditure and decreased levels of physical activity require assessment of caloric needs to achieve and maintain healthy body weight.

Smaller meals and portions require increased nutrient density.

Sensory changes of taste, smell, hearing, and vision may influence appetite and food choices by making food less appealing.

Drug–nutrient interactions need to be assessed due to higher risk of multiple medication and over-the-counter supplement use.

Denture problems, difficulty swallowing, or chewing impairment may restrict foods selected or eaten.

Social isolation, loneliness, and bereavement due to loss of spouse decrease interest in cooking and eating.

Income may be limited or fixed while healthcare and other expenses increase, resulting in food insecurity and economic problems.

Physical disability and cognitive impairments (depression and dementia) may make shopping and cooking difficult.

Lack of physical activity decreases muscle mass, which can affect mobility and strength.

Physiologic changes in digestion and absorption increase with age.

Table 9-2 ■ Counseling Awareness Issues in Older Adults

Managing Chronic Diet-Related Diseases

As people live longer, they often are diagnosed with a chronic disease condition. Examples of diet-related chronic diseases may include diabetes mellitus, elevated blood cholesterol (dyslipidemia), osteoporosis, cancer, heart (cardiovascular) disease, high blood pressure, or kidney disease. Many adults may have more than one chronic disease to address and integrate within their lifestyle. Diabetes, hypertension, and hyperlipidemia commonly occur in a cluster along with obesity. This combination of metabolic disorders is referred to as metabolic syndrome. This in turn increases the risk of cardiovascular disease. All of these diseases are related to lifestyle. A recent review of lifestyle intervention outcomes in type 2 diabetic overweight and obese adults required a decrease in at least 5% of body weight to reduce glycemic, lipid, and blood pressure to beneficial levels.[35] These treatment models included structured frequent and regular contacts with clients, self-monitoring assignments (i.e., food, physical activity, and/or blood glucose records), and learning problem-solving strategies. Any diet-related chronic disease requires innovative education strategies to keep clients motivated.

The chronic care model is often used in primary and specialty centers to deliver coordinated education through healthcare teams. This model works to integrate decisions in an organized manner to achieve higher outcomes than a single practitioner could deliver alone.[36] A nutrition professional is recommended as a fully involved collaborative team member, particularly in the management of diabetes mellitus and kidney disease. As an illustration of the importance of providing medical nutrition therapy for these disease conditions, the Center for Medicare Services (CMS) began to reimburse registered dietitians for medical nutrition therapy of these conditions in 2002. Reimbursement for other disease conditions and preventive care is still evolving.[37]

Education Strategies

Terms like "compliance" and "adherence" were often used to describe necessary health behavior changes to accomplish better health outcomes. A new emphasis has been placed on the concept of "self-management," where clients are considered members of the interdisciplinary team that cares for them. As a member of the team, they participate in goal setting and in identifying problem-solving strategies designed to address barriers to managing their treatment regimens. Common barriers include remembering to take medications, getting regular physical activity, monitoring blood glucose, managing a high pill burden, or affording the cost of diet-related foods.[38,39]

This emphasis on the client being considered the key player on the chronic disease management team is very effective for nutrition professionals to use when educating patients with chronic illness. The use of the electronic medical record may also increase the ability to access clients throughout the life span. Some healthcare systems are integrating access with education opportunities for health information. The nutrition and dietetics professional may be able to follow clients over time, removing the barriers of scheduling and location using evolving information technology advances in healthcare. An electronic reminder can be built into the electronic record system to remind clients to come for a scheduled clinic visit or remember to refill medications or complete a diet record.[40,41]

Specialty Care Strategies

Table 9-3 lists nutrition interventions recommended for care of clients with diet-related chronic diseases. The Academy of Nutrition and Dietetics regularly convenes evidence-based practice committees that examine the literature and publish recommendations for nutrition care in specialty areas of practice. Summaries of the evidence for medical nutrition therapy for chronic disease conditions such as type 1 and type 2 diabetes mellitus in adults and how to integrate the guidelines into the Nutrition Care

Referral to a registered dietitian nutritionist within 6 mo of diagnosis
Initial education visits (3–4) of 45–90 min each
Subsequent monitoring visits to assess need for additional follow-up
An annual visit to assess status and reinforce necessary lifestyle changes

Table 9-3 ■ Nutrition Intervention Recommendations for Diet-Related Chronic Disease

Process (NCP) have been published. Standards of practice and professional performance for all registered dietitians as well as for some specific diseases including diabetes, cancer, and kidney disease are revised at regular intervals, usually every 5 to 8 years, and are designed to provide clear roadmaps to provision of services to clients.[42,43]

Summary

Good nutrition is essential to the health, self-sufficiency, and quality of life throughout the life span. Nutrition professionals need to acquire the knowledge and skills necessary to counsel and educate people of all ages with a variety of food and nutrition challenges. Choosing food is a daily and highly personal activity. Some individuals will need to focus on maintaining the desire to eat just to reduce the risk of weight loss and undernutrition. Others will require extensive behavioral counseling to attain and maintain healthy body weight to reduce potential health risks.

The NCP, as presented in Chapter 1, is a complementary framework for nutrition care throughout the life span. The NCP concepts (assessment, diagnosis, intervention, monitoring, and evaluation) mirror the life span growth and change process. The nutrition counselor should assess and identify potential problems and their effects on nutritional status. The counselor should establish individualized plans for intervention that include adaptations for each life span group. They need to document how their education strategies reduce healthcare costs and achieve better health outcomes through prevention of disease or related complications throughout the life span.

CASE ANALYSIS 6

Develop written documentation for each client session of the family unit incorporating the NCP model as applicable.

Nutrition professionals deliver care as an essential role as a member of the interdisciplinary healthcare team throughout the life span. Prevention and treatment of chronic diet-related diseases offer an opportunity for nutrition counselors to become involved in long-term effective strategies to achieve the highest quality of life.

Review and Discussion Questions

1. List two goals of nutrition counseling for prenatal or pregnant women.
2. In counseling preschool-age and school-age children, what factors should be assessed? What educational and intervention strategies are recommended for children?
3. In dealing with adolescent boys and girls, what factors should be assessed?

4. What strategies are helpful in working with families?

5. What factors may have an impact on the diet and nutrition of older adults?

6. Identify three education strategies that support the self-management concept in chronic diet-related disease conditions.

Suggested Activities

1. Watch a child's television program. While doing so, note the number of food advertisements. Did these commercials make you want to consume the food item? Do they promote healthy eating?

2. Interview a nutrition professional who works with children or adolescents. Ask questions about the nutritional challenges encountered when counseling diverse populations.

3. Interview the mother or caregiver of a child. Ask what strategies she or he uses to encourage healthy eating habits and introduce new foods into the child's diet.

4. Plan a 15-minute presentation on nutritious snacks for a life span group of your choice. What types of instructional media would you use? Why?

5. Interview a teenager about his or her eating practices. Ask about food preferences. What factors influence food choices? How does the type of food the teen chooses to eat compare with what friends eat? Are foods chosen for health or weight reasons?

6. Buy a magazine read by adolescents. Assess the content of any articles on nutrition, food ads, weight control supplements, and the like.

7. Interview an older adult (age 65 years or older) about his or her food choices and eating practices. Ask about how the person purchases and prepares food, the number of meals eaten daily, and the intake of water and other beverages. Write a summary of your encounter using the NCP model.

8. Evaluate a patient education handout that is distributed in a public health community program for a specific life span group. Does the information in the handout give correct information? Is it written at the correct level for the population targeted?

9. Select a chronic diet-related health condition such as diabetes. Find a group of at least three education handouts appropriate for nutrition counseling. Compare them for content, focus, and client application. Discuss how you might use these materials in a sequence of ongoing counseling sessions and develop a set of recommendations for future materials you might require.

Education Skills

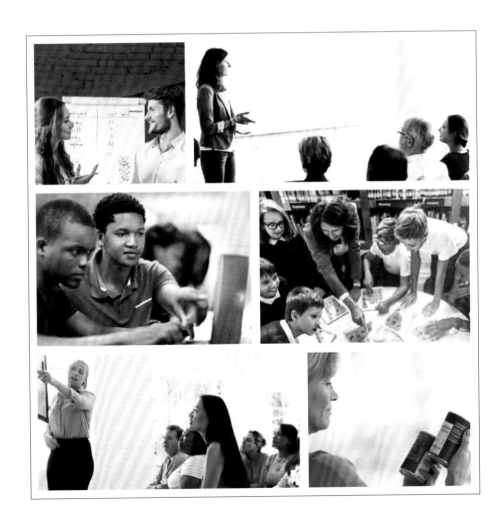

CHAPTER 10

Principles and Theories of Learning

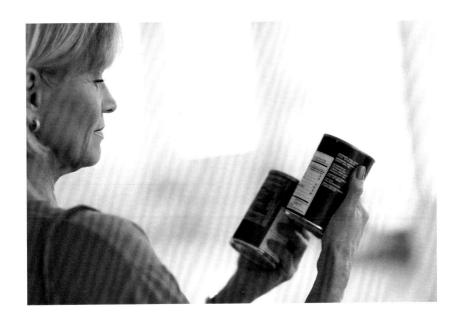

Objectives

- Compare and contrast learning theories and strategies.
- Differentiate between types of behavioral consequences.
- Specify strategies that enhance long-term memory.
- Describe several learning and teaching styles.
- Define the stages involved in the innovation–decision process.
- Identify the role of technology in learning.

John Richards has been referred for counseling because of his high blood pressure. He is 65 years old with acceptable body mass index and serum cholesterol levels within the normal range. Six months ago, his wife died. Since her passing, he has lived alone in the family home and has relied more on prepackaged meals and convenience foods. His physician recommended a diet restricted in sodium, with an increase in fruits and vegetables. If dietary changes are successful, he may not need medication.

All the foods that you regularly eat are ones that you learned to eat.[1]

—*Bee Wilson*

Introduction

The foundation for effective education is based on theory. Theoretical concepts are used in the planning, implementation, and evaluation of education. Nutrition education focuses on health promotion, the prevention of chronic diseases, and intervention and treatment. Achieving healthier lifestyles is a challenge for many.

Learning

What is learning? Learning may be defined as a change in a person as a result of experience or the interaction of a person with his or her environment. The changes may be in knowledge, skills, attitudes, values, and behaviors, and there are relatively permanent outcomes. Cognitive psychologists view learning as an "active mental process of acquiring, remembering, and using knowledge."[2] As you read this chapter, for example, you are learning. Other than learning by reading, the practitioner's challenge is to determine how to present people with the right stimuli and experiences on which to focus their attention and mental effort so that they can acquire new knowledge, skills, attitudes, and behaviors.

How do people learn? How do they retain what they learn? The field of educational psychology studies questions about the process of learning, including learner preferences and teaching delivery methods. Its major focus is on the processes by which knowledge, skills, attitudes, and values are transmitted between teachers and learners. Teachers must "learn about learning" before they can effectively teach.[1,2]

In the workplace, nutrition professionals provide learning opportunities in a variety of ways. They train and educate new employees and retrain experienced workers. They also participate in the delivery of educational programs for other health professionals, students, interns, residents, and paraprofessionals. Practitioners are concerned with discovering the most effective methods of teaching to influence the dietary behaviors of clients and the work behaviors of employees. Although theory alone does not guarantee effective education, applying theories to planning and implementing interventions does.

A major emphasis is on the education of clients. Effective client education includes the process of influencing behavior and producing changes in knowledge, attitudes, values, and skills required to improve and maintain health. Giving information (knowledge) or telling people what they should do is not sufficient to achieve changes in food practices. Counseling and education approaches that will promote changes in attitudes and behaviors benefitting health status are necessary.

Education takes place at different levels: the individual level, such as one-on-one or group classes; the social network, such as family; and the community level, such as society at large. Public health initiatives such as Eating Well with Canada's Food Guide and the United States Department of Agriculture's myPlate are two examples of community-level educational programs.[3,4]

Effective use of educational theory takes practice in helping people make changes in their eating practices and environments. Health behaviors are too complex to be explained by a single theory. To explain how people learn, psychologists have developed several learning theories. This chapter discusses behavioral learning theories and social cognitive theory, as well as memory, transfer of learning, adult learning or andragogy, learning and teaching styles, the adoption of innovations, and technology as a teaching tool. Many of these theories and strategies can be utilized together in the same intervention.[5]

The social and behavioral sciences provide many of the education models used by health professionals. These models can be found in other chapters of this book and include the Transtheoretical Model or Stages of Change Model and motivational interviewing in Chapters 5 and 6, behavior modification in Chapter 7, and social cognitive theory in Chapter 8. All of these can be applied to nutrition interventions. The educator must select the most appropriate strategies and methods for each situation.

CASE ANALYSIS 1

Identify the types of questions you would plan to ask Mr. Richards before educating him on the dietary changes he needs to make.

Behavioral Learning Theories

Behavioral learning theories are explanations of learning that are limited almost exclusively to observable changes in behavior, with emphasis on the effects of external events on the individual.[2] Theorists are interested in the way in which pleasurable or painful consequences of behavior may change the person's behavior over time. This approach is based on the belief that what we learn has readily identifiable parts and that identifiable rewards and punishments can be given to produce the learning.[6] The teacher's role is to arrange the external environment to elicit the desired response.[7]

Behavioral learning theories evolved from the research of several individuals, including Ivan Pavlov on classical conditioning; Edward Thorndike, who noted that the connections between stimuli and subsequent responses or behaviors are strengthened or weakened by the consequences of behavior; and B.F. Skinner's work on operant conditioning.[2] Other information on their research may be found in Chapter 7.

Based on the Pavlovian approach, association theory suggests that a stimulus event cues or elicits a response in the learner. Teaching or conditioning, therefore, involves arranging the stimulus and response events. This is a teacher-centered approach with passive learners.

Skinner's work focused on the relationship between behavior and its consequences. Skinner believed that many human behaviors are operants, not merely respondents. The use of pleasant and unpleasant consequences following a particular behavior is often referred to as operant conditioning.[2] Learning involves three related events: the stimulus, a response, and a reinforcer. The teacher must manage all three events. The desired target behavior must be followed by reinforcement for the behavior to continue. Thus, reinforcers, such as small objects, must be identified and given if the desired response is present. This is also a teacher-centered approach with a passive learner. Behaviorism does not explain every kind of learning as it disregards the activities of the mind.

In the following sections, four consequences of a behavior are discussed: positive reinforcement, negative reinforcement or escape, punishers, and extinction. In addition, shaping and the timing of reinforcement are examined.

Positive Reinforcers

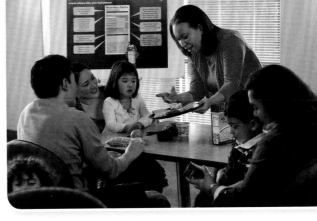

People learn through active involvement.
Source: US Department of Agriculture.

One of the most important principles of behavioral learning theory is that behavior changes according to its immediate consequences. Pleasurable consequences are called "positive reinforcers" or rewards and may be defined as consequences that strengthen and increase the frequency of a behavior.[2] Examples are praise for a job well done, good grades received in school, money in the form of a salary increase, and token reinforcers such as stars or smiley-face stickers on a chart. When behaviors persist or increase over time, one may assume that the consequences are positively reinforcing them. The pleasure associated with eating, for example, is a positive reinforcer, ensuring that people will consume their favorite foods again and again.

These reinforcers are highly personal, however, and none can be assumed to be effective all the time. The behavior of an employee who has a poor relationship with a supervisor, for example, may not be affected by the supervisor's praise. And the professional's praise of a client who has followed a dietary regimen may not matter to that specific individual. The person must value the reinforcer to increase the frequency of a desired behavior. The professional can explore the items that an individual considers positive reinforcers and can help arrange such reinforcement in the person's environment. Knowledge of results is also an effective secondary positive reinforcer. Clients and employees should know their stage of progress. If they know they are doing something properly, that knowledge reinforces the response.

The way in which praise is given is also important, and the person doing the praising must be believable.[2] The praise should recognize a specific behavior, so the person clearly understands why he or she is being recognized. "Good job" as a praise is not as effective as saying specifically, "Thanks for completing the extra project on time. I appreciate it."

Negative Reinforcers/Escapes

Reinforcers that are escapes from unpleasant situations are called negative reinforcers. These also strengthen behaviors because they enable the individual to withdraw from unpleasant situations.[2] Overeating may be reinforcing if the individual escapes, for example, feelings of loneliness, unhappiness, and fatigue. Or, an employee may escape the supervisor's wrath by behaving correctly. If some action stops, avoids, or escapes something unpleasant, the person is likely to repeat that action again when faced with a similar situation.[1]

Punishers

Negative reinforcers, which strengthen behaviors, should not be confused with punishers, which weaken behaviors. Unpleasant consequences, punishers, decrease the frequency of or suppress a behavior.[2] Punishment may take one of two different forms. One form involves removal of positive reinforcers that the person already has, such as a privilege. A second form involves the use of unpleasant or adverse consequences, as when a person is scolded for improper behavior. Punishment can make a person avoid the situation in the future, so scolding a client who has not lost any weight is not appropriate.

Extinction

What happens when reinforcers are withdrawn? A behavior weakens and eventually disappears, a process called extinction of a behavior.[2] If a person starts an exercise program or dietary change, for example, and there are not continuous positive reinforcers, that person may decrease the new behavior and eventually end it.

When behaviors are undesirable and the reinforcers for it can be identified and removed, the behavior also may become extinct. An employee's boisterous behavior, for example, may change if the supervisor and other employees ignore the person and do not respond with the attention he or she is seeking. Instead, the supervisor will want to reinforce positively nonboisterous behavior in this person.

Shaping

The decision of what to reinforce in a client or employee, and when, is also important. Does one wait until the desired behavior is perfect? No! Most people need reinforcement along the way to something new. Reinforcing each step along the way to successful behavior is called shaping, or successive approximations.[2,7] It involves reinforcing progress rather than waiting for perfection. When client or employee goals can be broken down into a series of identified steps or subskills, positive feedback may be given as each step or subskill is mastered or accomplished.

Timing Reinforcement

An important principle is that positive consequences that are immediate are more effective than those that are delayed. The connection between the behavior and the consequences is better understood in the person's mind.

As a result, the nutrition professional needs to identify with the client or employee not only what is positively reinforcing to that person but also a time schedule for dispensing that reinforcement for proper behaviors. This concept explains why it is difficult for people to change their eating behaviors. Usually, the positive consequences of the change, such as weight loss or better health, are in the future, whereas eating disallowed foods is positively reinforcing immediately. It tastes good or hunger is reduced. Eating is intrinsically reinforcing, that is, a behavior that is pleasurable in itself.[1]

The frequency of reinforcement has also been studied. In the early part of a behavior change, continuous reinforcement after every correct response helps learning. Later on, a variable or intermittent schedule of reinforcement is preferable. When rewards are overused, they lose their effect, so that after an individual has had some rewarded successes, rewards should be given less frequently. Table 10-1 summarizes some of the implications of the theories discussed in this chapter.

CASE ANALYSIS 2

What is your assessment of both motivating and challenging issues facing this client?

Theory/Model	Implications
Behavioral theory	Find out what reinforcers are valued
	Tell the person their stage of progress
	Use positive reinforcement
	Praise specific, not general, behaviors
	Reinforce progress on the way to mastery
	Use continuous reinforcement, then intermittent
	Ignore undesirable behaviors
	Avoid punishment
Social learning	Be a good role model
	Provide other good role models
	Avoid negative models
	Have new skills demonstrated and practiced

Table 10-1 ■ Implications of Learning Theories and Models

Theory/Model	Implications
Cognitive theory	Explore prior knowledge
	Gain and maintain attention
	Ask questions
	Use goal setting
	Use repetition and review
	Make information meaningful
	Organize information
	Link new information to the memory network
Learning styles	Identify preferences for styles
	Offer several methods or techniques of learning
Adult learning	Adults are self-directed
	Recognize prior experience
	Use participatory methods
	Orient learning to problems and projects
	Use goal setting

Table 10-1 ■ (continued)

Social Cognitive Theory

Social cognitive theory expanded the behaviorist view. Since the 1970s, Albert Bandura has been considered the father of the modeling theory. He believed that the observation of and imitation of other people's behavior, that is, vicariously learning from another's successes and failures, had been ignored. He maintained that people learned not only from external cues but also from observing models or "modeling." People who focus their attention on watching others are constructing mental images, analyzing, evaluating, remembering, and making decisions that affect their own learning. Professionals need to be aware of this and to be good role models. If we do not eat nutritiously and exercise regularly, for example, how can we expect others to do so?

When the media cover celebrities who are losing weight, many fans start on the same diet to model after their success. It is preferable, of course, if the model is an attractive, successful, admired, and well-known individual. Then people will imitate the behavior, hoping to capture some of the same success.

In group learning situations, clients and employees can learn from good role models. In demonstrating the operation of kitchen equipment to a new employee, part of the learning comes from watching the trainer. Then the employee imitates what he or she has seen. In group classes for individuals making dietary modifications due to heart disease, for example, people may be influenced to make dietary changes by modeling after the success stories of others in the group.

Individuals also learn vicariously from watching negative models. When we see that something does not work or we disagree with it, we decide not to imitate it. Seeing an obese person can trigger this type of reaction in some people. "I'll never be like that" may be a response. People judge behaviors against their own standards and decide which models to follow. Sometimes, employees model after others who take shortcuts and do not follow proper procedures. If the supervisor takes extra-long breaks and lunches, for example, employees may conclude that this behavior is permissible.

When the professional wants people to model knowledge or skills they are acquiring, it is important to have them practice and demonstrate the skill, not just rehearse it mentally. This shows whether or not they are modeling correctly. For example, the practitioner may want a client who is learning to make different food choices to plan several menus to model the new knowledge and skill. A new employee who can demonstrate the proper use of equipment is modeling correctly. If the individual is correct, feedback and positive reinforcement such as praise should be given; self-efficacy and motivation are then enhanced. If the person is only partially correct, using "shaping," one may give positive reinforcement for the correct portion and then assist in altering the rest. Mentoring another person is another example of using these principles as the mentor models and guides new roles and behaviors.

Each learner is more effectively counseled by a professional who has a familiarity with the learner's unique circumstances, learning style, and context. Each person is at a different developmental life stage with degrees of motivation. Family and social contexts vary. The professional can then personalize an intervention strategy for learning. A multicultural society requires the awareness of group customs, traditions, and acceptable counselor approaches (see Chapter 4, which discusses these aspects in detail).

EXAMPLE   "What can you eat for breakfast? In a restaurant? On trips?"
"What does the food label tell you?"

Cognitive Theories

Cognitive psychologists studying learning focus on mental activities, such as thinking, remembering, and solving problems that cannot be seen directly. Rather than observable changes brought about by external events, cognitive learning theories are explanations of learning that focus on internal, unobservable mental processes that people use to learn and remember new knowledge or skills.[2]

Which is easier to learn—the formulas for the essential amino acids or the United States Department of Agriculture (USDA) ChooseMyPlate food guide? Which is easier to remember—a phone number used yesterday for the first time or the food that was eaten for dinner last evening? The difference is between rote learning, which requires memorizing facts not linked to a cognitive structure, and learning and remembering more meaningful information without deliberately memorizing it. Both are necessary.

The cognitive view sees learning as an active internal mental process of acquiring, remembering, and using knowledge rather than the passive process influenced by the external environmental stimuli of the behaviorists.[2] Individuals pursue goals, seek information, solve problems, and reorganize information and knowledge in their memories. In pondering a problem, the solution may come as a flash of insight as people reorganize what they know.

The cognitive approach suggests that an important influence on learning is what the individual brings to the learning situation, that is, what he or she already knows.[2] Prior knowledge is an important influence on what we learn, remember, and forget. Remembering and forgetting are other topics in cognitive psychology. Table 10-2 compares the theories discussed in this chapter.

Discovery learning is an example of a cognitive instructional model. When people learn through their own active involvement, they discover things for themselves. This approach, using experimentation and problem solving, helps people to analyze and absorb information rather than merely memorize it.[2] The professional can provide problem situations that stimulate the client to question, explore, and experiment.

Memory

There are many theories of memory that explain how the mind takes in information, processes it, stores it, retains it, and retrieves it for use when needed. Cognitive perception theories see learning as an all-or-none event rather than an incremental process. Past perceptions are already stored in memory for future use. If the learner has no prior experience to draw upon (a perceptual deficit), a frame must be created with the help of the educator. With prior experience, a frame already exists. If the current

Category	Behavioral	Social Learning	Cognitive	Andragogy
Teacher's role	Arrange environment to get desired response	Serve as role model	Structure content or problems with essential features	Facilitator
	Arrange reinforcement	Arrange for other role models	Organize knowledge	Plan, implement, evaluate jointly
				Provide resources
Management	Teacher-centered	Learner-centered	Learner-centered	Learner-centered
Learner participation	Passive/active	Active	Active, solve problems	Active
		Imitate models	Test hypotheses	
Motivation	Rewards motivate	Both external and internal	Internal	Internal
	External		Use goal setting	
View of learning	Rote learning	Observation of others	Insight learning	Performing tasks
	Subject matter approach		Understanding	Solving problems
	Practice in varied contexts		Internal mental process	Goal-oriented
Strategy action	Stimulus–response	Social roles	Inquiry learning	Oriented to problem solving and task performance
	Behavioral objectives	Discussion	Discovery learning	
	Task analysis	Mentoring	Simulation	
	Competency-based	Role playing	Learning to learn	
	Computer-assisted learning			

Table 10-2 ■ Learning Theories and Strategies

257

frame is incorrect, a different frame must be created. Through the use of questions and listening, the nutrition professional can discover the learner frame of reference and build on it. Strategies must fit the client's frame of reference. Teaching involves managing real or vicarious experiences until the learner develops insight, outlooks, or thought patterns.[8] This is a teacher–student-centered approach with cooperative and interactive inquiry and problem solving.[7–9]

Other interventions are based in cognition–rational/linguistic learning theory.[7] Experiences become encoded in memory. As a result, people can organize, modify, or combine memories, resulting in new knowledge or higher levels of thinking. Reasoning skills allow analysis of experiences and prediction of future outcomes. Most behavior results from the cognitive analysis of knowledge, so thoughts are believed to precede a person's actions.[1]

The consumer information processing theory addresses processes by which a consumer takes in and uses information in decision-making. The theory points out that people have a limited capacity to process, store, and retrieve information at any one time. In making decisions, they seek only enough information to make a choice quickly. Thus, information should be organized, limited, and matched to the comprehension level of the individual, who can then process it with little effort. For example, people may look for the frozen dessert with the lowest fat content, store the information about their satisfaction with the product, and decide whether or not to purchase it again. Or, attitudes about a food such as carrots can be diversified to expand a consumer's processing of information and application to purchasing patterns.[10]

To enhance memory and reasoning, teaching requires providing labels for new experiences and structures. Problems may be treated as cognitive deficits requiring new structures. Clients with defeating self-statements and cognitive distortions, for example, require cognitive restructuring that rules out the current incorrect thought and introduces a new one (see Chapter 8).

The practitioner wants people not only to acquire information, skills, and attitudes but also to remember and use them. Since people are bombarded with information all day long from family, friends, coworkers, supervisors, newspapers, magazines, television, radio, and the Internet, how do they remember it all? They don't. Much is immediately discarded.

Psychologists agree that people must make sense of new

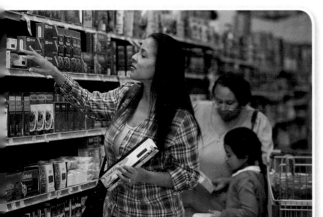

Children learn from family and peers.
Source: US Department of Agriculture.

information to learn and remember it. Some information enters working or short-term memory until it is used, such as the time of an appointment; then it is forgotten. Of course, nothing even enters short-term memory until the person pays attention to it, that is, focuses on certain stimuli and screens out all others.[2] Therefore, the nutrition professional needs to think of first obtaining and then maintaining a client's or employee's attention and focus. Otherwise, the individual may be thinking about something else.

There are various ways to gain a learner's attention, such as the use of media, bright colors, raising or lowering one's voice, using gestures, starting a discussion with a question, explaining a purpose, repeating information more than once, and saying "this is important." Gaining someone's interest in a topic at hand and indicating its importance to him or her as well as putting it in the context of what the person already knows are all helpful approaches. The professional should indicate how the information will be useful or important.[2]

Asking questions arouses curiosity and interest. The use of open-ended questions is an effective technique to solicit additional information. These questions typically begin with who, what, when, where, or why. Ask a new employee, "What do you know about the meat slicer?" Or, ask a new client with heart disease, "What do you know about saturated and trans fats?" Ask why they think learning this information is important to them. This forces the person to focus attention.

Working Memory

The human mind is like a computer. It receives information, performs operations on it to change its form and content, stores it, and retrieves it when needed.[2,7] Not all information or stimuli are selected for further processing, but some are focused on at a given moment.

As a person attends to something new and thinks about it, it enters the working memory. There are limits, however, to the amount of new information that can be retained at one time, perhaps five to nine items, and on the length of time it will be retained, probably 5 to 20 seconds.[2] Repeating something new over and over, such as the name of a person you have just met, helps to keep information in short-term memory longer. But if you meet five new people at once, this can be too much new information to handle.

Besides repetition, you may attempt to associate new information with information currently in long-term memory. Chunking, or grouping individual bits of information, also helps. For example, the telephone number 467 3652 becomes 467 36 52. Because of memory limits, it is helpful to give not only oral information but also written dietary guidelines to a client or a written task analysis to an employee, since details are forgotten quickly.

Long-Term Memory

Using technology, a person takes the input and "saves" it onto digital format to be retrieved later often by searching stored content. To move new information from working memory to long-term memory, a person uses similar principles to organize it and integrate it with information already stored in a network of interconnected neurons. Long-term memory involves three processes: encoding by attaching new information to other related memories, storage, and retrieval. Who cannot recognize the smell of a chocolate cake baking in the oven by retrieving the memory? Here, the professional needs to make it clear to clients and employees what is important and probably repeat it more than once. It takes time and effort to reflect, to grasp the implications, to interpret and experience, and to guide an internal representation of new knowledge in the brain.[2]

The ability to recall rote information is limited, whereas meaningful information is retained more easily. The implication for planning educational sessions for clients and employees is to make the information meaningful to the individual, present it in a clear and organized manner, and relate it to what the individual already knows and has stored in memory. The person can then connect it to other known information and apply it if necessary.

Which is easier to store and later retrieve—something one hears, something one sees, or something one both sees and hears? People retain visual plus verbal images and messages better. Some people use imagery to aid retention by picturing something in the mind.[2,11] Can you picture the USDA ChooseMyPlate food guide, or a food product label, for example?

There are various strategies to help people remember. The professional can summarize in the middle and at the end of a presentation. Repetition and review are helpful for retention. You may put an outline on a handout or project an image to organize information. Get people involved in talking with active instead of passive learning activities. Present information in a clear, organized fashion, not as isolated bits of information. Then, ask the person to translate the information into his or her own words or solve a problem with it, such as plan a menu or summarize what was said so that material provides personal significance.

People also remember stories, metaphors, and examples better than isolated facts. In teaching employees about food sanitation, for example, stories of actual outbreaks of foodborne illness are helpful. When teaching about modified diets, examples of actual client cases may be used. In a discussion of fiber with a client, examples of whole-grain breads and cereals, fruits, and vegetables may be discussed. Learning requires people to make sense of information, to sort it in their minds, to fit it into a neat and orderly pattern, and to use current information to help assimilate the new.[7,8,11]

Long-term memory requires connections of new knowledge to known information. Information is probably stored in networks of connected facts and concepts. Each piece of information in memory is connected to other pieces in some way. We remember things by association. The word "apple," for example, may be associated with fruits, red, or tree. You would be unlikely to associate it with a cat.

The following is an example of a partial knowledge network on water-soluble vitamins:

Water-Soluble Vitamins

Vitamin B			Vitamin C	
Niacin			Ascorbic acid	
Functions	Food sources		Functions	Food sources
	Vegetable	Animal		Vegetable	Fruit
	Cereal	Pork		Broccoli	Orange

If a person already has this network and learns something new about vitamin C—for example, that raw cabbage is a good food source of vitamin C—it is easy to file it into the existing network by association. If, however, a person knows nothing about vitamin C, it would be much more difficult to file the new information into long-term memory. The result is that it may be forgotten.

The following is an example of a knowledge network on food sanitation:

Germs/Bacteria

Salmonella	Clostridium botulinum	Staphylococcus
Food sources	Food sources	Food sources
Preventive measures	Preventive measures	Preventive measures

For food service workers, the term "germs" may be more meaningful and easier to store into memory than "pathogenic bacteria," since the latter term may be unfamiliar. It will be easier to add new information into an existing network if terms are recognizable and build upon previously learned concepts. Adding a new term such as "E. coli" (Escherichia coli) or "hepatitis A" will be more meaningful than a newer, broader term if a framework exists.

Nutrition educators need to spend time finding out what a person already knows, actively listening to the words he or she uses, identifying the topics in the knowledge networks, probing with the use of questions, and assisting the person with integrating new information into the existing network. Material that is organized well is much easier to learn and remember than material that is poorly organized. Our motivation to learn is intrinsic or internal as we seek to make sense of what is happening in our world.[6]

Organizing around concepts also helps the learner to categorize vast amounts of information into meaningful units. The following is an example of organizing information around the concept of meals:

Meals		
Breakfast	Lunch	Dinner
Time/place	Time/place	Time/place
Menu	Menu	Menu
Recipes/foods	Recipes/foods	Recipes/foods

Posing questions helps people learn by asking them to examine what they are hearing or reading.

When teaching about concepts, one needs to use a lot of examples. What mental picture or ideas does the client or employee have if the professional discusses "cholesterol," "saturated fatty acids," "blood glucose," "microorganisms," "grams" as a weight, "ounces" of meat, "quality improvement," and the like? Finding out what words or terminology people use in the content of their current knowledge network helps when selecting examples to use with them.

CASE ANALYSIS 3

What principles from the chapter would you use to enhance his memory of the changes you plan to tell him about?

Transfer of Learning

In human resource management as well as in other situations, the question frequently asked is "Did the training transfer?" In other words, can an individual take the knowledge, skills, attitudes, and abilities learned in the training situation, remember them, and apply them effectively on the job in a new situation or in a dissimilar one?[2,7] Transfer of learning cannot be assumed. It depends partly on the degree of similarity between the situation in which the skill or concept was learned and the situation to which it is applied. The implication is that one should teach people to handle the range of situations that they are likely to encounter most frequently at work (employees) or at home (clients). The practitioner needs to give many examples from the range of problems that the person may encounter in using the knowledge or skills learned.[12] When people actually use their new knowledge and skills to solve problems, transfer of training is confirmed.

For a client on a modified diet, for example, it is not enough to teach which foods to eat and avoid, but also how to transfer that information into planning menus, adapting current or using new recipes, choosing appropriate menu items in restaurants, and reading labels while shopping in the supermarket. Using knowledge or skills to solve problems, such as what to do in a restaurant, helps people apply what they learned. Can a person with diabetes, for example, convert the restaurant portion of a pasta serving into a serving from the exchange list or calculate the carbohydrate content? When grocery shopping, can the calories of a serving size be correctly identified?

Learning does not transfer automatically. For employees, learning is enhanced when teaching takes place in an actual or simulated environment. Cashiers, for example, need to be trained on the equipment they will be using in handling all types of transactions. When training does not transfer to the job, possible reasons are that trainees found the training irrelevant, that they did not retain it, or that the work environment or supervisor does not support the newly learned behavior.[13]

Since most people consider that it is "bad" to be wrong and "good" to be right, some people may avoid answering questions or solving problems for fear of being wrong, with the psychological discomfort this brings. The implication is that one should handle incorrect answers carefully, with every effort to preserve the person's self-image and avoid making the person feel embarrassed. If an answer is partially correct, concentrate on that part and encourage the person to elaborate more. If totally wrong, you may say, for example, "Perhaps I did not phrase my question well." Then you can rephrase it. Maintaining a relaxed atmosphere and demonstrating a nonjudgmental approach is desirable.

Andragogy

Besides behavioral and cognitive theories of learning, other theories have explored the differences between adults and children as learners. As a professional, understanding how adults learn will help you teach better. When you accept responsibility for teaching clients, patients, or employees, it is natural to think back to your own past experiences of being taught. Most educational experiences were the result of pedagogy, which may be defined as the art and science of teaching children.[13] The teacher was an authority figure, and students were dependents who complied with assignments and directions.

Adult education has challenged some of the basic ideas and approaches of pedagogy. Malcolm Knowles has focused attention on beliefs about educating adults and, instead of pedagogy, uses the term "andragogy." He maintains that the basic assumptions regarding adult learners differ from those regarding children. He sees adults as mutual partners in learning. Following are Knowles' major assumptions about adult learners[13]:

1. Adults become aware of a *need to know*. They seek to learn what they consider important, not what others think is important.

2. In adulthood, the *self-concept* changes from being a dependent learner to being a self-directed one. Adults have autonomy in the learning situation.

3. *Expanding experiences* are a growing resource for learning and can be shared with others.

4. *Readiness to learn* is based on the developmental issues in adults' lives. Learning should be relevant to their needs.

5. Adult learning is *problem-centered* rather than subject-centered, with a present-oriented focus and not a future-oriented one. Adults pursue learning that can be applied immediately to solve a problem.

6. *Adult motivation* to learn comes more from internal than from external sources.

Need to Know

Before learning something new, adults must become aware of a *need to know* about it.[7,13] They need to understand where they are now and see a need to reach a higher level of knowledge or skill. This may, for example, improve the quality of a client's health and lifestyle. For employees, it may mean that they will work more eagerly and productively.

Self-Concept

Childhood is a period of dependency. As a person matures, the *self-concept* changes, and the individual becomes increasingly independent and self-directed. Eventually, people make their own decisions and manage their lives.[7,13] Once people become adults, they prefer to be independent and self-directing in learning experiences. Any educational experience in which a person is treated as a dependent child is a threat to the self-concept. Negative feelings may result, and resentment, resistance, or anxiety will interfere with learning.

Experience

Compared with children, adults have more experiences and different kinds of *experiences* that they bring to new learning situations. This background is a resource for learning. Ignoring the adult's quantity and quality of experiences may be misinterpreted as a sign of rejection. Employees may have had previous work experience that can be built upon.

A client who has had diabetes for 5 years, for example, has a wealth of experience that should be recognized when the nutrition counselor discusses dietary changes. To ignore this prior experience and start from the beginning may annoy, bore, or possibly antagonize the client and may place obstacles in the way of the learning process. Teaching methods such as lectures are deemphasized in adult education in favor

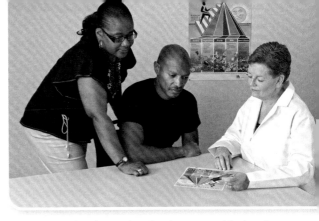

Adults are ready to learn when they have a need for learning. *Source: US Department of Agriculture.*

of more participatory methods that tap a person's wealth of experience, such as group discussion, problem-solving activities, role playing, and simulation. Practical applications that apply learning to the individual's day-to-day life are appropriate and useful.

Readiness to Learn

Readiness to learn differs for children and adults. Children are assumed to be ready to learn because there are subjects they ought to know about and there are academic pressures from teachers and parents to perform. Adults have no such pressures and are assumed to be ready to learn things required to perform their social roles in life—as spouses, employees, parents, and the like—or to cope more effectively in some aspect of their lives.

Education of adults should be appropriate to the individual's readiness or need to know something, and the timing of learning experiences needs to coincide with readiness. People seek information and are ready to learn when they are confronted by problems that they must solve. For example, new employees may be ready to learn about their job responsibilities, but not necessarily about the history of the company. Clients may not be ready to learn about dietary changes until they have accepted the fact that their medical conditions and future health require it.

Problem-Centered Learning

A child's learning is oriented toward subjects, whereas an adult's learning is oriented toward performing tasks and *solving problems.* These different approaches involve different time perspectives. Because children learn about things that they will use some time in the future, the subject matter approach may be appropriate. Adults approach learning when they have an immediate need to learn because they have a problem to solve or a task to perform. The implication is that learning should be applied to problems or projects that the person is currently dealing with. Adults learn what they want to learn when they want to learn it, regardless of what others want them to learn.

Motivation

Children are motivated primarily by external pressures from parents and teachers, by competition for grades, and the like. The more potent *motivators* for adults are internal ones, such as recognition, promotion at work, self-esteem, and the desire for a better quality of health and life.

From an examination of various educational theories, Knowles describes the appropriate conditions for learning to take place.[13] He suggests that learners should feel the need to learn something and should perceive the goals of any learning experience as their own personal goals. Before undertaking new learning, adults need to know why they need to learn it. Adults should participate actively in planning, implementing, and evaluating learning experiences to increase their commitment to learning, and the process should make use of the person's life experiences. The physical and psychological environment needs to be comfortable, as discussed in Chapter 11. The relationship between the professional and the learner should be characterized by mutual trust, respect, and helpfulness, and the environment should encourage freedom of expression and the acceptance of differences.[13]

The professional who accepts the assumptions of andragogy becomes a facilitator of learning or a change agent rather than a teacher. The practitioner involves the learner in the process of learning and provides resources for assisting learners to acquire knowledge, information, and skills, while maintaining a supportive climate for learning.

In summary, there is no single educational theory or model for practitioners to use to facilitate learning and behavioral change. However, the theory that the professional prefers will undoubtedly influence the way he or she teaches and the relationship with clients and employees. Individuals and groups are more likely to be motivated if the information presented emphasizes the personal consequences of behaviors, as mentioned in the Health Belief Model, and is appropriate to the individual's stage of change. Positive reinforcement appropriate to the needs and interests of the individual should be arranged.[1,2]

CASE ANALYSIS **4**

What would be your recommendation for follow-up?

Learning Styles and Teaching Styles

Both teaching style and learning style affect the learning process for the client or the employee.

Learning Styles

People have preferred learning styles. People's learning styles play an important role in how effectively they deal with new information. Each of us has a unique learning style and teaching style. Think for a minute about the ways you learn best or how you process and remember new information. If you recall your own school experiences, you preferred some teaching methods to others and processed and retained for a longer period of time material presented in your preferred style.

A unique learning style differentiates people in terms of preferences for content, methods of delivery, learning environment, and teaching techniques. Learning-style preferences are defined as "preferred ways of studying and learning, such as using pictures instead of text, working with other people versus alone, learning in structured or in unstructured situations, and so on."[2] Emphasis is placed on the learner and the learning environment.

Different styles of learning reflect the fact that learners differ in their preferences for and ability to process the content of various instructional messages. We perceive things through our senses. Brilliant individuals who do well learning new information from reading (visual learners), for example, may be all thumbs in a hands-on activity or experience enjoyed by others (tactile/kinesthetic learners). Some people learn well by listening to lectures, participating in group discussions, or talking things through (auditory learners, for whom their own discussion enhances remembering). These preferences influence how easy or difficult learning is for the individual, and therefore they have important implications for educators. People have been described as "hear-learners," who are thinking about the topic at hand; "see-learners"; "feel-learners," who make judgments based on feelings; and "do-learners," who prefer active experimentation.[14]

Components of style that influence learning include cognitive, affective, and environmental factors. Cognitive factors are the person's preferences in thinking and problem solving. Those who think through an experience tend more to abstract dimensions of reality. They reason and analyze what is happening. Others who sense and feel (affective) tend to prefer learning by way of more concrete, actual, hands-on experiences and are more intuitive. Some learn best by thinking through ideas; others learn best by testing theories and learn through self-discovery or by listening and sharing ideas.

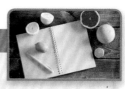

In addition to perceiving differently, people process information in different ways. Some are reflective, watching what is happening and thinking about it. Others are doers who prefer to jump right in and try. In learning to use a computer, for example, some prefer to read about it first and others just try different things. In a study environment, some require absolute silence to process information, others can block out sound, and still others prefer sound and turn on a radio or music when studying and learning. The learner's style preference may vary from situation to situation, affected by the subject matter or skill to be learned.

Learning styles are a function of personality.[7,15] One's personality can affect the preference for style of intervention. Extroverts, for example, enjoy a group environment for learning, whereas introverts prefer to listen, go away, and then try out the learning. Sensors need facts and details, whereas intuitives prefer the big picture and want to have a hand in getting there. Thinkers like brief, concise, logical information, and feelers want a way to change that will not affect themselves and others in a negative way. Judgers believe rules give structure to what they do, whereas perceivers find self-monitoring to be too structured.

Instruction can be improved and learners are likely to perform better if the professional identifies the learner's preferred learning style and makes the instructional environment compatible. Although people may have a mix of learning styles, many have a dominant style. To measure learning styles, researchers have developed a variety of inventories. Though perhaps helpful, they have been criticized for lacking reliability and validity.[2]

The instructor can attempt to diagnose the learning style by observing how people learn or by asking them questions about their preferences, such as "Do you prefer to read, to view, to listen, or to have actual experiences?" "Do you prefer to learn alone or in groups?" Whether training employees or designing adult nutrition education programs, professionals should offer new information in a variety of ways, since people learn in different ways—by thinking through ideas reflectively, by hands-on experiences, by solving problems, by experimentation, by trial and error, by viewing material, and by self-discovery. Since the preferred style varies with the situation, offering alternative techniques and methods that reflect the variety of ways in which people acquire knowledge and skills allows the learners to learn in their preferred mode at least some of the time.

CASE ANALYSIS 5

What learning style would be most successful for Mr. Richards?

Teaching Style

Teaching style is a related matter that affects learning significantly. Teaching style refers to the sum of what one does as a teacher—the preferred instructional methods, activities, organization of material, interactions with learners, and the like. People may be categorized as either teacher-centered or learner-centered.[16] The teacher-centered approach is associated more with Skinner and assumes that learners are passive and that they respond to stimuli in the environment. It is currently the predominant approach to education. In the learner-centered approach, such as Knowles' andragogy, individuals are assumed to be proactive and to take responsibility for their actions. Focus is on the learners and their needs rather than on the subject matter.

Some evidence suggests that teachers tend to select learning activities based on how they themselves prefer to learn, but instead they should be focusing on the learner's preferred style. Do you teach in the same way you were taught? Do you see yourself as the expert or as a facilitator? Good teachers seek to improve their styles through self-evaluation and adapt to the styles of learners.[17]

Educators Costa and Kallick[18] encourage the use of "16 Habits of Mind" (Box 10-1). These habits can be used by teachers and learners alike to assist in problem solving and outcome-oriented behavior. Encouraging these habits in clients with chronic disease states can be an effective action-oriented tool.

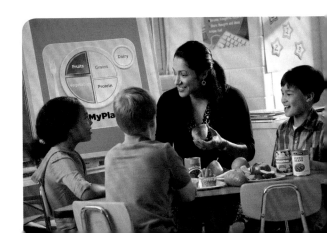

The learner-centered approach encourages active learning.
Source: US Department of Agriculture.

1. Persisting
2. Managing impulsivity
3. Listening with understanding and empathy
4. Thinking flexibly
5. Thinking about thinking (metacognition)
6. Striving for accuracy
7. Questioning and posing problems
8. Applying past knowledge to new situations
9. Thinking and communicating with clarity and precision
10. Gathering data through all senses
11. Creating, imagining, and innovating
12. Responding with wonderment and awe
13. Taking responsible risk
14. Finding humor
15. Thinking interdependently
16. Remaining open to continuous learning

Box 10-1 ■ Habits of Mind

From Costa A, Kallick B. *Learning and Leading with Habits of Mind: 16 Essential Characteristics for Success.* Alexandria, VA: Association for Supervision and Curriculum Development; 2008.

Diffusion of Innovations

The diffusion of innovations theory is important in the larger social environment of the community where people may, for example, rely on the mass media and the Internet as sources of information. This theory addresses how new ideas and practices are communicated and spread to members of the social system—in ways that may be either planned or spontaneous. The process by which adults adopt new ideas and practices, such as healthy eating patterns, involves five stages in the innovation–decision process[19]:

1. *Knowledge of the innovation.* A person becomes aware of a new idea, practice, or procedure.
2. *Persuasion.* A person forms a favorable or unfavorable attitude toward the innovation based on perceived characteristics of the innovation.
3. *Decision to adopt or reject.* A person engages in activities that lead to a choice to adopt or reject the innovation based on trial.
4. *Implementation of the new idea.* The person puts it into use.
5. *Confirmation of the decision.* A person seeks reinforcement of the decision already made and evaluates it over time.

An individual's response to nutrition labeling on foods, for example, and the USDA MyPlate food guide requires that he or she progress through a series of steps from knowledge of their existence, to forming a viewpoint about them as a source of information, deciding to adopt or reject their use, implementing and using them, through confirmation that he or she will continue with their use. Nutrition education and employee education are incomplete until stage 5 is reached. People learn only what they want to learn and adopt new behaviors to satisfy the basic needs of survival or to achieve some personal goal.

The characteristics of the innovation influence whether or not someone is persuaded in stage 2. Innovations are more readily adopted if they provide a relative advantage over current practices; if they are compatible with current beliefs, values, habits, and practices; if they are simple (degree of complexity) to understand and to use; if they can be tried (trialability); and if results can be observed (observability).[19] It may be unrealistic to expect new behaviors to be adopted from short-term educational endeavors. Short-term intervention should aim at the achievement of one or two goals for change rather than total change. The importance of a positive self-image and "self-view" is being revisited in the literature.[1]

CASE ANALYSIS 6

Develop written documentation for your session with this client. Incorporate the Nutrition Care Process model as applicable.

Technology as a Learning Tool

With new and emerging opportunities for professionals and consumers to utilize various forms of technology, such as smartphones and tablets, it is important to examine their role as a learning tool. Quintana and colleagues believe that the use of technology should be learner-centered, allowing for interaction between learners and teachers.[20] The use of a "scaffolding framework" technique in the design of software applications includes a three-tiered approach to facilitate learning. The software should allow the learner to engage in (1) sense making, (2) process management, and (3) reflection and articulation.[21]

SELF-ASSESSMENT 2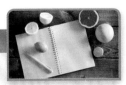

What is your experience using technology as a learning tool?

Summary

Effective education is based on theory. No single educational theory or model will facilitate learning and behavior change in all individuals; rather, an opportunity exists to adapt these theories to individual circumstances. This chapter focuses on several theories that seek to explain how people learn, including behavioral, social cognitive, and cognitive theories. These theories and the other topics explored in this chapter—andragogy, diffusion of innovations, technology as a learning aid, learning styles, teaching styles, and transfer of learning to new situations—provide dietetics practitioners with a variety of approaches to use in working with both clients and staff. A section on memory discusses how people remember new information.

Review and Discussion Questions

1. Compare and contrast the behavioral and cognitive theories of learning in terms of what is learned, the role of reinforcement, implications for use, and most suitable audiences.
2. Differentiate between the four types of consequences and their effect on behaviors.
3. What effect does the timing of reinforcement have?
4. How can you encourage persistence in a client's or employee's behavior?
5. What is modeling?
6. Can you remember today anything you learned yesterday?
7. What makes information easy for you to learn and remember?
8. What strategies enhance long-term memory?
9. How do adults differ from children as learners?
10. What steps are involved in adopting innovations?
11. What is meant by learning styles and teaching styles?

Suggested Activities

1. Match these types of consequences with the examples A through C (below):

    _____positive reinforcement

    _____negative reinforcement

    _____punishment

    A. "With the diet you are on, you should know better than to eat fried chicken and French fries."

    B. "Employees who learn the new procedures this afternoon will not have to take any work home to study this evening."

    C. "Congratulations on your success. I'm proud of you."

2. Extinction occurs as a result of which of the following?

    A. Not rewarding a response.

    B. Punishing a response.

3. According to cognitive learning theory, which of the following statements is true?

    A. Learning involves associations that are arbitrary.

    B. Learning involves specific information being organized into more generalized categories.

    C. Learning involves observing and modeling after others.

4. Cognitive educators believe that

    A. New information and knowledge should be presented in an organized fashion that considers prior knowledge.

    B. New knowledge and information should be presented separately from prior knowledge.

    C. It does not matter how new knowledge is presented as long as rewards are given.

5. Discuss in small groups each person's examples of experiences with positive reinforcement, negative reinforcement, punishment, and extinction.

6. Discuss in groups the techniques or methods that individuals use in enhancing their memories of new information.

7. Discuss in groups the different learning styles and environments people prefer for learning.

8. Role-play with a partner. One person serves as the teaching professional and the other assumes the client role. Utilize the diffusion of innovations theory for a label-reading educational session.

Planning Learning

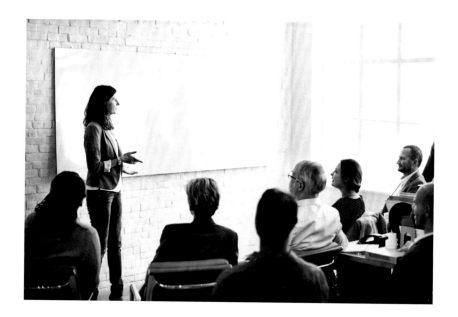

Objectives

- Differentiate between teaching and learning.
- Describe the necessary steps to planning effective educational sessions.
- Discuss the process of developing performance objectives.
- Write performance objectives using Mager's three components.
- Compare the three domains of learning and write objectives.

Paul Fisher is responsible for the school lunch program at a large urban high school with over 3,000 students. In the first 6 months on the job, he noted that some students did not eat a well-balanced diet and discarded portions of their meals, leading to a waste of food.

Before planning any nutrition education, he decides to identify what seems to be influencing students to select less healthful food choices.

If you're not sure where you're going, you're liable to end up someplace clsc.

—*Robert Mager*

Introduction

Nutrition professionals must be able to plan effective learning experiences. Globally, accredited higher education programs include competencies to prepare future practitioners for their roles in nutrition education, health promotion, and disease prevention. These include the ability to plan and deliver professional oral and written learning scenarios using current information technology while integrating appropriate planned education and behavior change theories to facilitate knowledge and skill application. Teaching is a major job responsibility of most areas of nutrition including clinical, community, education, consultation, management, and private practice.[1,2] Healthcare facilities accredited by the Joint Commission, the largest healthcare accrediting body in the United States, are required to provide the patient, family, or significant others with education specific to their needs along with medical record documentation.[3]

The primary goal of teaching is to promote learning. Learning activities occur in both individual and group scenarios. Learning locations comprise a wide array of informal and formal settings that may include inpatient or outpatient, acute or long term, assisted living and home care, public health and government programs, and health fairs and community events. Other settings may include academia, work sites, schools, health clubs, supermarkets, wellness promotion, the Internet, or other media outreach.

The learning audience comprises a wide variety of learners. These may include patients, clients, employees, parents, caregivers and family members, nurses and physicians, students, interns and residents, teachers, paraprofessionals, therapists, health department personnel, athletes, consumers, food service personnel, and the public.[3]

Managers provide learning to employees through training, continuing education, and staff development. Human resource orientation enables employees to know their job responsibilities. An employee's on-the-job performance must meet standards acceptable to the organization and requires periodic updating of knowledge and skills. It is the responsibility of the manager to ensure that training needs are recognized and met. The fact that an employee knows proper procedures, but may not always follow them, is an indication of the difficulty involved in getting a person to change.[4]

Nutrition educators teach clients and patients about normal nutrition and preventive health strategies as well as diet modifications necessitated by such medical problems as cardiovascular disease and diabetes. One day an educator may be teaching a 50-year-old man about fatty acids and cholesterol in foods, the next day teaching an 18-year-old pregnant woman about prenatal nutrition, and the next day teaching an athlete about nutritional needs before, during, and after exercise. Nutrition education cannot improve a person's health unless the results influence the purchase and consumption of foods and beverages and change eating behaviors.

The terms "teaching" and "learning" have different meanings. Some people have the mistaken notion that if they teach something, the audience or individual learns automatically and will transfer the learning to appropriate situations. An educator may explain to a pregnant woman about the United States Department of Agriculture (USDA) ChooseMyPlate food guide, tell her why it is important to use it in menu planning, and give her printed handouts. A passive learner may not participate in the learning. Individuals may be unable to connect the content of the learning process as it does not use their own food choices or menu planning. Knowledge alone cannot guarantee a change in food choices.

Teaching factual information should not be mistaken for education. The term "teaching" suggests the educator's assessment of the need for knowledge and the use of techniques to transfer knowledge to another person. Education is the process of imparting or acquiring knowledge or skills in the context of the person's total matrix of living. Education should assist people in coping with their problems and challenges as they adapt to circumstances.

Learning refers to the cognitive process through which people acquire and store knowledge, attitudes, or skills and change their behavior due to an educational experience. The change in behavior may be related to knowledge, attitudes, beliefs, values, skills, or performance.[5,6]

The principles and theories of learning are covered in Chapter 10. The purpose of this chapter is to discuss the process of planning learning as a model or framework to promote effective education.

Environment for Teaching and Learning

An educational environment has two components: the psychological environment and the physical environment. Both are important to enhancing teaching and learning.

Psychological Environment

The psychological climate for learning is important. A supportive and friendly environment with a tolerance for mistakes and a respect for individual and cultural differences makes people feel secure and welcome. Openness and encouragement of questions create a climate for learning. Address learners by their names and show respect for their opinions.

In group teaching and learning, participants should be encouraged to introduce themselves and to get to know one another at the first session. This promotes the synergy experienced by a cohort of learners. Collaboration and mutual assistance should be promoted. To promote learning, competition should be minimized to reduce feelings of anxiety. The educator who creates this informal, supportive, and caring environment for adult learners can obtain better results than one who creates a formal, authoritative environment. Many adults may not have experienced a formal learning situation outside of their early classroom education.[7-10]

Physical Environment

The physical environment should provide appropriate temperature, good lighting, ventilation, and comfortable seating to create conditions that promote learning rather than inhibit it. Noise from people talking or from the teaching setting may be distracting or interfere with a learner's attention. Everyone should be able to both see and hear each other. Facilitate interaction by seating groups of people in a circle or around a table where everyone has eye contact. Avoid seating people in rows where they only see the person's head in front of them.[11]

Steps to Effective Education

Successful educational efforts that meet the needs of the adult learner include several interactive steps. The following seven steps comprise a framework or model for planning, implementing, and evaluating learning:

1. Assessing learning needs of the individual or group (preassessment)
2. Writing performance objectives that are measurable and feasible and can be accomplished in a stated period of time considering the domains of learning

3. Determining educational content based on the learner assessment and the performance objectives

4. Selecting methods, techniques, materials, and resources appropriate to the objectives and the individual or group

5. Implementing the learning experiences (intervention) and provision of opportunities for the person to practice new information

6. Evaluating progress and outcomes performed continuously and at stated intervals, including reassessment of learning needs (postassessment)

7. Documenting the outcomes and results of education

The first three steps (steps 1–3) of planning learning are discussed in this chapter: (1) learner needs assessment, (2) performance objectives, and (3) content determination. Chapter 12 discusses the four additional steps (steps 4–7) of implementing and evaluating learning.

CASE ANALYSIS 1

List some initial methods to direct the planning and establishing of goals and objectives.

Conducting a Needs Assessment

The first step in education is to conduct a preassessment or needs assessment with the client or employee. Preassessment is a diagnostic evaluation performed by gathering data before instruction to establish a starting point. It serves to classify people regarding their current knowledge, skills, abilities, aptitudes, interests, personality, educational level, degree of literacy, age, gender, occupation, culture, lifestyle, health problem, and psychological readiness to learn (stage of change). Each person is unique.

A need for learning is the gap between what people know now and what they should know. This gap may also represent the difference between

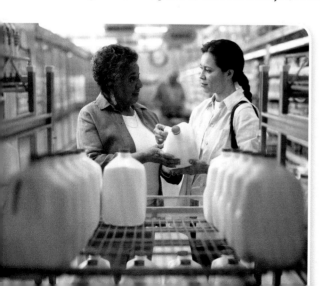

A needs assessment will compare what a person knows with what they need to know.

Source: US Department of Agriculture.

expectations of how employees should perform compared with how they actually function or perform.

$$\text{Desired knowledge, skill, attitude, or performance} - \text{Current knowledge, skill, attitude, or performance} = \text{Need for learning}$$

The goal is to assess the level of current knowledge and experience to identify the beginning level of learning content. For example, an educator counseling a client with long-term diabetes who knows how to count carbohydrates would begin the learning process at a more advanced level compared with a newly diagnosed client. It is essential to determine in advance how much the person already knows since it would waste everyone's time to repeat known information and could lead to boredom or lack of attention on the part of the learner.

The basis for educational planning is the preassessment of the client's or employee's needs balanced with what they need to know or do. Preassessment data are often a compilation of multiple sources that may include activities such as oral interviewing or records review. The initial conversation assesses the learner's intellectual and reading skills to understand the instruction.

The line of questioning should be based on what the person needs to know or would like to know. It is important to ask a variety of questions that address both a learner's self-evaluation and the educator's objective perspective of his or her knowledge.

EXAMPLE   "Have you been on a diet before?"
"What foods are good sources of potassium?"
"What is the relationship between your diet and your health?"
"Have you ever used a meat slicer before?"
"Please show me how you set tables at the restaurant where you worked previously."

Psychological preassessment is also necessary to understand the client's or employee's attitudes toward health and nutrition, willingness to change, motivation, and readiness to learn, which influence his or her behavior. Attitudes are thought to be predispositions for action and change. Despite our efforts, people often do not make the changes recommended by health professionals. Problems may not be caused by deficits in knowledge. Rather, the cause and solution may lie in the affective domain or in the individual's attitudes, values, and beliefs.[11,12]

Eating behaviors are the result of many motivations, and having nutrition information does not necessarily mean that it will be applied to better food choices. Motivation can enhance learning and behavior change as well as be a consequence of it. Extrinsic rewards—such as positive reinforcement or praise from peers, a promotion or salary increase for an employee, or a monetary incentive for participation—can influence learning. Intrinsic rewards for adults may be a better match to their learning interest. Adults tend to be highly pragmatic learners who want practical information leading to knowledge or skill about how to do something that *they* find important and valuable. The educator must identify the learner's environment, attitudes, values, and needs prior to delivering instruction.

For example, the hospitalized patient who has just learned of a confirmed diagnosis of chronic illness is likely to be more self-focused than knowledge-focused. The patient may be thinking "Why me?" "What did I do to deserve this?" "How will this affect my job? My lifestyle? My marriage?" The patient is more likely to have a longer term, rather than an immediate, need for nutrition information. A new employee may feel high levels of anxiety that may interfere with learning for the first few days on the job. Anxiety may arise whenever a superior trains a subordinate. "What does the superior think about me?" "I will appear to be dumb if I don't understand, so I had better pretend I do understand." Each of these feelings raises barriers to learning that must be recognized, reduced, or eliminated before teaching.[13-15]

In more formal situations, a preassessment questionnaire or test may be developed and administered to measure the knowledge gap. Pretest results are compared with posttest results after instruction has been completed. Preassessment is most necessary when the educator is unfamiliar with the knowledge, ability, and values of the learner. A survey questionnaire, a focus group, or a telephone interview survey may also be used.[16-19]

In the workplace, training and development programs are planned to meet current and future benchmarks of the organization. Training provides specific skills under the guidance of established personnel so that employees meet quality standards acceptable to the organization or as mandated by accreditation. Training is required on a continuous basis for both new and current employees accepting new assignments such as after a promotion or transfer.

Training needs assessment is the gap between current and desired performance: "What are the knowledge, skills, abilities, and attitudes that employees need to perform their jobs successfully?" Assessment data can be collected by directly observing the work, by structured interviewing of managers or employees about needs and problems, by seeing what is done correctly and especially what is not, by examining reports (accidents, incidents, grievances, turnover, productivity, and quality control and assurance), and by administering employee attitude surveys. This assessment deals with ends, not the means to the ends, which are determined later in the planning process.[12]

What approaches can he consider to assess the reasons why high-school students are not eating nutritiously? What information should he collect?

Developing Performance Objectives

Developing performance objectives means writing precise statements about what will be learned. They define the purpose of instruction and are helpful tools in planning, implementing, and evaluating learning. The educator needs to decide what is to be learned before selecting the optimal methods, techniques, and tools to accomplish it. The term "performance objectives" is used in this chapter, but the educational literature also interchangeably uses the terms "behavioral" and "measurable" objectives.

A well-stated performance objective communicates the intended outcome of instruction for the learner. It specifies the desired behavior or level of competence to be attained after instruction is complete. Writing performance objectives has many advantages. It results in less ambiguity regarding what is to be learned. Also, clear performance objectives make it possible to design and implement instruction, select appropriate instructional materials, and assess or evaluate whether or not the objectives are achieved. Both the teacher and the learner benefit from clearer instructions. When people know what they are supposed to learn, it does not come as a surprise. They should not be kept guessing about what should be learned or about what is important.

Objectives should focus on the person learning, not on the educator. The following objective is poorly stated: "The dietitian will teach the client about his diet." Note that this statement focuses on what the practitioner will do and not on what the client or learner will do. The following is preferred because it focuses on the client: "After instruction [when], the client [who] will be able to plan appropriate menus using the sodium-restricted diet as a reference [what]."

Mager wrote one of the most useful guides for writing performance objectives.[20] A key to writing measurable performance objectives is the selection

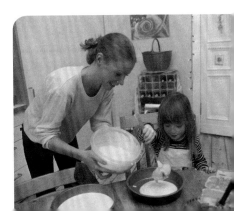

One should create an environment conducive to learning.

Source: US Department of Agriculture.

of the verb that describes the desired outcome. Some verbs are vague and subject to misinterpretation, as in the following objectives:

- To know (is able to know which foods contain potassium)
- To understand (is able to understand that foods high in potassium should be consumed daily when certain medications are prescribed)
- To appreciate (is able to appreciate the importance of following the dietary instructions)

It is not clear when using "to know" whether "knowing" means that the client will purchase foods high in potassium, be able to tell a friend which foods are high in potassium, or recognize them on a list. "Understanding" could mean being able to recall reasons, being able to read an article about it, or being able to apply knowledge to one's own situation. The meanings of "know," "understand," and "appreciate" are vague and unclear.

Instead, select verbs that describe what the person is able to do *after* learning has taken place. Note that the phrase "after learning [when], the individual [who] is able to [do what]" is understood to precede the phrase since one is describing what the person will be capable of doing. Another method involves starting with the action verb. The first two examples are rewritten from the unsatisfactory objectives in the previous list. Better verbs to use are summarized in Box 11-1 and include the following:

- To recall (is able to name five good food sources of potassium)
- To explain (is able to explain why foods high in potassium should be consumed)
- To write (is able to list the groups in the USDA myPlate)
- To compare (is able to compare the nutrient needs of an adult woman with those of a pregnant woman)
- To identify (is able to identify on the menu those foods that are permitted)
- To solve or use (is able to plan menus that include five servings of fruits and vegetables daily)
- To demonstrate (is able to demonstrate the use of the mixer or is able to select low-fat foods at the grocery store)
- To operate (is able to slice meat on the meat slicer)

Mager noted that three characteristics improve written objectives: (1) performance, (2) conditions, and (3) criterion. The "performance" tells what the learner will be able to do after an instruction is given. The second characteristic describes under what "conditions" the performance is to occur. Finally, a "criterion" tells how good the individual's performance must be to be acceptable. Table 11-1 summarizes the three-part system for writing objectives. Conditions and criterion may not be included in all objectives. In general, detailed information is important. The more that can be specified, the better the objective and the more likely that the learner will learn what was planned.[20]

CASE ANALYSIS ▸ **3**

What potential nutrition problems do you think he may have identified from what he has observed and gathered?

Verbs to Use		
Analyze	Discuss	Prepare
Apply	Distinguish	Produce
Assemble	Evaluate	Recall
Calculate	Explain	Recite
Cite	Identify	Recognize
Classify	Illustrate	Recommend
Compare	Interpret	Repair
Complete	List	Select
Construct	Measure	Solve
Contrast	Name	State
Define	Operate	Summarize
Demonstrate	Plan	Use
Describe	Practice	Write
Vague Verbs to Avoid		
Appreciate	Feel	Learn
Believe	Grasp	Like
Comprehend	Hope	Realize
Discern	Know	Understand

Box 11-1 ▪ Verbs Describing Performance

Part	Question	Client Example	Employee Example
Learner behavior	Do what?	Plans a menu for a day	Measures sanitizer in a bucket
Conditions	Under what conditions?	Given a list of permitted foods	When cleaning the work area
Criterion	How well?	With no errors	Using the exact concentration recommended

Table 11-1 ▪ Mager's Three-Part System for Objectives: Client and Employee Examples

Performance Component

The performance component of an objective describes the activity that the individual will be doing. The performance may be visible or invisible. An overt or visible performance may be seen or heard such as listing, reciting, explaining, or operating equipment. A covert or invisible performance requires that the individual be asked to do something visible or audible to determine whether the objective is satisfied and learning has taken place. In invisible performance, an "indicator behavior" is added to the objective:

- Is able to identify the parts of the meat slicer (on a diagram or verbally)
- Is able to plan a day's menu based on the USDA myPlate

Identifying is invisible until the learner is asked to identify the parts on a diagram or to recite them verbally, which are indicator behaviors. The major intent or performance should be stated using an active verb, and an indicator should be added if the performance cannot be seen or heard.

Conditions Component

Once the performance is clearly stated, it may be necessary to state whether there are specific circumstances or conditions under which the performance will be observed. The conditions describe the setting, equipment, or aids associated with the behavior. With what resources will the individual be provided? What will be withheld? Conditions are in parentheses in the following examples:

- (Given the disassembled parts of a meat slicer) is able to reassemble the parts in correct sequence.
- (Given a standard menu) is able to calculate the appropriate carbohydrate in the foods.
- (Given a list of foods including both good and poor sources of potassium) is able to identify the good sources.
- (Given a standard menu) is able to select low-sodium foods for a complete day.
- (Without looking at the diet instruction form) is able to describe an appropriate dinner menu.
- (Without the assistance of the practitioner) is able to explain the foods a pregnant woman should eat on a daily basis.

Although every objective may not have conditions, there should be enough information to make it clear exactly what performance is expected.

Criterion Component

A criterion may be added once the end performance and the conditions, if any, under which it will be observed are described. The criterion describes a level of achievement measuring how well the individual should be able to perform. Possible standards for measuring performance include speed, accuracy, quality, and percentage of correct answers.[21] A time limit can be used to describe the speed criterion. The following are examples:

- Is able to set a table (in 8 minutes or less)
- Is able to reassemble the meat slicer (in 5 minutes or less)
- Is able to complete a diet history (in 20 minutes)

For objectives that require the development of skill over a period of time, one must determine how much time is reasonable in the initial learning period as opposed to the time when the skill is well developed. A new employee cannot be expected to perform a task as rapidly as an experienced person.

When the person is expected to perform with a degree of accuracy, include this in the objective. Accuracy should communicate how well the person needs to perform for his or her performance to be considered competent. Examples include the following:

- Is able to set five tables (with no errors)
- Is able to identify good sources of potassium (with 80% accuracy), when given a list of foods including both good and poor sources
- Is able to plan a menu for a complete day (with no errors) when given a copy of a sodium-restricted diet
- Is able to calculate the carbohydrate in the diabetic diet (within 5 g)

Performance objectives should also indicate a quality indicator to assess what constitutes an acceptable performance. It is easier to communicate quality when objective standards are available to both the individual and the practitioner. Any acceptable deviation from the standards can then be determined. The following are examples of such standards:

- Is able to reassemble the meat slicer (according to the steps in the task analysis)
- Is able to measure the amount of sanitizer (according to the directions on the label of the container)
- Is able to substitute foods on a diabetic menu (using carbohydrate counting)
- Is able to pass the Commission on Dietetics Registration's credentialing examination (by attaining at or above the set criterion score)

CASE ANALYSIS **4**

Using one or more of the potential nutrition problems you identified in the prior case analysis exercise, write a performance objective.

Performance objectives are clear and measurable when they include the essential component of performance and optional components of condition and criterion to clarify quantity and quality.

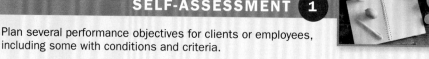

SELF-ASSESSMENT 1

Plan several performance objectives for clients or employees, including some with conditions and criteria.

Domains of Learning

Learning can be organized into domains, taxonomies, or classification systems to focus on precision in writing. There are three basic domains of objectives: (1) cognitive (knowledge), (2) affective (attitudes and values), and (3) psychomotor (skills). Each is a hierarchy from the simple to the complex. Figure 11-1 shows their interrelationship.

Cognitive Domain

The cognitive domain involves the acquisition and utilization of knowledge or information and the development of intellectual skills and abilities. A taxonomy of educational performance objectives in the cognitive domain,

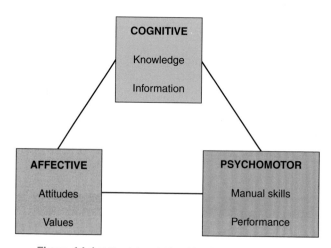

Figure 11-1 ■ The interrelationship of objectives.

published by Bloom and colleagues,[21-23] includes six major levels or categories and a number of subcategories:

1.0 KNOWLEDGE

    1.1 Knowledge of specifics

    1.2 Knowledge of ways and means of dealing with specifics

    1.3 Knowledge of the universals and abstractions in a field

2.0 COMPREHENSION

    2.1 Translation

    2.2 Interpretation

    2.3 Extrapolation

3.0 APPLICATION

4.0 ANALYSIS

    4.1 Analysis of elements

    4.2 Analysis of relationships

    4.3 Analysis of organizational principles

5.0 SYNTHESIS

    5.1 Production of a unique communication

    5.2 Production of a plan, or proposed set of operations

    5.3 Derivation of a set of abstract relations

6.0 EVALUATION

    6.1 Judgments in terms of internal evidence

    6.2 Judgments in terms of external criteria

The levels or categories are arranged in a hierarchy from simple to complex, from concrete to more abstract. The objectives in any one level are likely to be built on the behaviors in the previous level. The subcategories help to further define the major headings and make them more specific.

The educator needs to think beyond the simplest levels of knowledge and strive to write objectives at higher, more complex levels. Without examining the possibility of writing higher-level objectives, educators may tend to think only in terms of knowledge and comprehension, which are the easiest objectives to write (and learn). The learner may then be denied the opportunity of applying knowledge or using it in problem solving and will be reduced to memorizing facts. In nutrition education, for example, knowing facts is necessary at the lowest level (knowledge). Higher-level objectives will include the ability to analyze food labels, to synthesize all information learned so knowledge can be shared, and to evaluate nutrition information in making wise food choices. In the following discussion of the six levels in the taxonomy, examples of objectives are given.

Knowledge

At the lowest level in the cognitive domain, knowledge involves remembering information without necessarily understanding it. This includes the recall of specific bits of information, terminology, and facts, such as dates, events, and places, chronologic sequences, methods of inquiry, trends over time, processes, classification systems, criteria, principles, and theories. Table 11-2 suggests verbs describing performance in the cognitive domain.

> **EXAMPLE** Is able to list foods high in sodium.

Comprehension

The second level, comprehension, is the lowest level of understanding. It involves knowing what is communicated by another person and being able to use the information communicated. The use of information may include restatement or paraphrase, interpretation, summarization or rearrangement of the information, and extrapolation or extension of the given information to determine implications or consequences.

> **EXAMPLE** Is able to explain (verbally or in writing) why certain foods are not recommended on the diabetic diet.

Level	Verbs to Use
Knowledge	Cites, defines, describes, identifies, labels, lists, matches, memorizes, names, outlines, recalls, recites, repeats, reproduces, selects, states
Comprehension	Converts, defends, discusses, distinguishes, estimates, explains, generalizes, gives examples, paraphrases, predicts, recognizes, rewrites, selects, summarizes, translates
Application	Applies, assembles, calculates, changes, computes, demonstrates, designs, manipulates, modifies, operates, plans, practices, prepares, produces, shows, solves, translates, uses
Analysis	Analyzes, compares, differentiates, discriminates, distinguishes, identifies, illustrates, interprets, investigates, outlines, relates, researches, separates, solves, studies
Synthesis	Assembles, categorizes, classifies, combines, compiles, composes, creates, designs, diagnoses, explains, formulates, generates, manages, organizes, plans, recommends, revises, rewrites, summarizes, writes
Evaluation	Appraises, assesses, compares, concludes, contrasts, criticizes, critiques, discriminates, evaluates, judges, justifies

Table 11-2 ■ Verbs Describing Performance—Cognitive

Application

At the level of application, a person is able to use information, principles, concepts, or ideas in concrete situations. Knowledge is understood sufficiently to be able to apply it to solve a problem.

> **EXAMPLE**   Is able to plan a sodium-restricted menu for the day.

Analysis

Analysis entails the breakdown of information into its parts to identify the elements, the interaction between elements, and the organizing principles or structure. Relationships may be made among ideas.

> **EXAMPLE**   Is able to analyze the nutrition labeling on a food product for fat content.

Synthesis

Synthesis requires the reassembling of elements or parts to form something new. You may assemble a unique verbal or written communication, a plan of operation, or a set of abstract relations to explain data.

> **EXAMPLE**   Is able to explain the low-cholesterol diet accurately to a friend.

Evaluation

At the highest level in the cognitive taxonomy, evaluation is the ability to judge the value of materials or methods in a particular situation. Such judgment requires the use of criteria, which may be internal criteria, such as logical accuracy or consistency, or external criteria, such as external standards.

> **EXAMPLE**   Is able to evaluate a nutrition article from the daily newspaper.

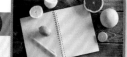

Plan several performance objectives in the cognitive domain on a similar topic.

Affective Domain

The affective domain deals with changes in attitudes, feelings, values, beliefs, appreciation, and interests. Often, the educator wants the learner not only to comprehend what to do but also to value it, accept it, and find it important. Attitudes and beliefs about food are widely recognized as important determinants of a person's food choices. We want people to value good nutrition and select healthful foods. When imparting information fails to bring about behavior change, the common response is to redouble efforts to teach facts and explain why something should be done. Instead, an examination of the person's attitudes and values should be pursued.

The affective domain involves a process of internalization from least committed to most committed. It categorizes the inner growth that occurs as people become aware of, and later adopt, the attitudes and principles that assist in forming the value judgments that guide their conduct. A learning goal for a pregnant woman would be to attain a level of basic knowledge (cognitive domain) about the proper foods to eat during pregnancy, but also to value the knowledge so much (affective domain) that she eats nutritious foods and practices good nutrition. Note that an objective in one domain may have a component in another. Cognitive objectives may have an affective component, and affective objectives may have a cognitive one.

Affective objectives are more nebulous and resist precise definition; therefore, evaluation of their achievement is more difficult. The practitioner may find it a formidable task to describe affective behaviors involving internal feelings and emotions, but they are as important as overt behaviors. Because affective objectives are more difficult to express, most written objectives express cognitive behaviors.

Krathwohl and colleagues[24] have published a taxonomy of educational objectives in the affective domain. It includes five major levels with subcategories:

1.0 RECEIVING (ATTENDING)

    1.1 Awareness

    1.2 Willingness to receive

    1.3 Controlled or selected attention

2.0 RESPONDING

    2.1 Acquiescence in responding

2.2 Willingness to respond

2.3 Satisfaction in response

3.0 VALUING

3.1 Acceptance of a value

3.2 Preference for a value

3.3 Commitment

4.0 ORGANIZATION

4.1 Conceptualization

4.2 Organization of a value system

5.0 CHARACTERIZATION BY A VALUE OR VALUE COMPLEX

5.1 Generalized set

5.2 Characterization

The ordering of levels describes a process by which a value progresses from a state of mere awareness or perception to the status of greater complexity until it becomes an internal part of one's outlook on life that guides or controls behavior. This internalization may occur in varying degrees and may involve conformity and high commitment or nonconformity. At higher levels, behavior may be so ingrained that it is unconscious rather than a conscious response. Responses may be produced consistently in the absence of external authorities and in spite of barriers. Thus, a client may eventually select healthful foods or an employee may wash his or her hands without thinking about it at the conscious level. Table 11-3 suggests verbs describing performance in the affective domain.

Level	Verbs to Use
Receiving	Asks, attends, chooses, describes, follows, gives, identifies, listens, replies, selects, uses
Responding	Answers, assists, complies, conforms, cooperates, discusses, helps, participates, performs, practices, presents, reads, recites, reports, responds, selects, tells, writes
Valuing	Completes, describes, differentiates, explains, follows, imitates, joins, justifies, participates, proposes, reads, selects, shares, supports
Organization	Accepts, adheres, alters, arranges, combines, compares, defends, discusses, explains, generalizes, identifies, integrates, modifies, organizes, prefers, relates, synthesizes
Characterization	Acts, advocates, communicates, discriminates, displays, exemplifies, influences, performs, practices, proposes, questions, selects, serves, supports, uses, verifies

Table 11-3 ■ Verbs Describing Performance—Affective

Receiving

At the lowest level of the affective domain, the learner is willing to receive certain phenomena or stimuli. Receiving represents a willingness to attend to what the teacher is presenting. The person may move from a passive level of awareness or consciousness to a neutral willingness to tolerate the situation rather than to avoid it and then to an active level of controlled or selected attention despite distractions.

> **EXAMPLE**   Is able to focus attention on instructions on a diabetic diet.

Responding

The second level is responding, which indicates a desire on the part of the learner to become involved in, or committed to, a subject or activity. At the lowest level of responding, the client or employee may passively acquiesce, or at least comply, in response to the professional or manager. At a higher level, a willingness to respond or voluntarily make a commitment to a chosen response is evident. Finally, a feeling of satisfaction or pleasure in response involves internalization on the part of the learner.

> **EXAMPLE**   Is willing to read diet materials with interest and ask questions.

Valuing

At the third level, valuing, the learner believes that the information or behavior has worth. The person values it based on a personal assessment. When the value has been slowly internalized or accepted, the client or employee displays a behavior consistent with the value. When something is valued, motivation is not based on external authorities or the desire to obey, but on an internal commitment. The learner will then demonstrate acceptance of a value, preference for a value, or commitment and conviction.

> **EXAMPLE**   Is able to select a nutritious meal from the cafeteria line.

Organization

At the level of organization, the learner discovers situations in which more than one value is appropriate. Individual values are incorporated into a total network of values, and at the level of conceptualization, a person relates new values to those he or she already holds. New values must be organized into an ordered relationship with the current value system. Perhaps a client has previously valued eating whatever he or she wants. Now the client has to learn a new value (different foods) and change an old one (some of the current eating choices).

> **EXAMPLE** Is able to discuss plans for making different, healthful food choices.

Characterization

The highest level, characterization, indicates that the learner has internalized the values for a sufficient time to control behavior and acts consistently over time. A generalized set is a predisposition to act or perceive events in a certain way. At the highest level of internalization, beliefs or ideas are integrated with internal consistency.

> **EXAMPLE** Is able to select only those foods permitted on the diet at almost all times.

Behavioral change in the affective domain takes place gradually over a period of time, whereas cognitive change may occur more rapidly. Affective change may take days, weeks, months, or years at the higher levels.

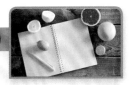

SELF-ASSESSMENT 3

Plan a performance objective for each level in the affective domain on a similar topic.

Psychomotor Domain

The psychomotor domain involves the development of physical abilities and skills. Knowledge and attitudes are interrelated and may be necessary to perform these skills. For example, a person cannot drive a car or operate a meat slicer (tasks requiring manual skills) without some basic knowledge of the equipment. Table 11-4 suggests verbs describing performance at the various levels of the psychomotor domain. The performance of physical ability proceeds to increasingly complex steps. Following are Simpson's

Level	Verbs to Use
Perception	Attends, observes, perceives, recognizes, watches
Set	Demonstrates, positions, prepares, senses, touches, uses
Guided response	Calculates, computes, cuts, imitates, performs, practices, repeats, replicates, tries
Mechanism	Assembles, calibrates, cleans, disassembles, operates, performs, practices, prepares, repairs, uses, washes
Complex overt response	Cooks, demonstrates, executes, interviews, masters, performs
Adaptation	Adapts, changes, develops, modifies, organizes, produces, solves
Origination	Instructs, operates, originates, uses

Table 11-4 ■ Verbs Describing Performance—Psychomotor

seven levels and selected subcategories; there are other similar psychomotor domain category systems[25,26]:

1.0 PERCEPTION
    1.1 Sensory stimulation
        1.1.1 Auditory
        1.1.2 Visual
        1.1.3 Tactile
        1.1.4 Taste
        1.1.5 Smell
        1.1.6 Kinesthetic
    1.2 Cue selection
    1.3 Translation
2.0 SET
    2.1 Mental set
    2.2 Physical set
    2.3 Emotional set
3.0 GUIDED RESPONSE
    3.1 Imitation
    3.2 Trial and error
4.0 MECHANISM

5.0 COMPLEX OVERT RESPONSE
    5.1 Resolution of uncertainty
    5.2 Automatic performance
6.0 ADAPTATION
7.0 ORIGINATION

Perception

The lowest level of the psychomotor domain is perception. It involves becoming aware of objects by means of the senses—hearing, seeing, touching, tasting, and smelling—and by muscle sensations or activation. The learner must select which cues to respond to in order to perform a task and then must mentally translate the cues received for action.

> **EXAMPLE** Is able to recognize a need to learn how to use the meat slicer.

Set

Set is the second level and suggests a readiness for performing a task. This may involve mental readiness to start the task, physical readiness to correct body positioning to accomplish the task, and emotional readiness by having a favorable attitude or willingness to learn the task.

> **EXAMPLE** Is able to position oneself to use the meat slicer.

Guided Response

The third level of the psychomotor domain is guided response. The professional or trainer guides the employee during the activity by emphasizing the individual components of a more complex skill. The subcategories include imitation of the practitioner, trial and error, and feedback until the task can be performed accurately. Performance at this level may initially be crude and imperfect.

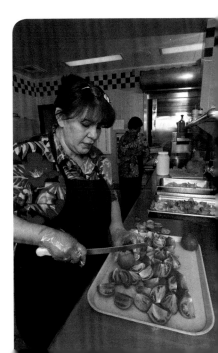

Objectives for learning should be planned around what the employee needs to know and do.

Source: US Department of Agriculture.

> **EXAMPLE**   Is able to practice the steps in using the meat slicer under supervision.

Mechanism

Mechanism, the fourth level, refers to habitual response. At this stage, the learner demonstrates an initial degree of proficiency in performing the task, which results from some practice.

> **EXAMPLE**   Is able to use the meat slicer properly.

Complex Overt Response

The fifth level, complex overt response, suggests that a level of skill has been attained over time in performing the task. Work is performed smoothly and efficiently without error. Two subcategories are resolution of uncertainty, in which a task is performed without hesitation, and automatic performance. Performance is characterized by accuracy, control, and speed.

> **EXAMPLE**   Is able to demonstrate considerable skill in using the meat slicer with a variety of foods.

Adaptation and Origination

Adaptation requires altering manual skills in new but similar situations, such as in adapting slicing procedures to a variety of different foods on the meat slicer. The final level, origination, refers to the creation of a new physical act, such as slicing something that has not been done before.

An understanding of the psychomotor domain, which may be helpful to recall the process of learning to drive an automobile: responding to the physical and visual stimulation, feeling mentally and emotionally ready to drive, learning parallel parking by trial and error under the guidance of an instructor, developing a degree of skill, and finally starting the car and driving without having to think of the steps. With time, sufficient skill is developed so that the person can adapt quickly to new situations on the road and create new responses automatically.

SELF-ASSESSMENT   **4**

Plan a performance objective for each level in the psychomotor domain in a similar subject area.

Determining the Content of Learning Plans

A close examination of the learning objectives helps to identify the content of the learning plan. Each objective states what the learner will be able to do when instruction is complete and defines the content to be taught. The preassessment may have eliminated certain objectives as unnecessary; those that remain are used in planning content.

Using the taxonomies ensures that the objectives of learning are applied to the needs of the learner. Some people may need to start at the lowest level in the taxonomy, whereas those who have already mastered the lower level objectives are ready for those at higher levels. The taxonomies assist the educator in thinking of higher levels of knowledge that may be more appropriate for the learner. They also serve to remind the educator that there are interrelationships among the three domains. Although clients can plan menus using their diets, it is also important they think that the food choices are important enough to their health to follow them. Employees need not only to know proper sanitation procedures but also to value them if they are going to practice optimum sanitary procedures regularly.

CASE ANALYSIS 5

What approaches to nutrition education might he try with high-school students eating lunch in the cafeteria? Using the performance objective you wrote, what domain(s) of learning should be used in the learning plan?

Organizing Learning Groups

Learning may take place individually or in groups. Groups are advantageous in that they save time and money and provide opportunities for people to share experiences. Those who are successful in making dietary changes can model behaviors and discuss information with those who have been unsuccessful in coping. The more complex the information to be learned, the greater is the need to discuss it in groups. However, an experienced employee who needs to be trained in a new technique would derive greater benefit from an individual non–group-focused learning plan that does not waste time reviewing steps he or she has already mastered.

Even when a single learner is involved, the educator should consider whether or not other learners should also be present. In nutrition counseling and education, the individual responsible for purchasing the food and preparing the meals should be present. When a child is placed on a modified diet, such as a diabetic diet, usually the mother or caregiver requires instruction as well, since her cooperation is essential to the child's successful adherence to the diet and management of the disease.

The preassessment should show differences in knowledge levels and should assist in making grouping decisions. Frequently, all new employees are grouped together for initial orientation and training. This is an example of grouping by similar learning needs rather than by age, educational level, amount of experience, or job title. Grouping by general learning content often requires division into more than one learning group based on employees' job content and application. Wait staff, for example, may require sessions on sanitary dish and utensil handling, whereas cooks may need classes on sanitary food handling.

Another consideration is whether supervisors should be taught in the same classes as their employees. One disadvantage of such a grouping is that the employees may be reluctant to participate by asking questions when the superior is present. Setting the size of the group will affect the learning plan. Larger groups of 30 to 50 or more will decrease the ability for individual participation compared with small groups of 10 to 15.[11,12,27]

Summary

This chapter has explored the initial steps in planning learning. After needs assessment has been completed, performance objectives should be written in the cognitive, affective, and psychomotor domains. Decisions need to be made about whether learning should be organized by individuals or groups. The content of instruction is determined from an examination of the objectives. The steps taken to plan learning will increase the effectiveness of the learning process. Chapter 12 explores the remaining steps in the framework for education.

Review and Discussion Questions

1. How do you define teaching and learning?
2. What are the three parts of Mager's learning objectives? What question does each answer?
3. What are the three domains of learning objectives? What are the levels in each domain?
4. How are the objectives in the three domains interrelated?
5. What training topics would be appropriate for food service employees in the three domains? For healthcare educators?
6. What are some guidelines for arranging physical and psychological environments?
7. What are the steps to education?
8. What are the reasons for conducting a preassessment or needs assessment?

Suggested Activities

1. Make a list of questions you would ask in the preassessment of knowledge of some subject with which you are familiar.
2. Write three performance objectives using active verbs to describe behavior.
3. Write examples of performance objectives containing conditions and a criterion.
4. Write examples of objectives in various levels of the cognitive, affective, and psychomotor domain. Note overlap from one domain to another.
5. Decide which of the following performance objectives are measurable:
   A. Presented with a menu, the client will be able to circle appropriate food selections according to his or her diet.

B. At the close of the series of classes, the clients will be more positively disposed toward following their diets.

C. After counseling, the client will know which foods he or she should eat and which not to eat.

D. The client will be able to explain the diabetic diet to her husband.

6. Examine the following objectives and decide whether each concerns primarily the cognitive, affective, or psychomotor domain.

A. All dishwashing staff will be able to complete the meal service cleanup within 1 hour of close of service.

B. Given a series of objectives, the student will be able to classify them according to the taxonomies in the chapter.

C. At the end of the session, clients will request more weight control classes.

CHAPTER 12

Implementing and Evaluating Learning

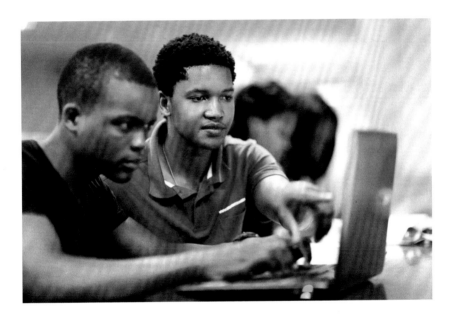

Objectives

- Explain the advantages and disadvantages of various educational methods and techniques.
- Discuss the educational methods and techniques appropriate in the cognitive, affective, and psychomotor domains.
- Compile a task analysis.
- List the ways in which instruction can be organized and sequenced.

- Identify the purposes of an educational evaluation.
- Explain several types of evaluation.
- Prepare a lesson plan.
- Compare and contrast formative and summative evaluations, norm-referenced and criterion-referenced evaluations, and reliability and validity.
- Plan, implement, and evaluate an educational presentation for a specific target audience.

Susan Grey, RD, has decided that there is a need for prenatal nutrition classes in the outpatient clinic. Many of the patients are teenagers with limited incomes who are on suboptimum diets. The clinic nurse is also interested in cooperating to reduce the time she spends in individual counseling with patients.

I hear and I forget, I see and I remember, I do and I understand.

—*Confucius*

Introduction

How does the educator or trainer successfully educate clients and employees? With clients, the practitioner seeks to promote health and reduce the risk of chronic disease. With employees, the manager seeks to enhance their ability to do their jobs. The initial three steps in planning learning, as discussed in Chapter 11, include a preassessment of the learner's current knowledge and competencies; the development of performance objectives in the cognitive, affective, and psychomotor domains; and the determination of educational content based on the performance objectives.

This chapter continues with the discussion of the implementation and evaluation of the learning plan. The final four steps begin with the selection of appropriate learning activities for the cognitive, affective, and psychomotor domains. These planned learning activities are implemented along with opportunities to apply theory through application and practice. An evaluation of the outcomes of learning is then completed, and if necessary, an evaluation is repeated at intervals to assure mastery of the learning plan. Finally, documentation of the educational process is completed.

Selecting Techniques and Methods

Various techniques and methods of educational presentation are available to deliver the learning plan to the audience. Techniques are the ways that the instructor organizes and presents information to learners to promote the internal processes of learning.[1] They establish a relationship between the teacher and the learner and between the learner and what he or she is learning. These include activities such as lectures, discussions, simulations, and demonstrations. All are not equally effective in facilitating learning, and each has its advantages and disadvantages, and uses and limitations as summarized in Table 12-1.

Teaching Method	Strengths	Weaknesses
Lecture	Easy and efficient. Conveys most information. Reaches large numbers. Minimum threat to learner. Maximum control by instructor.	Learner is passive. Learning by listening. Formal atmosphere. May be dull, boring. Not suited for higher-level learning in cognitive domain. Not suited for manual learning.
Discussion (e.g., panel, debate, case study)	More interesting, thus motivating. Active participation. Informal atmosphere. Broadens perspectives. We remember what we discuss. Good for higher-level cognitive, affective objectives.	Learner may be unprepared. Shy people may not discuss. May get side-tracked. More time-consuming. Size of group limited.
Projects	More motivating. Active participation. Good for higher-level cognitive objectives.	Size of group limited.
Laboratory experiments	Learn by experience. Hands-on method. Active participation. Good for higher-level cognitive objectives.	Requires space, time. Group size limited.
Simulation (e.g., scenarios, in-basket, role-playing, critical incidents)	Active participation. Requires critical thinking. Develops problem-solving skills. Connects theory and practice. More interesting. Good for higher-level cognitive and affective objectives.	Time-consuming. Group size limited unless on computer.
Demonstration	Realistic visual image. Appeals to several senses. Can show a large group. Good for psychomotor domain.	Requires equipment. Requires time. Learner is passive, unless can practice.

Table 12-1 ■ Strengths and Weaknesses of Teaching Methods

In deciding on the method that will be most effective, the instructor may be guided by several factors. These may include the educational purpose, learner preference or style, learner needs, group size, facilities available, time available, cost, and one's previous experience or the degree of success with the techniques. One must consider what is effective for different populations, such as those from different cultural and ethnic groups, socioeconomic groups, educational and literacy levels, and age groups so that desired outcomes are reached.[2]

The domain of the performance objectives may suggest which approach is most appropriate since methods and techniques differ for cognitive, affective, and psychomotor domains. All factors being equal, the practitioner should select the technique that requires the most active participation of the learner and includes strategies for effective behavioral change. Studies show that the more actively a person is involved in the learning process, the better the retention.[3] Figure 12-1 shows that reading and hearing information are not as productive as both seeing and hearing or, better yet, discussing information or doing something with it.

Lectures

The lecture is the presentation technique that is most familiar to people. It is a traditional passive method of informing and transferring knowledge—the lowest level in the cognitive domain—from the teacher to the learner. It is especially useful in situations with a large number of learners, a great deal

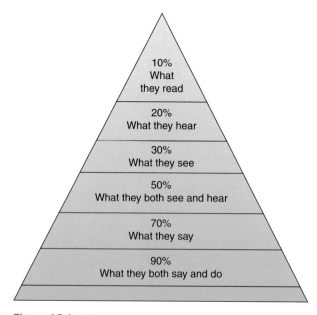

Figure 12-1 ■ What people remember.

of information to be communicated, and a limited amount of available time.[4] Examples are a class on sanitation for food service employees or on cholesterol and fat in relation to heart disease for work site employees or medical center clients.

In spite of the advantages of efficiency, a major drawback of lectures is that there is no guarantee that the material is learned and remembered or that food choices and eating behaviors will change. This is because the individual is a passive participant whose learning depends on listening skills. Lecture may be the least effective technique for use with adults.

Although well-educated people may respond positively to lectures because of long experience with this approach, those with less education or those from other cultures may learn better with other methods.[5] Their attention to lectures may wane quickly as they tune out, especially if the lecturer is not an effective speaker or if the lecture is dull. Lectures seldom meet the requirements of adult education because they lack self-directed learning and problem-solving approaches. Lectures are improved by limiting the number of concepts presented, using examples and summaries frequently, and adding focused visual aids. Lectures can become more interactive by providing ample time for interactive discussion along with written handouts to reinforce what was heard.

Discussion

Discussion tends to promote active participation by learners. This technique can be used on a one-on-one basis or in a group. Interactive discussion helps participants to examine their own thinking and internalize knowledge through the exchange of ideas and verbal responses. The instructor can guide the discussion by raising open-ended questions, posing problems, or highlighting key issues so that clients or employees make comparisons or work to draw conclusions.

Group discussion is greater when the participants are fairly well acquainted or have a common interest. With a series of classes on weight reduction, for example, clients could discuss and share what they have done to change their food choices, recipes, and shopping habits. The basis for discussion may be common experiences, written case studies, or topics that were preannounced so that the group can interact. For best results, seating should be arranged in a circle so that everyone can see and hear other participants. The instructor should facilitate but not dominate the discussion. Smaller groups of 10 to 15 people offer more opportunity for participation as learners explore their thoughts, values, and experiences; think critically; and influence others.

Facilitated discussions, such as those presented by debates and panels, may be more appropriate for a large group. In this scenario, the educator should plan content and discussion topics that attract the audience's listening interest, although very few learners may actually get a chance to actively participate due to time and group size constraints.

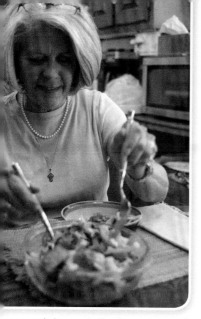

A demonstration is one approach to presentations.

Source: CDC/Amanda Mills.

Discussion is more time-consuming than lecture, but it can be more interesting for learners, and thus more motivating. The learning plan should include higher level cognitive and affective objectives. The key points raised in the discussion should be summarized intermittently by the instructor to increase the learner's acquisition and retention of information since we remember what we say out loud.[6]

Simulation

Simulations of real-life situations are active ways to develop learner knowledge, skills, behaviors, and competencies. Several means of representation may be used such as scenarios, "in-basket" exercises, critical incidents, and role-playing. These methods involve learning by actively doing something—in other words, experiential learning rather than learning by listening or watching. Active learner involvement enhances optimum transfer of learning.[7]

Simulation may be based on scenarios or models of real-life problem situations. Clients on sodium-restricted diets, for example, could look at restaurant menus and determine what they should order. Learners use a process of inquiry in exploring a problem and developing decision-making and evaluative skills. Food service employees could discuss food temperatures and Hazard Analysis Critical Control Points procedures through preparation, holding, service, and leftovers.[8]

In-basket exercises test the person's ability to handle day-to-day challenges. The instructor can describe a critical incident by providing written memos, notes, requests, or reports to simulate a supervisor's decision-making ability in handling problems that arrive in the in-basket on the desk each day. Simulated emergencies such as fires and electrical blackouts or unusual incidents can be used. The learner has to provide a solution in handling the situation or problem.

Role-playing, in which two or more people dramatize assigned parts or roles simulating real-life situations, is another possibility. Role-playing allows learners to practice new behaviors in relatively safe environments, and it can be used to work through real problems. Role-playing is followed by a discussion of the problem, ideas, feelings, and emotional reactions such as the handling of an employee disciplinary problem or learning to say no when offered disallowed foods. Though time-consuming, simulations may be helpful in providing opportunities for individuals to make a connection between theory and practice, to engage in critical thinking as active participants, and to develop problem-solving and coping skills. Simulation may be used with cognitive, affective, and psychomotor objectives.[1,9]

Demonstration

A demonstration may be used to show how something is done or to explore processes, procedures, equipment operation, techniques, ideas, or attitudes. This technique is used to combine knowledge and skill with cognitive and psychomotor objectives. Learning to prepare low-fat recipes and learning how to use a meat slicer are examples of instances in which demonstration is appropriate. Usually, the learner observes as the instructor makes the presentation or models the skill, although a participant volunteer may be used. The demonstration may be a dramatic learning experience if it holds the individual's attention and may be appropriate for any type of learning objective.[10]

If skills are demonstrated, the person will need ample opportunity to practice the task or skill soon after and evaluate the performance after passively watching the instructor. Job instruction training (JIT), discussed later in this chapter, is an example of the use of demonstration to achieve mastery.

Visual and Audio-Assisted Instruction

According to an old Chinese proverb, "one picture is worth more than 1,000 words." An effective media presentation can enhance learning by providing variety and improving memory through visual and audio stimulation. Self-directed and instructor-directed computer programs can be used with a wide variety of learners when matched to the learning situation. An audiotape can be used to hear language or dialogue. A videotape could illustrate an unfamiliar setting or piece of equipment. The newest vehicles for delivering innovative training include podcasting, cell phones, computer-interactive videoconferencing, and other electronic devices. Media is considered an adjunct to learning and should not be considered the total learning experience.[11,12] (Chapter 14 discusses media in more detail.)

CASE ANALYSIS ❶

Develop a lesson plan for the prenatal nutrition class. Which teaching method(s) would you select for this audience?

Techniques for Different Domains of Learning

For learning in the cognitive domain, most of the preceding techniques may be effective. There are additional factors to consider in fostering learning in the affective and psychomotor domains. Because learners represent different learning styles, there is an advantage to using mixed methods rather than only one method.[1,13]

In the affective domain, the educator seeks to influence the learner's interests, attitudes, beliefs, and values. This requires ongoing contacts rather than a single session. At the lowest level in the affective domain, receiving and awareness, audiovisual materials or guided discussion can begin to present the relationship between food choices and obesity. At higher levels, where the adoption of new attitudes and values is important, the individual must participate more fully in discussion of food choice options. Commitments that are made public are more likely to be adopted than those that are kept private, and attitudes are acquired through interpersonal influences.[14]

Using multiple instructional strategies that influence deeper level learning of nutrition and the modification of attitudes is more likely to promote behavior change. Promoting the active involvement of participants and interpersonal interaction in a group can help. Different types and dimensions of these techniques can address the variety of learning styles more effectively than a single teaching method.

The problem-solving process in which the instructor presents a puzzling situation or problem is an example of multiple-step learning. The learner or learner group may be asked to calculate the daily fat or sodium allowance from food labels. The steps require the learner to identify and clarify the problem, form hypotheses, gather data, analyze and interpret data, select possible solutions, test solutions, and finally draw conclusions and select the best solution to the problem. People learn how to solve problems, evaluate possible solutions, and think critically. Clients can be guided through this process so that they learn to solve their own nutrition problems.[3,10,14]

Modeling is also a method of influencing a person's behavior. People learn by observing others and then imitating them in unfamiliar or new situations. The teacher should behave as the learner is expected to behave, modeling the desirable attitude or behavior. People are more likely to accept new behaviors, such as healthful food choices or routine hand washing, when they meet and have discussions with people who have successfully adopted them.[15]

Skills in the psychomotor domain are learned with direct experience and practice over time. The instructor may begin with a demonstration, but then the learner needs to practice the skill under supervision. "Coaching" is a term that describes the assistance given to someone learning a new skill; it can apply to an educational experience as well as a sport. Coaching suggests a one-on-one, continuous, supportive relationship from which a person learns over time. It is perhaps the best method for on-the-job training of employees. After the demonstration, the trainer can give encouragement, promote confidence, and offer guidance as the trainee performs the task. Coaching takes into consideration different learning abilities and needs, allows actual practice, and provides people with immediate feedback regarding their performance.[13,16,17]

Task Analysis

A task analysis is a written sequential list of the steps involved in performing any task from beginning to end and includes the knowledge, skills, and abilities needed as well as the conditions under which it is performed and the proper method of performance. Usually, the major steps are numbered, and each step describes what to do. Many job-related tasks involve the psychomotor domain; thus, actions are listed in the analysis. It is often necessary, however, to have some background knowledge from the cognitive domain in performing the task. Balancing a checkbook, for example, is both a manual and an intellectual skill, as is operating a computer.

After the sequential steps are listed, each one should be examined to see whether any explanations from the cognitive domain need to be added. If step one, for example, is to plug in the meat slicer, a key point is to have dry hands to avoid the danger of electrical shock. If a final step in the wait staff's task analysis for bussing dirty dishes includes washing hands, an explanation may be added regarding the transfer of microorganisms to clean food and utensils. In food service, sanitation and safety statements are frequently needed. Other explanations of reasons why a step is necessary or notes on materials or equipment may be important to add. There are many ways to complete a task analysis.

Employees need to learn the skills related to their jobs, and clients may need to develop skills in menu planning and food preparation using a new dietary regimen, such as sodium restriction. Regardless of the kind of skill involved, the learner needs to be able to perform the skill initially and then to improve the skill through continued practice. After grasping the basics of playing tennis, driving a car, or baking a cake, for example, a person requires repeated experience to develop these skills.

If available, a job description may be used as a starting point in determining job content, but job descriptions do not give information that is specific enough for determining the content of training. All the tasks included in a job should be listed individually. If the job description is unavailable, it may be necessary to interview employees or observe their work to determine the job content. Wait staff, for example, complete a number of tasks during the day, such as greeting customers, taking their orders, placing orders in the kitchen, serving the courses of the meal, bussing dishes, setting tables, receiving payment for services, and maintaining good public relations. Each is a separate task making up the total job, and each task or set of actions can be defined in task analyses.

Once it is written, the task analysis should be used by both the trainer and the trainee. The trainer may examine the task analysis to construct learning objectives that describe the behavior expected at the end of training. In assessing the person's need for instruction, the gap representing the difference between the skill described in the task analysis and the individual's current skill must be addressed. A demonstration should show what to do and then allow the person to perform the task. The task analysis may be used as an ongoing reference since it describes what to do in sequence. Using the task analysis in coaching or in supervised on-the-job training facilitates the learning of skills.

After mastering the basic skill involved and being able to recognize the correct sequence of procedures, the individual needs repeated practice to improve the skill. With time and practice, improvements in speed and quality of work should develop.[1,18,19]

Job Instruction Training

A great deal of employee training takes place not in the classroom, but on the job. New employees require orientation and training with either an experienced worker or a supervisor. Current employees may need retraining periodically, may be assigned new tasks, or may receive promotions that require the development of new skills and abilities.

A four-step process entitled job instruction training (JIT) was delineated for rapid training of new employees. It may be used to teach skills and is based on performance rather than subject matter. The four steps are (1) preparation, (2) presentation, (3) learner performance, and (4) follow-up.

This is similar to tell, show, do, and review. Before instruction, a task analysis should be completed and the work area arranged with the necessary supplies and materials that the employee is expected to maintain.[17] Box 12-1 summarizes the main points.

CASE ANALYSIS   **2**

What instruction materials, audiovisuals, and/or handouts would you plan to use in the prenatal class?

Preparation

The first step prepares the employee psychologically and intellectually for learning. Since a superior may be the trainer, the setting is important. Any tension, nervousness, or apprehension in the subordinate employee must be overcome because it may interfere with learning. A friendly, smiling trainer puts the person at ease by creating an informal atmosphere for learning in which mistakes are expected and tolerated. The trainer states the job to be learned and asks specific questions to determine what the individual already knows about it. Motivation for learning increases when employees become interested in their jobs. Finally, the trainer should be sure that the employee can physically see what is being demonstrated.

Step I: Prepare the learner

1. Put the learner at ease.
2. State the job.
3. Find out what the individual knows about the job.
4. Develop interest.
5. Correct the person's position.

Step II: Present the operation

1. Tell, show, and illustrate.
2. Explain one important step at a time.
3. Stress key points.
4. Instruct clearly, completely, and patiently, but no more than the learner can master.
5. Summarize the operation in a second run-through.

Step III: Try out performance

1. Have the learner do the job.
2. Have the learner explain key points while performing the job again.
3. Make sure that the learner understands.
4. Continue until you know that the learner knows the job.

Step IV: Follow-up

1. Put the learner on his or her own.
2. Designate where to obtain help.
3. Encourage questions.
4. Taper off.
5. Continue with normal supervision.

Box 12-1 ■ How to Instruct

Presentation

The second step presents and explains the operation as the employee is expected to perform it. The trainer shows, tells, and illustrates the operation one step at a time using a prepared task analysis. Key points should be stressed. The instruction should be carried out clearly, completely, and patiently, with the trainer remembering the employee's abilities and attitudes.

Since the ability to absorb new information is limited, the trainer needs to determine how much the learner can master at a time. It may be 5 to 10 steps with key points, or it may be more. It may be 15 minutes or 1 hour of instruction. Overloading anyone with information is ineffectual, since the information will be forgotten. After this initial instruction, the operation or task should be summarized and performed a second time.

Performance

The third step, performance, tests how much the employee has retained, as he or she tries out the operation using the written task analysis as a reference. The employee does the job while the trainer or coach stands by to assist. This is a form of behavior modeling. Accuracy, not speed, is stressed initially. As the employee completes the task a second time, the trainer should ask the employee to state the key points. To be sure of understanding, the trainer should ask such questions as "What would happen if . . .?" "What else do you do . . .?" and "What next . . .?" Employees may need to repeat the operation 5 times, 10 times, or however many times are needed until they know what to do. The trainer continues coaching and giving positive feedback, encouragement, and reassurance until the employee learns the operation.

Follow-Up

Follow-up occurs in the fourth step as supervision tapers off. At first, the employee is left alone to complete the task. The individual should always know, however, where to obtain assistance if it is needed. Any additional questions ought to be encouraged in case problems arise. Normal supervision continues to ensure that the task is done as instructed, since fellow workers may suggest undesirable shortcuts.

Mager pointed out that when the learner's experience is followed by positive consequences, the learner will be stimulated to approach the situation, but that when adverse consequences follow, the learner will avoid the situation.[20] A positive consequence may be any pleasant event, praise, a successful experience, an increase in self-esteem, improvement in self-image, or an increase in confidence. Adverse conditions are events or emotions that cause physical or mental discomfort or that lead to loss of self-respect. They include fear, anxiety, frustration, humiliation, embarrassment, and boredom. In influencing learners in the affective domain, as well as the other domains, the dietetics professional should positively reinforce learner responses.

Sequence of Instruction

Since there is a great deal to learn, instruction requires some type of organized sequence. Sequence of instruction is characterized by the progressive development of knowledge, attitudes, and skills. Learning takes place over time, and the process should be organized into smaller units. Since the ultimate outcome is able performance or behavioral change, it is important to consider how meaningful the sequence is to the individual, not the teacher or trainer, and whether or not it promotes learning. Mager provides several recommendations for sequencing. Instruction may be arranged from the general to the specific, from the specific to the general, from the simple to the complex, or according to interest, logic, or frequency of use of the knowledge or skill.[20]

In moving from the general to the specific, an overview or large picture should be presented first, followed by the details and specifics. For example, one would present an overview of the reasons for the diabetic diet and the general principles of the diet before presenting the details. With a new employee, a general explanation of the job should precede the specifics. After the individual has digested some information, it is possible to consider a specific-to-general sequence.

Material may be organized from the simple (terms, facts, and procedures) to the complex (concepts, processes, theories, analyses, and applications) so that the individual handles increasingly difficult material. If the taxonomies are used in writing objectives for learning, the hierarchy of the taxonomies provides a simple-to-complex sequence.

Another possibility is sequencing according to interest, or from the familiar to the unfamiliar. One may begin instruction with whatever is of most interest or concern to the individual. Initial questions from patients, clients, employees, or other audiences suggest such interest and should be dealt with immediately so that they are free to concentrate on later information. "How long will I have to stay on this diet?" "Can I eat my favorite foods?" The information that the person desires is a good starting point for discussion.

Similarly, if the learner perceives a problem, the instructor can start with that problem rather than with a preset agenda. As learning proceeds, the individual may develop additional needs for information or goals for learning that may be addressed. Generally, people who have assisted in directing their own learning tend to feel more committed to it.

Logic may suggest the sequence. Certain things may need to be said before others. Safety precautions may need to be introduced early, for example, when discussing kitchen equipment. Sanitary utensil handling may be important to discuss with wait staff before discussing how to set a table.

Frequency of use of the knowledge or skill may also dictate sequence. The skill used most frequently should be taught first, followed by the next most frequently used skill. If training time runs out, at least the learner has learned all except the least frequently used skills. The instructor should teach first what people "need to know" rather than the "nice to know" information. Finally, even though learners may have been practicing individual elements of the job, they need practice on the total job. This practice may be provided in the actual job situation or through simulation.[9,17]

Evaluation of Results

Evaluation is key to successful education. Accountability to measure effectiveness in terms of outcomes is necessary in both clinical and managerial arenas. Expected outcomes should be defined before starting the intervention rather than later. Nutrition education or employee training that does not show improvement cannot be considered effective. Evaluation is important for continuous improvement and refinement of education.

Evaluation connotes judgments about the value or worth of something compared with a standard. Everyone makes these judgments daily, both consciously and unconsciously. "The food tastes good." "The television show is worth watching." "She is not motivated." Our thoughts turn to evaluation automatically as we compare something with some standard and pass judgment.

Educational evaluation consists of a systematic appraisal of the quality, effectiveness, and worth of an educational endeavor, such as instruction, programs, or goals based on information or data. That it is systematic suggests that advance planning has taken place and that the process will provide data on the quality or worth of the educational endeavor.

Consider not only what to evaluate but also when to evaluate and how the evaluation will be done. An evaluation plan involves several steps: defining objectives or outcomes; designing the evaluation based on objectives; choosing what to evaluate; deciding how and when to collect data to obtain timely feedback; constructing a data collection instrument or method; implementing the data collection; analyzing results; reporting them; and setting a course of action.

Although the terms "measurement" and "evaluation" are sometimes interchanged, their meanings are not equivalent. Measurement or "educational assessment" is the process of collecting and quantifying data in terms of numbers on the extent, degree, or capacity of people's learning in knowledge, attitudes, skills, performance, and behavioral change. Testing is one kind of measurement. Measurement involves determining the degree to which a person possesses a certain attribute, as when one receives a score of 85 on a test. However, such a measurement does not determine quality or worth. These systems require experimental designs, data collection, and statistical analysis of the data. The term "assessment" can also mean estimating or judging the value of the data collected, as in nutrition assessment.[21,22]

Evaluation, on the other hand, is based on the measurement of what people know, think, feel, and do. Evaluation compares the observed value or quality with a standard or criterion of comparison. Evaluation is the process of forming value judgments about the quality of programs, products, goals, and the like from the data. One may evaluate the success of an educational program, for example, by measuring the degree to which goals or objectives were achieved. Evaluation goes beyond measurement to the formation of value judgments about the data. To be effective, evaluation designs should specify not only what will be evaluated but also when it will be evaluated, such as the score difference between a pretest and a posttest.

Purpose of Evaluation

Careful evaluation should be an integral part of all nutrition education programs and employee training programs. There are several purposes of evaluation. One cannot make judgments about effectiveness without it. Program evaluation may be used for planning, improvement, and justification. As a system of quality control, it can determine whether the process of education is effective, identify its strengths and weaknesses, and determine what changes should be made. To determine accountability, one needs to know whether people are learning, whether trainers are teaching effectively, whether programs accomplish the desired outcomes, and whether money is well spent. In times of limited financial resources, accountability requires an examination of cost–benefit ratios. Is the program useful and valuable enough to justify the cost? Is there evidence that training is changing employee behavior on the job and contributing to the bottom line? It is important to determine whether the learning objectives were accomplished and whether the individual learned what was intended or developed in desired ways.

Evaluation helps nutrition professionals make better decisions and improve education. It is helpful in making decisions concerning teaching, learning, program effectiveness, and the necessity of making modifications in current efforts or even of terminating them. Evaluation provides evidence that what you are doing is worthwhile. Plans for evaluation should be made early in the planning stages of an educational endeavor and not after it has begun or is completed. One evaluation system is the "logic model" that uses categories of input, activities, and outcomes to describe a flow process throughout the education or intervention process.[23]

With employees, training evaluation should show improved job performance and financial results. Another question often asked is "Does training transfer?" One needs to determine whether the skills and knowledge taught in training are applied on the job. If they are, this demonstrates the value of the training to the organization, and the effectiveness of the method of training. If not, change is needed.

As with other parts of his adult education model, Malcolm Knowles suggested that evaluation should be a mutual undertaking between the educator and the learner. He recommends less emphasis on the evaluation of learning and more on the rediagnosis of learning needs, which suggests immediate or future steps to be taken jointly by the dietetics professional and the client or employee. This type of feedback from evaluation becomes more constructive and acceptable to adults. Thus, evaluation may be considered something you should do with people, not to people. If problems are apparent, then solutions may be found jointly by the professional and the individual.[24]

Formative and Summative Evaluations

Formative and summative evaluations are two types of evaluations used to improve any of three processes—program planning, teaching, or learning. Formative evaluation refers to that made early or during the course of education, with the feedback of results modifying the rest of the educational endeavor. Summative evaluation refers to an endpoint assessment of quality at the conclusion of learning.

Formative Evaluation

Formative evaluation is a systematic appraisal that occurs before or during the implementation of a learning activity for the purpose of modifying or improving teaching, learning, program design, or educational materials. It is often qualitative in nature, with data collection by observation, interviewing, and surveys. It can help to diagnose problems in student learning and in teaching effectiveness. It pinpoints parts mastered and parts not mastered and allows for revision of plans, methods, techniques, or materials.

Formative evaluation may be performed at frequent intervals. If the learner appears bored, unsure, anxious, quizzical, or lost, or if you are unsure of the person's abilities, for example, it is appropriate to stop teaching and start the evaluation process. Ask the person to repeat what he or she has learned. In diabetic education, if formative evaluation shows that the person does not understand the concept of carbohydrate counting, he or she will not be able to master more complex behaviors such as menu planning. Having located the problem that carbohydrate counting is not understood (comprehended by the client), the educator can change approaches to try to overcome the problem. Perhaps, an alternative explanation that is clearer or simpler or a concrete illustration is indicated. During group learning, a collaborative member may be able to provide an explanation that an individual understands better than the explanation of the educator.[25]

Before nutrition messages and educational materials are designed and implemented, formative evaluation or market research activities, such as focus group interviews and structured discussions with members of the target audience, are designed and implemented. This type of qualitative evaluation helps the educator to learn about individuals' thoughts, ideas, and opinions and tells whether recipients are likely to ignore, reject, or misunderstand the message or accept it and act on it.

Formative research is essential for tailoring intervention strategies. The moderator of a focus group uses open-ended interviewing strategies with groups of 8 to 15 people. The focus group approach has been used to assess consumer preferences, to plan and evaluate nutrition education interventions, and to pretest print materials. It can answer questions about readability, content, and applicability.

Failure to learn may not always be related to instructional methods or materials per se, but may derive from problems that are physical, emotional, cultural, or environmental in nature. By performing an evaluation after smaller units of instruction, the educator can determine whether the pacing of instruction is appropriate for the patient, client, or employee. Frequent feedback is necessary to facilitate learning. It is especially important when a great deal of material has to be learned.

Mastery of smaller units can be a powerful positive reinforcement for the learner, and verbal praise may increase motivation to continue learning. When mistakes are made, they should be corrected quickly by giving the correct information. Avoid saying such things as "No, that's wrong." "Can't you ever get things right?" "Won't you ever learn?" Positive, not negative, feedback should be given. Approach the problem specifically by saying, for example, "You identified some of the foods that are high in sodium, which is very good. Now let's look a second time for others."

Summative Evaluation

Summative evaluation has a different purpose and time frame from that of formative evaluation. Summative evaluation is considered final, and it is used at the end of a term, course, or learning activity. The purpose of summative evaluation is to appraise results, quality, outcomes, or worth using quantitative approaches. It may include grading, certification, or evaluation of progress, and the evaluation distinguishes those who excel from those who do not. Judgment is made about the learner, teacher, program, or curriculum with regard to the effectiveness of learning or instruction for the target population. This judgment aspect creates the anxiety and defensiveness often associated with evaluation.

Evaluation should be a continual process that is preplanned along with educational sessions. Evaluation preassessment determines the individual's abilities before the educational program, and progress should be evaluated continually during and immediately after the educational program. Follow-up evaluation at regular intervals may measure the degree to which the person has forgotten information or has fallen back to previous behaviors.[26]

Norm- and Criterion-Referenced Methods

Besides formative and summative evaluation, there are norm- and criterion-referenced interpretations. In norm-referenced results, the group that has taken a test provides the norms for determining the meaning of each person's score. A norm is like the typical performance of a group. One can then see how the individual compares with the results of the group, whether above or below the norm. In criterion-referenced results, a

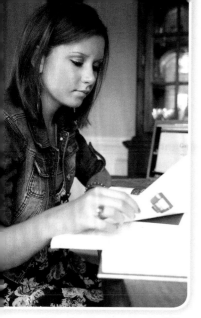

Educational outcomes should be assessed.

Source: CDC/Amanda Mills.

standard is used as a basis for the level of proficiency required. Instead of comparing learners with each other, the instructor compares each individual with a predefined, objective standard of performance of what the learner is expected to know or to be able to do after instruction is complete. A criterion-referenced measurement ascertains the person's status in respect to a defined objective or standard, and test items, if tests are used, correspond to the objectives. If the learner can perform what is called for in the objective, he or she has been successful. If not, criterion-referenced testing, which tends to be more diagnostic, indicates what the learner can and cannot do, and more learning can be planned.

Some instructors may believe that a test should not be too easy, but the degree of difficulty of a test may not be as important as whether a person can perform. The instructor may believe that some of the questions have to be difficult so that a spread of scores is produced to separate the brightest from the rest, the As from the Bs and Cs. Some tests are developed with the intent that not everyone will be successful and variation in individual scores is expected. Students are graded in a norm-referenced manner by comparison with other individuals on the same measuring device or with the norm of the group. A norm-referenced instrument indicates, for example, whether the individual's performance falls into the 50th percentile or the 90th percentile in relation to the group norm. This method is not as appropriate for affective and psychomotor objectives.

With criterion-referenced evaluation, everyone can do well by attaining a minimum standard. Instruction has been successful when learners reach a defined level of expertise. The registration examinations for dietitians and for dietetic technicians are examples of criterion-referenced tests.

Formative evaluation is almost always criterion-referenced. The instructor wants to know who is having trouble learning, not where they rank compared with others. Summative evaluation may be either norm- or criterion-referenced.[27]

Types of Evaluation and Outcomes

After considering the purpose (why) and timing (when) of evaluation, the educator should resolve the question of what to evaluate. Several types of evaluation can be used in measuring effectiveness. These are (1) measurement of participant (client, employee) reactions to programs;

(2) measurement of behavioral change; (3) measurement of results in an organization; (4) evaluation of learning in the cognitive, affective, and psychomotor domains; and (5) evaluation of other outcomes.[27] The evaluation of health education is usually focused on one or more types: knowledge, attitudes or beliefs, change in behavior, and other measures.

Participant Reaction to Programs

The first type of evaluation deals with participant (employee, client) reactions to educational programs and whether or not they are favorable. Preferences may vary by age of the participants, cultural or ethnic group, gender, socioeconomic status, and other variables. You need to decide what should be evaluated. Were participants pleased and satisfied with the program, subject matter, content, materials, speakers, room arrangements, physical facilities, and learning activities? When a program, meeting, or class is evaluated, the purpose is to improve decisions concerning its various aspects, to see how the parts fit the whole, or to make program changes.

The quality of learning elements, such as objectives, techniques, materials, and learning outcomes, may also be included. Hedonistic scales or happiness indexes, such as smiley faces or numerical scales, have been used to determine the degree to which participants "liked" various aspects. Although these judgments are subjective, they are not useless, since learners who dislike elements of a program may not be learning.

Behavioral Change

A second type of evaluation is the measurement of change in behavior. Did employee or client behavior or habits change based on the learning? In measuring behavior, the focus is on what the person does. In employee training, for example, you may assess changes in job behaviors to see whether transfer of training to the job has occurred. Continual quality improvement has influenced the need for this type of evaluation. It is necessary to know what the job performance was before training and to decide who will observe or assess changed performance—the supervisor, peers, or the individual. This type of assessment is more difficult to measure and can be done selectively.

The ultimate criterion for effectiveness of nutrition education is not merely the improvement in knowledge of what to eat, but also changes in dietary behaviors and practices as the individual develops better food habits. Is the person consuming more fruits and vegetables, for example? These changes are difficult to confirm and often depend on direct observation, which is time-consuming; on self-reports; and on indirect outcome measures, such as weight gained or lost in a person on a weight reduction diet, reduction in blood pressure in hypertensive persons, or better control of blood sugars in diabetes mellitus.[14,26,27]

Organizational Results

Professionals involved with employee training gather a third type of evaluative data to justify the time and expense to the organization. Management may want to know how training will positively benefit the organization in relation to the cost. Results in terms of the following aspects may be attributed, at least in part, to training: improved morale, improved efficiency or productivity, improved quality of work, better customer satisfaction, less employee turnover, fewer accidents or worker's compensation claims, better attendance, dollar savings, number of employee errors, number of grievances, amount of overtime, and the like. Did changing employees' behavior on the job improve business results? If not, it is not useful.

Learning

Whether learning has taken place is a separate question, even if the program rated highly on entertainment value. The learning of principles, facts, attitudes, values, and skills should be evaluated on an objective basis, and this task is more complex. If the learning objectives are written in terms of measurable performance, they serve as the source of the evaluation. To what degree were the objectives achieved by the learner?

Whether a person has succeeded in learning can be determined by developing situations, or test items, based on the objectives of instruction. A program is ineffective if it has not achieved its objectives. It is important for the test items to match the objectives in performance and conditions discussed in Chapter 11. If they do not match the objectives, it is not possible to assess whether instruction was successful, that is, whether the learner learned what was intended.

Mager pointed out that several obstacles must be overcome to assess the results of instruction successfully. Some obstacles are caused by poorly written objectives, whereas others result from attitudes and beliefs on the part of instructors who use inappropriate test items.[20]

One of the problems in evaluation results from inadequately written objectives. If the performance is not stated, if conditions are omitted, and if the criterion is missing, it will be difficult to create a test situation. If these deficiencies are discovered, the first step is to rewrite the objective. Mager suggested a series of steps to select appropriate test items[27]:

1. Note the performance (what the person will be able to say or do) stated in the objective. Match the performance and conditions of the test item to those of the objective.
2. Check whether the performance is a main intent or an indicator. If the performance is the main intent, determine whether it is covert (invisible) or overt (visible, audible).

3. If the performance is covert, such as solving a problem, check for an indicator behavior, a visible or audible activity by which the performance can be inferred.
4. Test for the overt indicator in objectives containing one rather than the main performance.

The first step is to see whether the performance specified in the test item is the same as that specified in the objective. If they do not match, the test item must be revised, since it will not indicate whether the objective has been accomplished. If the objective states that the performance is "to plan low-fat menus" or "to operate the dish machine," for example, the test should involve planning menus or operating the dish machine. It would be inappropriate to ask the learner to discuss the principles of writing menus or to label the parts of the dish machine on a diagram.

In addition to matching performance, the test should use the same specific circumstances or conditions that are specified in the objective.

> **EXAMPLE** (Given the disassembled parts of the meat slicer) is able to reassemble the parts in correct sequence.

The conditions are "given the disassembled parts of the meat slicer." The practitioner should provide a disassembled machine and ask the employee to reassemble it. An inappropriate test would be to ask the learner to list the steps in reassembling the meat slicer or to discuss the safety precautions to be taken.

If the learner must perform under a range of conditions, you may need to test performance using the entire range. If a client eats at home and in restaurants, the dietetics professional must determine whether the person is capable of following the dietary changes in both environments. If students are learning to take a diet history, they should be taught to handle the range of conditions, including people of different ages, socioeconomic levels, and cultural groups. Not every condition will be taught and tested, but the common conditions that the individual will encounter should be included in the objectives and in testing.

The main intent of an objective may be stated clearly or it may be implied. The main intent is the performance, whereas an indicator is an activity (visible, audible) through which the main intent is inferred:

> **EXAMPLE** (Given a copy of a sodium-restricted diet) is able to plan a menu for a complete day.

In this example, the main intent is to discriminate between foods permitted and omitted on the diet, and the indicator is the ability to plan menus. You can infer that the client knows what is permitted and what is not if accurate sodium-restricted menus are planned. Test for the indicator in objectives that contain one. This, of course, does not prove that the person will change eating behaviors.

Covert actions are not visible, but are internal or mental activities, such as solving problems or identifying. If the performance is covert, an indicator should have been added to the objective, as explained in Chapter 11, and the indicator should be tested.

> **EXAMPLE**   Is able to identify the parts of the slicer (on a diagram or verbally).

For this example, the employee should be provided with the indicator, a diagram of a meat slicer, and asked to identify the parts.

Although some performances are covert, others are overt. Overt actions are visible or audible, such as writing, verbally describing, and assembling. If the performance is overt, determine whether the test item matches the objective.

> **EXAMPLE**   Is able to reassemble the parts of the meat slicer.

The employee should be provided with the parts of the meat slicer and asked to reassemble them. Performance tests are appropriate when skills are taught. If the employee is being taught to use equipment, the evaluation should be to have him or her demonstrate its operation. If a student is learning interviewing skills, an interview session is indicated as the evaluation.

The discussion so far has used examples of objectives in the cognitive and psychomotor domains. Affective objectives describe values, interests, and attitudes that are thought to predispose dietary changes. While the cognitive and psychomotor domains are concerned with what individuals can do, the affective domain deals with what they are willing to do. These changes are covert or internal and develop more slowly over a period of time. Evaluation of their achievement is more difficult and needs to take different forms.

Attitudes are inferred based on the evidence of what people say or do. To assess whether the individual has been influenced by education, the professional may conduct a discussion and listen to what the individual says or observe what he or she does, since both saying and doing are overt behaviors. In measuring attitudes and values, the person needs the opportunity to express agreement rather than deciding on right or wrong answers. A self-reported attitude survey may be used, for example. Statements can be given to which the person responds on a 5-point scale, from "strongly agree" to "strongly disagree." To evaluate change in the learner's behavior, the practitioner attempts to secure data that permit an inference to be made regarding the person's future disposition in similar situations. In the affective domain, this is a more difficult task.

It is conceivable that the individual may display a desirable overt behavior only in the presence of the practitioner. The attitude toward following a diabetic diet or an employee work procedure may differ depending on the dietetics professional's presence or absence. Since time is required for change in attitudes and values, evaluation may have to be repeated at designated intervals. To determine realistically how the person is disposed to act, the measurement approach needs to evaluate volitional rather than coerced responses.

Other Outcomes

An outcome is a result and can be defined as what does or does not happen after an intervention. The criterion of nutrition education program effectiveness has generally been improvement in knowledge, in awareness, and in dietary behaviors or physiologic parameters, or both. This criterion can be measured in many ways depending on the application and outcome data available. For professional education programs, the use of hard copy and electronic portfolios representing evidence of skills and competency is one way to assess outcome measures.[28–30]

SELF-ASSESSMENT 1

You have just discussed sodium restriction with a man diagnoses with hypertension. How can you assess what he has learned?

Outcomes should have clear interpretations related to the dietitian's intervention in improving nutrition and health status. They may be of several types: (1) physiologic or biologic measures, (2) behavioral change based on self-report, (3) diet-related psychosocial measures, and (4) environmental or other measures of dietary behavior. Biologic indicators are changes in clinical or biochemical indices, such as serum lipid levels in cardiovascular disease, hemoglobin or serum albumen level in pregnancy, and glycosylated hemoglobin level in diabetes. Eating behavior changes such as decreasing fat intake or increasing fiber intake are based on self-reports, which can be subject to bias. Psychosocial outcomes include increased nutrition knowledge, attitude change, or self-efficacy for behavior but do not prove the change in food choices. Other changes are in body mass index or weight, increases in the level of physical activity, decreased blood pressure, or reduction in risk factors for disease and improved health (both long-term goals).

Care must be taken in interpreting some of these results, since they may reflect variables other than education. Stress, for example, can affect a person's blood sugar even when the diabetic diet is followed. In nutrition education interventions, behavior has been measured in different ways ranging from observable food choices to dietary intakes. These may include reports by teachers or parents of children's food preferences, such as refusing a food, willingness to taste a new food, and selecting a more nutritious food when other choices were available. Actual food choices and consumption, plate waste, and self-reported intake can be used to evaluate dietary intake. Other measures include 24-hour dietary recall, food records and food frequency questionnaires, changing food preparation practices and recipes, or percentage of participation after an intervention.

Physical measures can include laboratory values, blood pressure, weight indices, urinary output, and physical activity status. Mean maternal weight gain, infant's birth weight, and Apgar scores at birth can be used to evaluate pregnancy outcomes and the health of newborn infants.[24]

Organizational changes include changes in school lunch menus, such as to lower fat and sodium, or food choices and nutrition information offered at the worksite. Data can be collected on the number of work-related injuries or food sanitation incidents after safety training.

Data Collection Techniques

There are many techniques for collecting evaluation data: paper-and-pencil tests, questionnaires, interviews, visual observation, job sample or performance tests, simulation, rating forms or checklists, individual and group performance measures, individual and group behavior measures, and self-reports. As measurement devices that will be analyzed statistically, they require the use of specific experimental designs. Regardless of the particular instrument or technique used, it should be pretested with a smaller group before actual use. Since comparisons are desired, it is usually necessary to collect preliminary data on current performance or behaviors.[21]

Tests

Tests, especially written tests, are probably the most common devices for measuring learning. Tests sample what one knows, and schools depend heavily on them. Multiple-choice, true–false, short answer, completion, matching, and

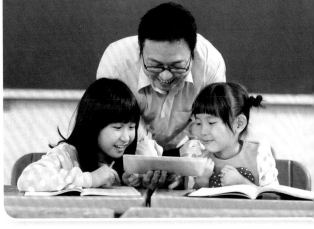

essay questions are used to measure learning in the cognitive domain. These tests are appropriate when several people are expected to learn the same content or material. Sometimes, both a pretest and a posttest are used to measure learning. This method assists in controlling variables, but be careful not to attribute all the changes noted on the posttest to the learning experiences since other factors may have been involved.

Visual aids assist learning.
Source: CDC/Amanda Mills.

CASE ANALYSIS **3**

What evaluation or outcome measures do you suggest for the prenatal class?

Although tests are appropriate with school-aged children, adults may respond less favorably. The practitioner should avoid evoking childhood memories associated with the authoritarian teacher, the dependent child, or the assigned degree of success and failure based on right or wrong answers. In one-on-one situations, the practitioner could ask the individual to state verbally what he or she learned as though telling it to a spouse or friend. Alternatively, a self-assessment instrument may be used.

Questionnaires

Questionnaires may be preplanned and are often used to assess attitudes and values that do not involve correct answers. Questions may be open-ended, multiple-choice, ranking, checklist, or alternate response, such as yes/no or agree/disagree. In evaluating behavioral change on the job, trainees and supervisors can both complete a questionnaire.

Interviews

Interviews conducted on a one-to-one basis are another form of evaluation. They are the oral equivalent to written questionnaires used to measure cognitive and affective objectives. Before the interview, the instructor should preplan and draw up a list of questions that will indicate whether learning has taken place. After instruction, evaluation may consist of asking the learner to repeat important facts. An advantage of an interview is that the evaluator can put the person at ease and immediately correct any errors. Another advantage is that the interviewer can probe for additional information. Although this method is time-consuming, it is appropriate for people with low literacy or those less educated. Focus group interviews, mentioned earlier, are an example of a qualitative, formative evaluation.

Observation

In many cases, visual observation is an appropriate method of evaluating learning. The behaviors to be observed should be defined, and an observation checklist may be helpful. When employees are under direct supervision, systematic ongoing observation over a period of time is a basis for evaluating learning. The supervisor can observe and report whether the employee is operating equipment correctly or following established procedures properly. If the employee has been taught sanitary procedures, for example, the professional can see whether or not they are incorporated into the employee's work. Evaluate the performance, using what was taught as a standard. If discrepancies are found, further learning may be indicated.

Performance Tests

When direct observation is not possible or would be too time-consuming and costly, a simulated situation or performance test can be observed. Performance tests are appropriate in the cognitive and psychomotor domains. You can ask a wait staff member to set a table, a cook to demonstrate the meat slicer, or a client to indicate what to select from a restaurant menu. The client could be given a list of foods and asked to differentiate those appropriate for his or her diet. With permission from the learner, audiotape or videotape may be used to record the teaching session. The instructor and learner may discuss the results together and plan further learning to correct any deficiencies. The observer needs to delineate which behaviors are being observed and what is to be acceptable behavior.

Rating Scales and Checklists

Rating scales and checklists have been used to evaluate learner performance and teacher effectiveness. Categories or attributes such as knowledge level or dependability are listed and should be defined in detail to avoid ambiguity. Emphasis should be placed on attributes that can be confirmed objectively rather than judged subjectively. A 5- or 7-point scale is used, allowing a midpoint, and the ratings should be defined, for example, from "excellent" to "poor" or from "extremely acceptable" to "very unacceptable." The list should include as a possible response "No opportunity to observe."

Rating scales are subject to several errors. Two evaluators may judge the same individual differently. To avoid error, definition of the terms and training of evaluators are essential. The ratings may suffer from personal biases. In addition, some raters have the tendency to be too lenient. Error may result if the rater is a perfectionist. Some evaluators tend to rate most people as average, believing that few people rank at the highest levels. Another possible error is the "halo" error, in which an evaluator is so positively or negatively impressed with one aspect of a person that he or she judges all other qualities according to this one impressive aspect.

Performance Measures

In employee training programs, individual and group performance measures may be assessed. These may include work quality and quantity, number of errors, days of absenteeism, number of grievances, and other types of problems that affect work performance.[17]

Self-Reports

Self-reports, self-evaluation, and self-monitoring are another approach to evaluation. In the affective domain, written questions or statements are presented and the individual supplies responses. "What changes, if any, have you made in your food choices?" "What are you doing differently?" Self-reports, such as a 3-day food record, have been used to measure behavioral change. Responses may be distorted or biased if the individual can ascertain the acceptable answer.

All methods of evaluation have advantages and limitations, which need to be considered. Although evaluation may not provide proof that an intervention and education worked, it does produce a great deal of evidence.

CASE ANALYSIS   4

What type of evaluation(s) would you use for the prenatal nutrition class?

Reliability and Validity

The concepts of reliability and validity are essential to the measurement of the effectiveness of nutrition education outcomes and employee learning. Validity indicates whether we are measuring what we intend to measure. There are different types of validity, such as content-related, construct-related, and criterion-related (concurrent and predictive) validity, all of which help to "defend" the validity of the instrument. Content-related validity, which is the simplest and perhaps the most important, refers to whether the test items or questions correspond to the subject matter or purpose of instruction or to the knowledge, skills, or objectives they are supposed to measure for a specific audience by culture, age, literacy level, and the like. If one is interested in determining knowledge of dietary fiber, for example, are the questions appropriate in content?

Reliability refers to the consistency and accuracy with which a test or device measures something in the same way in each situation or over time. For example, if a test is given twice to the same students to sample the same abilities, the students should be placed in the same relative position to others each time if the test is reliable. Methods for determining the reliability and validity of tests may be found in the educational literature.[27]

In all cases, keep in mind that the measuring device should assess whether the learner has attained the requisite knowledge, skill, or competence needed and whether behavior has changed. Pretesting evaluation instruments with the intended audience is essential. If the learner has not attained the intended knowledge or skill, additional learning may be indicated.

After the data from evaluation are collected, they should be compiled and analyzed. The statistical analysis of data is a lengthy subject of its own beyond the scope of this book. Future plans or programs may be modified based on the results of the evaluation. Results should be communicated through evaluation reports to others such as participants, management staff, decision makers, and future learners.[21,27]

Lesson Plans and Program Plans

A lesson plan is a written summary of information about a unit of instruction. It is prepared and used by the instructor. Various formats for lesson plans are available, but the content is essentially the same. A lesson plan is a blueprint that describes all aspects of instruction. It includes the following[20]:

- Preassessment of the participants or needs assessment
- The performance objectives identified
- The content outline (introduction, body, conclusions)
- How the content will be sequenced
- A description of the activities participants will engage in to reach the objectives
- Instructional procedures (techniques and methods)
- Educational materials, visual aids, media, handouts, and equipment
- Amount of time allotted or scheduled
- Facilities to be used

- Method of evaluating whether the learner reached the objectives, outcomes, or other results
- References

Once written, a lesson plan is a flexible guide to instruction that can be used with many different individuals or groups. A series of lesson plans or activities may be grouped into a larger unit of instruction covering a longer time frame, such as a whole day or several days. The term "program planning" is also used. A plan for a longer program would include essentially the same components as a lesson plan, with the addition of the names of speakers or others responsible, and cost considerations. Sample lesson plans are found in Boxes 12-2 and 12-3.

I. Target audience: New wait staff
II. Objective: When setting tables, wait staff will be able to handle dishes and utensils in a sanitary manner.
III. Time allotted: 15 minutes
IV. Preassessment: Question new employees to determine what they already know about sanitary dish and utensil handling.
V. Content and sequence:
   1. Wash hands. Handling of flatware by the handles.
   2. Handling of cups by the base or handle and glassware by the base.
   3. Handling plates and bowls on the edge without touching the food.
   4. Use a tray.
   5. The hands and skin as major sources of disease-causing bacteria and their transmission to food and utensils.
   6. Proper bussing of dishes to avoid contamination of the hands.
   7. Hand washing.
VI. Learning activities:
   1. Demonstration and discussion of proper handling of dishes and utensils when setting tables, serving food, and bussing tables.
   2. Discussion of hand washing.
   3. Actual practice by new wait staff.
VII. Materials: Dishes, utensils, tray, handout of important points to remember.
VIII. Evaluation: Whether or not dishes and utensils were handled properly during the actual practice; continued observation of the employee's performance on the job.

Box 12-2 ■ Sample Lesson Plan on Sanitary Dish Handling

I.   Target audience: Pregnant women

II. Objective: To be able to identify foods and quantities of foods that will meet the daily calcium needs for pregnancy and plan menus using these foods.

III. Time allotted: 30 minutes

IV. Preassessment: Question audience about which foods contain calcium and how much of these foods should be eaten daily during pregnancy. Determine any previous pregnancies and what was eaten.

V.   Content and sequence:
1. Total daily calcium needs, with the important functions of calcium during pregnancy.
2. Dairy foods as a source of calcium, with quantities of calcium in each.
3. Other foods as good sources of calcium, with quantities of calcium.
4. Calcium sources for lactose-intolerant individuals.
5. Have audience suggest breakfast, lunch, dinner, and snacks that meet the need for calcium.
6. Questions from the audience.
7. Have each person plan her own menu for tomorrow.

VI. Learning activities: Group discussion of food sources of calcium. Show actual foods and food models for portion sizes. Group planning of a day's menu followed by each individual planning, something appropriate for herself for the next day's menu.

VII. Materials: Actual food samples, food models, paper and pencils for menu planning, chalkboard or flip chart for writing menus, handout with good sources of calcium and the amount of calcium in each, including the daily recommended intake for pregnancy, and a sample menu.

VIII. Evaluation: The menu planned by each individual. Discussion with individuals during their follow-up prenatal visits.

Box 12-3 ■ Sample Lesson Plan on Calcium in Pregnancy

Documentation

Nutrition professionals are accountable for the nutrition care they provide in all settings, including in consulting and private practice and at the work site. Accepted standards of practice for quality control and accreditation agencies, such as the Joint Commission on Accreditation of Healthcare Organizations, mandate that dietetics and nutrition services be documented and communicated to other health professionals providing care.[31] Patient records also provide evidence in malpractice suits and are important to the denial of legal liability. This is increasingly important when transferring information to others over the Internet.[32]

Documentation provides a developmental history of nutrition services to clients. Measurement and documentation of desired outcomes—medical, clinical, educational, and psychosocial—are essential. The information communicated demonstrates what services have been delivered that contribute to healthcare delivery and that these services provide the patient or client with a specific benefit that will offset the cost of the service.

The usual place for documentation is in the medical or client's record. The Academy of Nutrition and Dietetics implemented a nutrition documentation process using categories of Problem, Etiology, and Signs or Symptoms that endeavors to standardize language used in the nutrition care process. Chapter 1 covers these systems in more depth.[33] Documentation of employee education and training programs is also essential. Records should be kept of all information included in employee orientation. The use of an orientation checklist is helpful in ensuring that everything the employee needs to know has been communicated to him or her. Records should be kept on file showing the date and content of ongoing training sessions, such as in-service programs, and off-the-job experiences, such as continuing education.[1]

CASE ANALYSIS 5

What documentation would you plan to use for the prenatal class?

Summary

This chapter has examined the selection and implementation of learning activities in the cognitive, affective, and psychomotor domains. Task analysis and JIT were described. Finally, the evaluation process in which data are collected and analyzed to determine the success of educational endeavors was outlined.

1. Develop a lesson plan for a prenatal nutrition class.
2. What audiovisual materials would you suggest?
3. What handout materials would you recommend?
4. How long should the presentation be?

Review and Discussion Questions

1. What are the advantages and disadvantages of the educational methods and techniques?
2. What methods and techniques are appropriate for objectives in the cognitive domain? The affective domain? The psychomotor domain?
3. Explain how a task analysis would be used with JIT.
4. In what ways may educational instruction be organized or sequenced?
5. What are the purposes of evaluation?
6. Differentiate the following: formative and summative evaluation; reliability and validity; criterion-referenced and norm-referenced evaluation.
7. What are the major types or levels of evaluation? If you had to describe each to someone desiring to evaluate employee training, what major elements of each would you emphasize?
8. If you had to evaluate a diabetes education program, what would you do? How would you go about it?
9. What are the parts of a lesson plan or program plan?
10. What should be documented in the medical record?

Suggested Activities

1. Complete a task analysis for using a procedure or a piece of equipment (coffee urn, meat slicer, dish machine, mixer, oven, grille, broiler, etc.), listing the sequential steps and key points.
2. Using the JIT sequence and a task analysis, teach someone to use an unfamiliar piece of equipment.

3. Plan learning using one of the techniques in the chapter (other than lecture), such as discussion, simulation, or a demonstration. Carry out the plan.

4. Develop one or two performance objectives on a topic of interest for a target audience defined by age, sex, socioeconomic status, and educational level. The audience may be pregnant women, mothers, schoolchildren, adolescents, adult men or women, elderly, employees, executives, sports figures, or a person with a chronic disease. Plan the preassessment, content, techniques for presentation, teaching aids and handouts, and evaluation methods. Carry out the educational plan.

5. Develop one or two visual aids to use in teaching.

6. Give a pretest of knowledge on a subject. Instruct the learner on the subject. Follow up with a posttest to examine results.

7. Locate a logic model for an existing education program. Compare this evaluation method with another method presented in this chapter.

8. List three ways in which you might evaluate whether an employee learned from a training program. List three ways in which you might evaluate whether a patient comprehended instruction regarding a diabetic diet.

CHAPTER 13

Delivering Oral Presentations

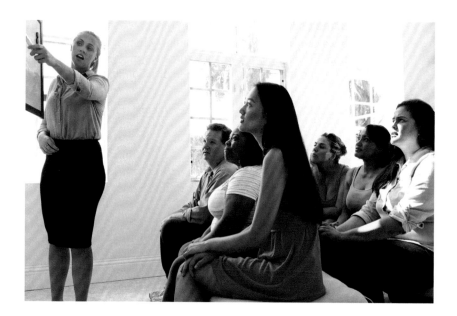

Objectives

- Describe the process of presentation preparation.
- List the three components of a presentation and their content.
- Discuss effective speaker delivery techniques.
- Identify challenges and postulate ideas to overcome barriers.
- Outline special issues when presentations involve media.
- Deliver a presentation to others and complete a postpresentation critique.

, RD, works in a corporate wellness program. She has noticed that some employees who eat in the work place cafeteria make less than optimum food choices for lunch. Others go out to a nearby fast-food restaurant. She is asked by management to give a 30-minute presentation on healthy, nutritious lunches.

There are always three speeches, for every one you actually gave. The one you practiced, the one you gave, and the one you wish you gave.

—*Dale Carnegie*

Introduction

Presenting effective information in an oral format is a cornerstone of communication. Most practitioners will be required to give an oral presentation to share their expertise multiple times during their careers. This important professional skill is included in the Standards of Practice and Standards of Professional Performance of the Academy of Nutrition and Dietetics as well as practitioner competencies from Australia, Canada, and other countries.[1–5]

The presentation skills discussed in this chapter apply to a wide variety of professional venues involving students, clients, peers, and employees. Formats involve both small and large group settings. As is true for so many of the other skills discussed in this book, the confidence needed to deliver a message orally and articulately cannot be achieved by reading alone. Mastering the ability to communicate a message to an audience is an acquired skill that begins by having the courage to apply the techniques in real situations. The goal of delivering an effective message is to produce a desired outcome such as changing behavior, understanding new information, appreciating new trends, or developing new skills.

There is a large body of literature on the general subject of oral communication, presentation planning, and public speaking.[6–9] The purpose of this chapter is to provide information on how to create and deliver effective oral presentations. This process includes preparation, organization, delivery, and evaluation. Other chapters in this book cover planning the learning process (Chapters 11 and 12) and creating audiovisuals (Chapter 14). These are necessary complementary skills for effective oral communication.

Write a brief abstract for Joan summarizing the work place presentation.

Preparation of an Effective Presentation

The key to an effective oral presentation is preparation. The speaker must assess the needs of the planned presentation through a series of audience, program, and content analysis activities. This philosophy incorporates both an inside and an outside viewpoint of audience and speaker goals. The program planner can often provide input supplemented by the presenter's own preparation analysis.[6-10]

Audience Analysis

The first step is an audience analysis. This step is necessary if the speaker is to maintain the delicate balance between what the audience expects to learn and what the presenter wants them to learn. Collect information about the planned audience. This may include data such as age, gender, educational level or occupation, years of experience, and present knowledge of the topic. What is the audience's goal in attending the presentation? Are individuals volunteering to attend or is this a mandatory training session? What is their perceived value of the sessions? Did they pay to come and listen or is this a free event? The presentation will be more successful and focused if many of the audience's goals and expectations are incorporated in the program.[7,10]

Program Analysis

The second step is program analysis. The speaker needs to know the setting and overall structure of the program. Will there be only one presenter or multiple speakers? There will be more flexibility regarding content and delivery style if you are the only presenter. If the presentation is part of a larger program, find out which are the topics and speakers that both precede and follow your presentation. Ask for the learning objectives and planned content of the entire program. This will ensure that you complement, rather than duplicate, the information to be presented.

Consider the position of the presentation in relationship to scheduled meal and refreshment breaks. Assess what instructional media are available for use. Ask if handouts are expected, submission deadlines, and how they will be provided to the audience. Some programs require that handouts be posted in advance electronically or printed for on-site presentation. Determine time constraints. Evaluate the allotment of presentation time in relation to the time required for audience questions.

Collect information on the physical layout and location of the venue. Will there be a podium and microphone? Where do the presenters sit while other speakers present? How will the room be set up? Will the audience be seated in chairs or at tables? What will be the potential distractions? Can audience members enter and leave the room? Will they be eating lunch or drinking beverages during the presentation? Discuss the expectations of the sponsoring organization and the presenter's role in the overall program. The goal is to anticipate all program setting issues that may be present as part of your preparation so you can be ready to address their effect.[8-10]

Content Analysis

The third step is content analysis. The key to holding the attention of an audience is to be coherent and to communicate with focused messages. An audience has limited time to absorb the speaker's ideas. The secret to brevity and simplicity is to know one's objectives before planning the talk. The content of the presentation needs to match the learning objectives. What does the speaker want to accomplish? What changes are intended in the knowledge, attitude, or behavior of the audience? Will they perform a task or recall some information? A common mistake made among untrained presenters is to attempt to cover too much in the time allotted. Inexperienced speakers often feel the need to parade their expertise and overload the audience with information. For example, the content of a presentation on food safety should vary depending on whether it is given to seasoned employees, or new employees, or a combination of the two groups.

In contrast to reading, which allows a person to go back to reconsider an idea, listening requires ongoing concentration. When the brain begins to feel overloaded and saturation sets in, it protects itself by shutting down or wandering elsewhere. You have probably had the experience of pretending to be listening to an overly meticulous speaker while your mind was elsewhere, having lost interest in the speaker's message. The content of an oral presentation needs to be limited to a few major points, generally formatted as three to five learning objectives. The listener can absorb focused content particularly when it is reinforced through details, examples, and a variety of media. Too much information and too many different points defeat the purpose. Listeners are more likely to give their full attention when they know where the presentation is going and are able to follow the presenter's reasoning. They are more likely to grasp examples and internalize them with greater ease.[7,10-12]

Components of an Effective Presentation

The three main organizational components of a presentation are the introduction, body, and summary. Most people are not aware that the organization of a presentation is critical to the response of the audience. An audience might retain about the same amount of information after hearing an organized presentation compared with a disorganized presentation, but only attendees at the organized presentation would consider its message seriously or possibly change their attitude toward the subject matter. An audience that hears an organized speaker is more likely to infer that the speaker is competent. An organized presentation gives the audience a sense that he or she knows exactly where the talk is going by structuring the talk with a defined beginning, middle, and end.[6-8,10-12]

Title and Speaker Introduction

Two important pieces precede the presentation itself: the creation of the presentation title and format of the speaker introduction. The title, as the initial impression, sets the stage by providing an interest level to the audience of the presentation. The title should be engaging but informative. It should prompt a degree of curiosity without deterring from the actual purpose of the presentation. The program organizer may suggest a title early in the process. The presenter should strive to have input into the final decision as a method of ensuring an initial energy level of audience expectation. For example, compare the following title options of "Diabetic Management" or "Innovative Methods to Improve Diabetic Management." The audience anticipates the active learning setting and value that the second option suggests.[7]

The introduction of the speaker should provide the information necessary for the audience to establish his or her credibility with the subject matter in a concise manner. The goal is to highlight only the pertinent information relevant to the audience rather than share the speaker's entire life history. The speaker introduction is most effective when it weaves professional information with a personal touch to connect the audience with the speaker. The speaker should provide a brief written introduction to the presenter to help link the content to the audience's recognition of the speaker's professional expertise. For example, the introduction could begin with pertinent educational and work experience. The introduction could continue with a suggested phrase such as "You may have read Mary's current article on this subject in the June issue of the *Journal of the American Medical Association* . . ." or "You will be interested to know Mary engages in the physical activity philosophy she will share today by being an avid walker herself . . . ."

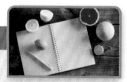

SELF-ASSESSMENT 1

How would you be introduced if you were asked to give a talk on nutrition? Write out an introduction for yourself.

Each of the three main organizational components of the actual presentation serves a specific function. The introduction begins the presentation by providing basic information to create interest. The body presents the actual data, details, and substance of the topic. The summary concludes the presentation and provides a take-home message for the audience. Generally, the introduction and summary sections should each take about 5 to 10 minutes of presentation time. The body should comprise the remainder of allotted time to cover the material while allowing for audience questions after the summary.[7-12] A detailed discussion of each component follows.

Introduction to the Presentation

The introduction serves as a transition to the body of the talk. The introduction content describes to audience members how the topic relates specifically to their needs. Start with an opening sentence or two that will set the stage for the general purpose of the presentation and gain listeners' attention. Follow with additional information to maintain the audience's interest, providing data to support the topic, or briefly describing the scope of the problem. This information heightens listeners' perception of the value of the presentation to them personally. Finally, the introduction outlines the specific learning objectives.

The objectives direct the listeners to the body of information that will follow. The speaker should engage the audience by "promising" a specific outcome (i.e., what listeners will know) at the end of the presentation. This may include ways to better control their health, provide more nutritious meals to their families, or become more food secure. Other ideas may convey how to be in a position in which others think better of them or respect them more, or feel they have the knowledge to develop and apply new skills in their job. The learning objectives prepare the audience to be attentive to the forthcoming message. Not every human need can be related to every topic, but as many as possible and as appropriate should be incorporated during the introduction.

An opening statement to consumers who come for a free presentation on the topic of heart disease might be: "You are here today to learn more about heart disease and how to make changes in your eating lifestyle to reduce your risk." This statement will start the connection. Brief statistics could then follow, showing the number

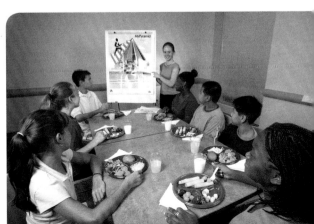

The professional enhances the presentation with visuals.
Source: US Department of Agriculture.

of heart disease deaths that occurred within the last year that were diet-related. The learning objectives continue the introduction by previewing the information in the body of the presentation. "Today I intend to discuss three specific points. First, we will examine the relationship of diet to heart disease. Second, I will discuss how to read food labels for the fat and cholesterol content of foods, and finally, I will provide guidelines on how to apply your new nutrition heart-savvy knowledge when eating out."

Not only does the introduction help the audience to listen to the talk with an expectation of what is to come, but the organization itself adds to the "halo effect" and increases the audience's perceptions of the speaker's credibility. The speaker should return to the learning objectives within the body of the presentation, if possible, to remind audience members of how the listening process is fulfilling their own needs.

CASE ANALYSIS 2

Write an introduction for Joan to use in her presentation?

Body of the Presentation

The body of the presentation expands the points mentioned in the introduction by providing the actual information and data. Presenters need to have a rationale for the way they decide to organize this major section to achieve the learning objectives. The body of the presentation also should ensure that audience members fully understand the content message, believe the speaker, and are comfortable enough with the speaker to share their objections in the event that they are confused or wish to challenge the presenter. Audience members expect to be able to do something differently after a presentation. Examples are to start reading food labels, to try a new recipe, to purchase a different food at the store, to eat breakfast, or to change the way they train other employees.

The speaker needs to construct the message clearly and concisely by presenting the information in a logical order. The content level is critical. It is necessary to direct the level of information from the baseline knowledge of the audience to a higher level that can be accomplished within the time allotted. This can be challenging when the audience has various levels of knowledge and expertise. The audience's understanding is enhanced by designing and incorporating media and participative experiences that include a wider scope of content than is covered in the presentation time. For example, a reference or simple handout of the principles of a heart-healthy diet that will not be discussed in depth during the talk may be given in addition to a specific handout focusing on the heart-healthy fats covered in depth during the body of the talk. In this way, the speaker meets the needs of both the audience members who need more information on the basic concept and those with advanced knowledge.

The presenter increases validity of the content and speaker credibility when he or she provides references, documentation, and sources along with the information presented. Finally, the speaker needs to develop a rapport with the audience during the body of the presentation by pacing the information through the presentation. Audience members should feel confident about the information presented and feel comfortable asking questions at the end of the presentation. If the speaker moves too quickly from one point to another, audience confusion and frustration may result. The breadth and depth of the content should match the time allowed. It is the responsibility of the speaker to end the presentation at the specified time, with enough time for questions. It is unfair to both the audience and the next speaker to take more time than planned due to poor organization or preparation.[7–12]

CASE ANALYSIS   3

What are the objectives of Joan's presentation?

Summary of the Presentation

The summary and conclusion signal the audience that the presentation is "winding down" and about to end. This transition needs to be gradual and smooth. When possible, review the initial learning objectives to remind the audience they have participated in achieving the overall goals of the presentation.

Concluding remarks such as "I guess that is all I have to say," "Thank you for listening," or "How about some questions?" are abrupt and sound haphazard. Remember that the speaker's credibility is influenced by the audience's perceptions of how well he or she has organized the presentation. Verbal clues such as "In conclusion . . .," "To summarize . . .," or "Before concluding, I want to leave you with one more thought . . ." are helpful in letting the audience know that the presentation is about to terminate. Many speakers use a final quote or anecdote to reinforce an important point one last time, display their contact information if not already provided on the handout, or use a standard slide with a question mark to set the stage for audience questions.

Be proactive in asking whether your listeners have any questions. Of course, people are often hesitant to ask questions. The speaker should prepare a few for the audience. You could ask for a reaction from a participant who has been paying attention. You might say, "I noticed that you smiled when I was discussing the list of foods to avoid. Would you be willing to share what food will be most difficult for you to give up and some ideas you may have for an acceptable alternative?" After responding to the first question, which was generated by the presenter, it is often simpler to get others to respond when asked "What *other* questions or comments do you have?"[7-12]

Remember to bring business cards and to remain after the presentation to speak with people who may want to share comments or ask questions. Speakers who have maintained good eye contact and have prompted the inference of warmth through smiling almost always find themselves interacting with audience members who wish to engage them after the presentation. This is frequently a chance to develop contacts for additional speaking engagements, and it is therefore an opportunity for the best kind of face-to-face public relations. When a long line of people is waiting to talk and time is limited, encourage the remaining people to use your business card information to contact you. Be sure to follow up as promised.

CASE ANALYSIS 4

How should Joan handle the conclusion of her presentation?

Implementation of an Effective Presentation

Using some basic techniques, described in the next paragraphs, speakers can create and deliver an effective presentation.

Audience Connection

Audiences identify with speakers who appear worthy and knowledgeable. Speakers, therefore, should subtly let listeners know during their presentation that they are qualified. For example, one might say, "... in an article I wrote last year for the *Journal of the Academy of Nutrition and Dietetics* ..." or "of the several hundred patients I have worked with in the past." Audiences tend to be more attentive when they believe that the person speaking to them is able to relate to their circumstances or demonstrate any connection they may have with a particular group. For example, you might say, "I have lived in this community for 15 years ..." or "I was once 25 lb overweight myself ...." If one gives it some thought, almost all audiences have some traits with which the speaker can identify.[10-12]

Presenters are evaluated by the audience and the audience's perceptions add to the ambiance from the moment they enter the room. Whenever possible, presenters should arrive early and make an effort to meet people. Their own self-confidence, whether real or feigned, will relax the audience and increase attendees' perceptions of the speaker's desire to share information. Presenters should never volunteer negative information regarding their own stress or fear of speaking. The audience wants to learn and enjoy. When they are aware of the speaker's fragility or stage fright, they tend to become nervous themselves in sympathy.[8-12]

If the presenters are waiting to be introduced and are seated among the audience or on a stage, they should be aware that audience members will be watching their every move. This starts before beginning the presentation. Speakers must be careful to smile, look confident, and extend themselves to others. After the speaker is introduced, the way he or she walks up to the podium is critical. The pose that the speaker assumes during the presentation is also influential. During those first moments, an initial impression is being created. The speaker should walk confidently while looking and smiling toward the audience. Before uttering the first words to the audience, a good technique is to spend a long 3 seconds just looking out at the audience. Try to smile and establish eye contact with several people. This allows them to infer poise, confidence, and the speaker's desire to connect with them.[10,13]

Trained speakers see almost everything from their position in front of the room. If they are alert, they may see people who are beginning to fidget. They can interpret and act on such feedback. Speakers might decide consequently to give the audience a brief interaction, such as responding to a question by asking audience members to raise their hands. They might heighten their own movements to regain attention. They might engage in a new activity, perhaps one that involves audience participation. They might see some people coming in late, looking awkwardly for a seat. This gives them the opportunity to publicly welcome them and ask others to move over to provide seating. The audience will begin to send signals and participate when they realize the speaker is sensitive to them.[8,9]

Although individual situations may make it difficult to adhere to this structure, a general rule is to plan on at least 10 minutes for audience interaction when the speaker-allotted time is 60 minutes. When speaking for more than an hour, audience participation activities during the presentation are essential to keep the audience engaged and invested. The highly acclaimed TED (Technology, Entertainment, and Design) talk format uses an 18-minute time frame.[10]

Use of Visuals

Media are a direct extension of the speaker and consequently reflect directly on the speaker's credibility. Media may include computer-generated slides, video or audio clips, handouts, flip charts, and even actual props such as food. Media that are prepared, designed, and implemented with

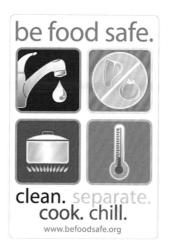

Figure 13-1 ■ Select simple messages to support oral presentations.
Source: Partnership for Food Safety Education

high professional standards set the stage for a superior presentation. For example, a speaker who uses slides in large print with attractive clip art, rather than a black-and-white lettering with small print, allows the audience to infer that he or she is an experienced and considerate presenter (Figure 13-1). Even the quality and color of the paper used in handouts can add or detract from the overall impression.[10–12] More information on creating effective media is found in Chapter 14.

CASE ANALYSIS 5

What media could Joan plan to use in her presentation?

Delivery Techniques

The written text and the oral presentation are entirely different. There is no objection to a presenter initially writing out the entire talk. This involves carefully organizing the information to be presented using whatever systematic order seems appropriate, such as topics, steps, or other framework. However, once the talk is written, the speaker needs to recognize that the written manuscript represents the "science" of a presentation, whereas the actual delivery represents the "art." Each time it is delivered, the presentation should be somewhat different. Use unique words, examples, or anecdotes to suit particular audiences and situations. The choice of words in spoken language also tends to differ from that in written language.

Sentences in oral speech tend to be simpler, shorter, and more conversational, including common words and contractions. In comparison, a written manuscript may be more erudite and academic. The only way for speakers to develop this art is to rehearse from a simple outline and not a manuscript. It is also essential to rehearse in front of real people who will react and comment, rather than in front of inert settings such as mirrors, walls, or car windshields.

Never read or memorize! There are other good reasons for not rehearsing from a manuscript. The speech tends eventually to become memorized and that can be deadly. Once a speech is memorized, speakers tend to become more speech-centered than audience-centered. They tend to become more concerned about whether they can remember each line exactly as it is written on the manuscript. Speakers become less concerned about whether the audience is enjoying, learning, listening, and understanding. Another problem that arises from manuscript speaking is that it is *dull!* Because the speaker's facial expressions and vocal intonations are not spontaneous, the monologue tends to sound memorized and can easily become boring to listeners.[7,8,10–13]

One of the least effective practices that presenters can do is to admit to an audience self-doubt: scared, ill prepared, missing material, sick with a cold, or lack of confidence. The audience does not know what it may be missing and is generally much less critical of speakers than speakers are of themselves. The speaker must act confidently, even when he or she does not feel it internally. Speakers experience themselves in the situation from the inside out. The audience experiences them from the outside in. This means that if asked whether they are nervous or anxious, speakers should always answer "No!" Audience members see only the tip of the iceberg when they observe the speaker. They usually do not feel the intensity of the speaker's anxiety. Audiences are commonly unaware of it unless it is brought to their attention through the speaker's own confession.[12–14]

The feelings commonly referred to as "stage fright" may date back to the dawn of the human race, when our prehistoric ancestors had to survive by living in caves and sharing the food supply with other beasts. Faced by a predator, our ancestors had a genuine use for a sudden jolt of energy, which gave them the power to do battle or run (i.e., fight-or-flight response). The vestiges of this power, stemming from the secretions of the adrenal gland, still manifest themselves today when people sense danger. Who hasn't felt that ice block in the stomach while being reprimanded by the boss or experienced sweaty palms and racing heart while walking into a room full of strangers? Occasionally, one still reads newspaper accounts of a person exhibiting superhuman strength under conditions of fear or danger, as in the father who lifts a car off his child who has been pinned under the wheels. This is an example of the power that comes with the adrenaline jolt. When a person is unable to fight, run, or in some other way utilize this surge, he or she may become overwhelmed by the internal feelings themselves.

The best safeguard against stage fright is adequate preparation and rehearsal. The more one practices in front of *live people*, the less nervousness one exhibits. Other ways of dealing with these feelings include being active during the presentation and "acting" calm and confident. If presenters know they are going to be full of extra energy because of their excess adrenaline secretions, they should address this in their planning. Energy can be incorporated during the presentation by activities such as passing out materials, using a pointer, or any other activity that involves motion. Motion is a release for tension and anxiety. It allows the audience to infer enthusiasm from the speaker's movement rather than fright, nervousness, or tension. It may not work for everyone, but many people can learn to control their public behavior if they visualize themselves as acting.[10-13]

All movement should be meaningful. Do not pace. Presenters should look for opportunities to break the invisible barrier between themselves and their audience. Walking toward the audience, walking around the audience, walking in and out of the audience, and walking among the audience are all acceptable ways of delivering a presentation. What is not acceptable is pacing back and forth, particularly with eyes down, as the speaker pulls his or her thoughts together before uttering them. Movement into an audience is a communication vehicle in itself. When presenters penetrate that invisible barrier between themselves and the audience, they are nonverbally indicating their desire to connect, to be closer, to better sense what it is the audience is feeling about the speaker and the content. In fact, as speakers walk among the audience, the audience can begin to be seen from a different perspective. The speaker may gain new insights into how better to clarify particular points and issues from this experience.[10,13,15]

Environmental Control

Take control of seating the listeners before everyone settles down. It may be their boardroom, gymnasium, or meeting hall, but it is the presenter's "show." Make conscious decisions about whether or not to pull the group into a circle, half-circle, rows, sitting around tables, and so forth. When it is possible to know beforehand which persons are the most influential, their seats should be reserved and placed in the best position to see, hear, and appreciate visual aids as well as the speaker. Box 13-1 provides a final checklist for presentations.

Presenters do best when they omit all barriers between themselves and their audience. Avoid using a podium, if possible. Sometimes, due to the room setup or requirements of other speakers, this cannot be avoided but the speaker can stand next to the podium. Use of a table, which can feature handouts and other materials, is preferred. Adults generally do not learn optimally through lecture the method. Unless the speaker is extraordinarily talented, a straight lecture presented from behind a podium should be avoided. When delivering a message while standing in front of a group

Customizing and completing this checklist before presentations will help avoid last-minute problems.

· Do I have my presentation notes?
· Do I have all my supporting materials?
· Are handouts available for each of the attendees?
· Will the facility be unlocked and open?
· Are the tables and chairs arranged as requested?
· Do I understand how to operate the lighting system?
· Do I understand how to control the temperature of the room?
· Do I know the location of the electrical circuits?
· Is all the media equipment required in place and working?
· Do I have presentation accessories? (i.e., timer, business cards, laptop, laser pointer)
· Do I have backup accessories? (i.e., extra bulb, extension cord, marker, laser pointer)
· Do I have the type of audio system I require? Is it working?
· Have I switched my smartphone to silent during the presentation?
· Will there be a sign to announce the presentation location?
· Will someone be introducing me, and have I given all the information I want shared with the group?

Box 13-1 ■ Checklist for Oral Presentations

without a barrier, the speaker is more disposed to stop the talk to respond to the verbal or nonverbal feedback of listeners. Gestures and movement, too, can be expansive and visible without the lectern barrier.[6-8]

Practice the use of the media in relationship to the speaking location. Evaluate the use of media with the available lighting and determine if a change in the lighting settings is necessary or possible. Check the arrangements for distribution of the handouts, if applicable. Identify the person who is responsible for introductions and verify the information as necessary.

Determine the options in microphone use. Whenever possible, try to use a clip-on or wireless system, which allows more movement than a positioned microphone at a podium. Ask for a glass of water to be provided during the presentation. Drinking from a bottle of water is distracting.

A presenter should be familiar with the site and equipment.

Be rigorous about time constraints. Bring a small travel clock or timer with large numbers to help monitor time available or locate a clock if present. Turn off any personal electronics. Calculate prior to the presentation actual transition times between the introduction, body, and summary of the presentation. The presenter can also designate a member of the program committee or a colleague in the audience to signal when to begin stating the conclusion.

CASE ANALYSIS   6

What implementation approaches would you recommend with Joan's audience?

Voice and Diction

Vocal inflection and variation add interest and the impression of speaker enthusiasm. For some people, controlling this variation is simple and natural; for others, it is a challenge. Nevertheless, the presenter needs to attend to voice modulation. The goal when speaking in front of a group is to sound natural and conversational. However, what sounds natural and conversational when standing in front of a large group is not the same as what sounds conversational in a small face-to-face group. "Natural and conversational" from the presenter's point of view is exaggerated. The highs need to be a bit higher and the lows need to be a bit lower. What may sound to the presenter's ear as phony and theatrical generally sounds far less so to the listener. The good news is that this trait can be fairly easily and quickly developed, even in those who recognize a problem in this area. It requires risking sounding foolish and exaggerated in front of trusting others until adequate reinforcement has convinced the presenter that the increase in vocal variation is really an advantage. In any case, a delivery that is of narrow range or monotone is difficult to respond to for more than a few minutes.[10,13,15]

When talking in front of a group, the speaker should generally attempt to speak more slowly than in ordinary conversation. What is an appropriate rate during a small face-to-face discussion is probably too fast for a group presentation. For some reason, there seems to be a correlation between the speech rate of the speaker and the size of the audience. What might be easily grasped at a more rapid rate in face-to-face conversation is not understood as quickly in large groups. Speaking at a slower rate also allows the presenter to scan the audience while speaking to see if he or she is being understood. This also allows one to see if some people need an opportunity to disagree, to see if he or she needs to talk louder, or to increase the variation because some listeners look bored.

Professional speakers attend to their diction, particularly when pronouncing words such as "for," "can," "with," "picture," "going to," and "want to." In ordinary conversation, one is not likely to judge negatively a speaker who mispronounces common words and engages in sloppy diction, saying, for example, "fer," "ken," "wit," "pitcher," "gunna," and "wanna," for the words listed above. However, when that speaker is in front of an audience, these mispronounced words often stand out and lead to negative inferences regarding the speaker. Professionals who present themselves in front of groups must attend to their diction because they risk losing credibility if it is poor.

Once speakers have become conscious of their diction and have decided to improve it, several steps are required. First, speakers can ask trusted others who are often around them to listen critically and to stop them each time a diction error occurs. Second, after they learn of the common diction problems, speakers need to train themselves to hear the errors. It is difficult to critically evaluate ourselves during speech. Like learning to ride a bicycle or use a computer, this learning and training task is uncomfortable at first, but improvement comes quickly. Third, speakers need to recognize that working on diction is an ongoing task. Professional speakers never stop listening to the way their words are coming out and continually plan ahead to pronounce them correctly. When necessary, phonetically clarify difficult words or phrases on small cards. Guard against stumbling or mispronunciation by practicing these challenges over and over until they flow easily.[10,12,15]

Gestures and Body Language

It is good practice to keep your hands away from your body and from one another. Allow them to be free to gesture. Avoid holding anything in them while talking unless it is a useful prop like a laser pointer or a visual aid. A laser pointer or a computer mouse should selectively illustrate important points. Audiences are distracted when laser points move in a wild or circular manner repeatedly on the screen. Presenters often feel awkward with their hands hanging loosely at their sides. Perhaps if they could see themselves on videotape in this posture, they would realize that it is natural looking, but even more important, they would probably see that one tends not to stay in that position. If hands hang loosely at the presenter's sides, eventually the hands begin to rise and gesture spontaneously to emphasize important points.

It is risky to begin a presentation holding a pen, paperclip, rubber band, or other instrument not directly related to the presentation. Unconsciously, the fingers begin to play with the instrument, and the audience becomes fascinated with watching to see what the speaker will do. Presenters need to train themselves to keep their faces animated, using a variety of facial expressions. For many of the same reasons expressed earlier, it is important that speakers use all the communication vehicles available to them to maintain the audience's attention. Facial expression is itself a communication vehicle. When it is lively, animated, expressive, and changing regularly while the speaker reacts to the feedback coming toward him or her from the audience, it enhances the verbal message and allows the audience to go on unconsciously inferring the speaker's audience-centeredness. This is easier for some people to do than for others; however, everyone can improve. Because it is not easy for a speaker to "act" expressive, it does not mean that this person cannot grow considerably in the ability to look expressive.[10-13]

Eye contact is a vehicle of communication. Use eye contact to see everyone and respond to the nonverbal feedback. When speakers have the opportunity to present themselves and their ideas to an audience, they want the audience to understand them, to believe them, and to follow their recommendations. A speaker has the best chance of being successful in achieving these goals when able to interpret the audience's ongoing reactions. Presentation speaking is often considered a one-way form of communication in which the speaker talks at the audience as they listen. Effective speaking is actually a two-way situation in which audience and speaker communicate with one another constantly and simultaneously.[9]

Facial expressions are important. Presenters must remember to smile and look as if they are enjoying the experience of sharing information. Smiling can be rehearsed and may feel phony, but it needs to be built into the design of the presentation. Speakers do not need to be constantly grinning, but they do need to maintain an expression of interest and engagement with their audience. The easiest way to convey these impressions is by smiling naturally and often during the presentation. Unfortunately, it is not easy to smile when one is unsure of the material. All the preceding techniques can be implemented only after the speaker has sufficiently mastered the content and has consciously, through rehearsal, developed skills.

Professional Appearance

Professional dress suggests to the audience one's status as a speaker by providing a sense of confidence. Ironically, this means selecting appropriate clothing that does not attract attention and that the audience will not remember! A well-tailored business suit for men paired with a neutral color shirt (off-white or light colors for camera work) and a tie that complements in a similar color tone are good choices. Women can choose skirt

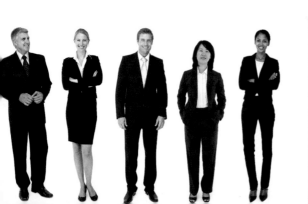

Professional appearance is important.

or pant suits and neutral or pastel business tops. If you are speaking from a raised stage, consider the view "upwards" from the audience viewpoint. Comfortable, polished shoes are important with stable heels to prevent loss of balance with movement. Bright colors, large patterns, unusual designs, casual styles, light-reflecting or noisy jewelry, and dangling earrings all may distract from the speaker's message by drawing too much of the audience's focus away from the oral message.[13,15–18]

CASE ANALYSIS   7

What should Joan wear to this presentation?

Evaluation Methods

Effective speakers use feedback from every presentation they give to fine-tune their skills. Standard program evaluations often rate the speaker on the planned learning objectives. More in-depth program evaluations may add information on effectiveness and presentation traits. Ask the program planner to provide a copy of the audience evaluation of the presentation. Obtain an audiotape or videotape. Some speakers tape their presentations or ask a trusted audience member to do so on their behalf.[7]

CASE ANALYSIS   8

What method(s) could be used to evaluate the effectiveness of the presentation?

Adaptations

Although workshops and media interviews rely on many of the general presentation guidelines that are outlined, each of these situations warrants specific adaptations to be successful and effective in its own arena.

Group Workshop Format

Workshops are oral presentations of longer duration with multiple topics. Workshop leaders should plan on using techniques that involve all participants. Open communication should occur between the leader and the participants as well as among the participants themselves. This portion of the chapter on presentation skills deals specifically with tips for leading and planning a group workshop format. More information can be found in Chapter 15 on group learning strategies.

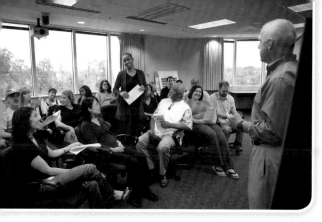

A presenter should arrange the seating area in advance.
Source: CDC.

Strategies to encourage participation include dividing the larger group into smaller groups, giving smaller groups time to get to know one another, and then assigning each small group sets of activities related to the workshop topic. These small group activities may include such things as case studies, role-playing, questionnaire completion, brainstorming, or discussion. Participants can also become involved through the use of digital audience-response systems where they can express their opinions anonymously yet their merged responses can be shared for further discussion as a group. Occasionally, participants may be asked to complete preworkshop assignments, such as filling out a questionnaire, reading material related to the workshop, or performing some other task. Reactions to these tasks can be processed among the participants in small groups.[7]

Media Interview Format

Increasingly, public health and dietetics interventions depend on effective health communication. This may include the influence of media politics, the accuracy of media reporting, the use of media for health education and advocacy, and the availability of training in media relations for staff members. An organization's image and credibility are clearly influenced by both the manner and content of its media spokespersons. This portion of the chapter on presentation skills deals specifically with tips for presenting oneself or one's organization in the media.

When given the opportunity to present information through the mass media, one needs to understand the power of the media to influence and the inferences that listeners or viewers make. This effect is based not only on the speaker's presentation and speaking skills but also on the speaker's manner. After grasping the enormous persuasive power of mass media, a presenter can train to use it to his or her advantage. However, if the presenter is unaware and makes no special adaptations for the media, the presentation will be unsuccessful—even though the content is excellent.[10–13]

Presenter's Style

When communicating through the mass media, speakers need to remember that in more than 50% of listeners, interpretation of the message is influenced not by the content but by the form—the speaker's manner, energy, and level of enthusiasm and the vehicles and media used for transmission.

It is best to present the information directly in a conversational manner with only a brief outline as a guide. Speakers who paraphrase, quote, or read directly from a manuscript ordinarily will not convey the same tone of confidence, integrity, passion, and sincerity that a person who is speaking for himself or herself will be able to demonstrate. To demonstrate passion, for example, the speaker needs to know the material thoroughly, have strong feelings about it, and allow himself or herself to emulate the message and not read just empty words.[9–15]

Airtime is expensive and interviewers may interrupt or give signals to wind up the comments. When invited to be interviewed or share information through the mass media, speakers need to verify how much time they will be allotted and plan accordingly. When time is limited, the speaker needs to decide ahead of time what points are most essential, have these points highlighted, and express them first. If additional time is provided, he or she can then elaborate or add additional information.[10,11,13,15]

Chances of being selected for a media presentation increase if videotaped clips or focused content outlines are submitted. Once something is taped, the performance becomes a permanent record that can appear anywhere or anytime in the future, so preparation and focus are key components of success.[10]

Often, radio and television interviewers do not have time to become well informed regarding the specifics of their guests' causes. Always maintain a professional manner. Being short with an interviewer may well be interpreted as arrogance and reflect negatively on the speaker's cause. Keep the message simple. It would be wise to rehearse and tape answers and then listen carefully. Use commercial breaks to clarify the direction of the conversation.

Humor is a powerful communication vehicle, but not all people have the gift. Interviewees should be particularly careful about trying to be funny. It may make them look foolish unless they are confident they have the special gift. When, however, the material itself is genuinely funny and has been tried successfully in other audiences, the use of humor can be considered.

Often television and radio programs conduct preinterviews to determine whether the guest is articulate and interesting enough to hold the audience. This is the time to do your best. Just because the host is being kind and polite does not mean that he or she will not decide to omit the least interesting or articulate guests.

After presenting in the mass media several times, one becomes adept at processing the experience while it is happening. Presenters need to develop a third eye to monitor themselves in the media and send back messages to themselves about how they are doing during the presentation or interview. Because the human mind whirls several times faster than speech speed, it is possible to see and hear yourself while talking and to modify accordingly. The rule generally is that for the mass media, one's natural behavior should be exaggerated somewhat larger than life but without being outrageous. Speakers need to behave in a way that generates inferences of self-confidence, sincerity, and even charisma.

Hand gestures on television should be carefully controlled; they tend to be distracting on the screen. Speakers need to sustain interest through their dynamic voice, cadence, inflections, pauses, tone, and facial expression. Although large expansive gestures generally don't work well, variety and variation do work.

Handling Questions and Problems

Very few nonprofessional presenters are able to improvise and come off looking professional. Answers to questions that the interviewee expects to be asked should be rehearsed and not read from notes. If asked a question you can't answer, the smartest thing to do is admit it. Continue by offering to locate the answer and forward it to the appropriate people with a clear deadline. One could also say: "While I can't exactly answer that, I can tell you that . . . ." This brings the discussion back to the presenter's main message. Part of the self-monitoring process should include the interviewee judging the length of his or her own answers. Avoid long-winded answers or monologues. They tend to bore listeners and irritate the interviewer. Keep the response focused. Dress is a communication vehicle itself. The best advice is to dress conservatively and in good taste and to avoid being flashy or drawing attention through clothes.[10,13,15,16–18]

When one is representing an organization, often the same questions will be asked over and over, day after day. Remember, this is the first time many in the audience may be hearing this message; presentations need to sound fresh each time, even though it may be the speaker's 20th time in 2 days answering the same questions.[9]

Bored listeners and viewers change channels. Guest interviewees and presenters need to prepare themselves with interesting anecdotes and aphorisms. Personal experiences tend to hold attention. The deadliest mistake is to become too intellectual or abstract.

When several guests are on the same panel or are involved in a simultaneous interview, someone may attempt to dominate or interrupt. Be prepared to assert yourself if this occurs. Push back into the conversation and say something like "Let me finish my point" or "Hold that thought while I finish one point." This should be done with a smile and kind voice, but it should, by all means, be done. Listeners and viewers respect the person who stands up for himself or herself—politely. Never become defensive to a member of the audience or another panelist. The speaker should simply look to the moderator to move the program on.

If you feel offended publicly, grin and bear it rather than reacting emotionally. You can say "I don't agree" or "Let's look at this from another perspective," but do not snap back a retort. This response may portray you as being weak or overly sensitive, rather than competent and qualified.

Speakers should avoid mentioning the time, place, or date of the live broadcast. If a media clip is not "dated," it has a better chance of being used again by other affiliates who may need material.

There may be times when the speaker thinks he or she has been invited to talk about a specific cause, but once there the interviewer steers to other topics. When this happens, it is the speaker's responsibility to get his or her original message across even if the host isn't considerate enough to afford the right opportunities. If questions become inappropriate or are about topics that you would rather not discuss, simply say, "I would rather not discuss that." Don't waffle or use "double-talk." Credibility is destroyed when listeners infer deception.

Final impressions count, especially in the media. The speaker should use the final public moments to leave a positive impression of a composed, assertive, and controlled person. Privately, before leaving, the speaker should look for the producer and director and thank them personally as well. A firm handshake and looking people in the eye while talking add a separate nonverbal message itself, apart from the verbal one being expressed.[10-15]

Summary

The suggestions provided in this chapter need to be practiced rather than memorized. Presenters need to involve participants in their presentations. Straight lecture without interaction among participants is less effective in bringing about change than lecture with discussion.

Developing presentation skills and handling the myriad of problems that can occur with media or interviewers constitute a process that occurs over time. Presenters get better and better with each subsequent opportunity or practice.

Review and Discussion Questions

1. What are the three analysis processes used when preparing a presentation?
2. What are the major components of an effective presentation?
3. Describe and analyze several experiences you have had as an audience member.
4. Why is it important for a presenter to proofread all materials used in the presentation?
5. What does it mean to be audience-centered?
6. How can presenters overcome challenges such as nervousness, fear, and stage fright?
7. Why are a presenter's verbal and nonverbal expressions important?
8. What is the difference between a presentation and a workshop?

Suggested Activities

1. Design and deliver a 10-minute presentation on some issue related to foods, nutrition, or dietetics, such as safety of the food supply, a new food product, fiber in foods, reduced fat or calories in foods, snacks, restaurant meals, or sodium.
2. Design and deliver a presentation intended for a group of parents of obese children. A minimum of two visual aids should be used. Included with the 20-minute presentation should be five full minutes of audience–speaker interaction.
3. Design and deliver a 30-minute presentation intended for a group of people who have recently learned they have diabetes. A minimum of three visual aids are required, including flip chart and handout material. Plan on at least 8 minutes of interaction with the audience; this should

be prompted by the speaker's perceptions of the nonverbal feedback emanating from the audience.

4. Design and deliver a 60-minute presentation intended for a group of people who have paid to be taught or trained by you in an area related to your specialty in the area of dietetics. Develop whatever aids seem appropriate.

Note: If possible, all presentations should be videotaped. Presenters should provide reaction sheets to the audience and later write a critique of the taped presentation responding to their own subjective reactions, the critique sheets of the audience, and the instructor's comments.

CHAPTER 14

Using Instructional Media

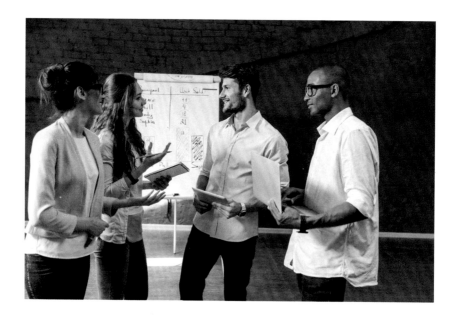

Objectives

- Describe key points for utilizing and/or creating instructional media.
- Explain the difference between asynchronous and synchronous education.
- Evaluate instructional media for intended audiences.
- Measure literacy and numeracy level of educational materials.
- Identify key technology trends in media.

Julie gathered her flip chart and markers and headed for her office door at 9:00 AM. She was conducting an employee training session on proper handwashing that began at 9:00 AM. As she entered the training room, she said to the 20 participants, "Oh well, I'm here. Let's begin by watching a short video."

Julie tried to login to the classroom computer without success. She realized she would not be able to show the DVD disk she had also brought. Frustrated and embarrassed, Julie said, "Nothing in this room works right." Julie called the Media Center from the training room using her cell phone, but no one answered. She turned to the group and said, "I was in a hurry this morning, and I forgot my handouts for the session. It will just take me a few minutes to go back to my office to get them." She then left the room.

The commonality between science and art is in trying to see profoundly, to develop strategies of seeing and showing.

—Edward Tufte

Introduction

Instructional media is a broad term used to describe a wide array of visual materials. Formats vary from simple traditional tools such as food models or flip charts to more sophisticated digital technology such as webinars or podcasts. The use of visual media when presenting information to any audience greatly enhances the delivery of your message. Communication is more effective when an audience is engaged in the process of learning through visual connections. This chapter examines and evaluates the types of instructional media most commonly available, offers suggestions for effective use, and discusses the evolving application of digital media technology.

Benefits of Visual Media

"A picture is worth a thousand words." How true! Four pictures, therefore, are worth 4,000 words. The more information you want your audience to remember, the more visual assistance is needed. When people can see materials rather than merely hear them or read about them, they remember more. Visual media are especially helpful to groups with limited reading ability, literacy or numeracy issues, and language challenges.

A large body of evidence documents that individuals remember less of what they read (7%–10%) or hear (20%–38%) and remember most from what they see or do (55%–80%).[1] Although the estimates vary, the trend is clear. Using visual media helps enhance learning and retaining information. Talking alone, whether about healthy eating or sanitation principles, only gets limited results. Active participation is the key to learning.[2,3]

Visual media are part of the instructional input. Visuals enhance written and oral communication methods and make them more interesting. Pictures and sounds have the power to compel attention, to enhance understanding, and to promote learning in a shorter time frame than by using solely verbal explanations. But a strong presentation does not overly rely on visual aids. The presenter should be able to convey the message without visuals if necessary.

Planning Use of Visual Media

Planning what instructional media to use is part of the overall program planning for any learning situation. Answers to the following seven questions will help your thinking:

1. What are the objectives or aims of the session? What should audience members learn or be able to do?
2. What methods or activities (i.e., lecture, discussion, individual counseling, simulation) will facilitate accomplishing the objectives? Where can media provide reinforcement of the methods and activities?
3. Who is the audience? What is the size of the audience? What are the characteristics of the learner (i.e., age, gender, educational and literacy level, language preference, cultural or ethnic group)?
4. What is the learner's current level of knowledge of the topic? A presentation to a lay group, for example, would need different visuals than a presentation to a group of professionals. New employee training may need a different approach compared with an audience of long-term employees.
5. What purpose(s) do the visuals serve? Is it to generate interest in the subject; to affect attitudes, emotions, or motivation; to entertain; to present information; to attract and hold attention; to involve the learner in mental activity promoting learning; or some combination of these purposes?
6. How can you concisely organize and sequence the points to be made while emphasizing them with visuals? How are the key messages being reinforced? Can you break down the learning into key steps and assess knowledge at each step?
7. How will you evaluate the effectiveness of the total presentation, including visuals?[4,5]

The instructional media selected depend on the goals, the size of the audience, the physical facilities, the equipment and time available, as well as the learning style of the audience.

CASE ANALYSIS **1**

Using the questions above, what information might apply to Julie's audience?

Before discussing types of visuals, let's identify key principles for all visuals.

Art and Design Principles

The quality and effectiveness of media may depend to a great extent on art and design principles. A practitioner does not have to be a great artist, but some understanding of simple principles improves results. First and foremost, the visual must be large enough for all participants to see. Know basic parameters on the physical conditions where your presentation will occur and the type of presentation before selecting and/or creating the visuals.

Simplicity and Unity

The presenter should try to convey only one idea at a time, since too many ideas confuse the audience. Decide what should be at the center of attention or interest and then build around it. Focus on it immediately and reinforce the message. The inclusion of three main messages is enough for most presentations.

Wording and Lettering

Be concise and use the fewest words possible. Use an image when you can. Working on conciseness of wording should help to organize the thoughts that the presenter wants to get across. Titles and labels are placed at various locations. Headings or headlines need to clarify the emphasis and should be in larger print.

Standardizing the size of the lettering (type size) and the kind of lettering (fonts) conveys a more professional appearance. Times Roman and Gothic are more readable than some stylized script fonts (see Box 14-1 for examples of fonts). The size must be large enough to be read by the reader who is sitting the farthest away. Limit the number of fonts to one or two. Type size also needs to be considered in handouts. For handouts, a minimum of 12-point type size is recommended; for the elderly, a 14- or 18-point type size. Dark colors on light backgrounds provide an effective contrast.[4]

10 point type

12 point type

14 point type

18 point type

24 point type

36 point type

48 point type

Times New Roman

Century

Courier New

Freestyle Script

Arial

COPPERPLATE GOTHIC BOLD

Rockwell

Lucida Handwriting

Box 14-1 ■ Type Styles, Fonts, and Print Sizes

For slides, the number of words should be limited to 20 to 36 per slide. The "rule of six," is to use not more than six lines and not more than six words per line with type size of 24 points or higher.[4] Capital letters are appropriate for short titles of five to six words or less, but not advised for longer sentences (i.e., ALL CAPS ARE MORE DIFFICULT TO READ WHEN USED IN LENGTHY TITLES). Traditional use of capital and lower case is preferable for longer titles, allowing space for readability (i.e., A Combination of Upper and Lower Case Letters Allows the Reader to Comprehend Material). You may wish to number lists or use bullets (•), underline words for emphasis, or add stars to key points.[4,5]

Color

Color can enhance visuals and demand attention. A noted color design consultant, Laura Guido-Clark, uses the principle that "within 90 seconds of viewing an object or environment, you base up to 90% of your subconscious judgment on color alone."[6] You should combine colors that are pleasing aesthetically and do not clash. It is best to decide on the focus of the visual and select the color for that element first. Colors have subtle meanings for individuals. In most Western countries, red and orange are considered "hot," whereas green, blue, and violet are considered "cool" colors.[4] Colors closest to nature, such as blue and green, may feel fresh and are most pleasing to the widest audience. The presenter should start by considering the background color. If it is light, any bright colors may be used. With a dark background, lighter shades are needed for contrast and the print must be larger to be readable. Select a color or theme and only change it for major reasons. Look for standardized templates, such as found in PowerPoint, that provide preselected color palates that are balanced.

Images

Visual images can illustrate difficult concepts well. This includes proportions, relationships, similarities, and differences. An illustration evokes a visual picture of a procedure or technique. A cartoon can add fun to the presentation and increase the viewer's memory of a concept. The use of a flowchart or logic model can visually illustrate a process. As with the other principles, the food and nutrition professional should consider the layout of the illustration and its effect on the audience understanding. Is it too crowded? Confusing? Is the image serving its purpose to enhance the text rather than distracting from it? A complex table or chart may be better as a handout than as a slide. Reduce to a simplified format or break up your message into several slides. Select relevant images in a purposeful manner. If inserting audio or visual elements, try to limit them to 60 to 90 seconds or less.

Balance and Emphasis

There are two kinds of balance, formal and informal. Informal balance is asymmetrical and more attention-getting and interesting than symmetrical balance. Formal balance occurs when one half is the mirror image of the other half. Bear in mind that our society reads from left to right and top to bottom, so that is the way most audiences will view any visual.[4] Figure 14-1 illustrates balance.

Multiple Formats

Consider preparing multiple instructional formats. Have a plan to deal with media and equipment that do not work or are too small for the space.

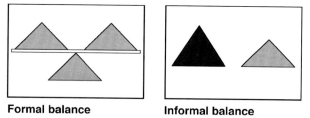

Formal balance **Informal balance**

Figure 14-1 ■ Formal and informal balance.

Bring a printed copy of any digital presentation. Always be prepared to deliver the presentation without the assistance of media.

CASE ANALYSIS 2

How could Julie have been prepared for use of multiple instructional media?

Copyright and Permission

Obtain necessary permissions for any images or recordings you are planning to use. Some web-based images and reference materials can be used freely as part of the public domain. Other materials clearly show copyright information when downloaded and have limitations on their use.[3,4]

Asynchronous or Synchronous Learning

Instructional information may be delivered in a synchronous or asynchronous manner. In synchronous learning, all the participants are learning at the same time. This may be one on one, as a small group, or as a large group. Traditionally, synchronous learning was done in one location in an office, classroom, or conference room. Today, synchronous learning can occur at two or more sites via many methods such as videoconferencing, with distributed accompanying printed materials or live webinar interactive Internet presentations. Asynchronous learning is "anytime learning." Reading a journal article, watching a podcast from a web site, and participating in an e-mail discussion based on your schedule are examples of asynchronous learning. Asynchronous learning gives learners much more freedom over their approach to learning. They can read, listen, or watch the material until they are comfortable with it. Both types of education should be designed so the learner must actively participate in the process whether by participating with others or by completing tutorials and quizzes.

Computer-based learning modules are common in many work sites. Computer-based instruction can be used in various ways. It provides time flexibility and a consistent message.[2,7] Learners read or listen and complete practice or comprehensive tests. This method is particularly good for learning facts such as remembering medical terminology or practicing skills such as calculating a parenteral nutrition solution. The clients or employees are given rapid feedback on how well they comprehend the material. Tutorials, games, and simulations may augment the learning.

Today, the technology and teaching methods have advanced to the point that very interactive facilitated learning between teacher and student can occur via the computer. Computer-based distance education is a rapidly growing instructional media format. An online distance education class generally has all the components of a traditional class: textbooks, readings, assignments, and tests. The class discussion is replaced by a web-based discussion facilitated by the teacher. The lecture is replaced by readings, visual lectures, and audio or video streaming. The students and faculty generally need high-speed Internet connections.[8,9]

For "just-in-time" patient, client, or employee education, many institutions are using stand-alone computer kiosks (terminals). This touch-screen approach allows access to information from convenient locations with visual and audio components. Clients can get information when they need it. It does not replace, but rather augments, the food and nutrition professional's message.[10-12]

These two types of learning can be used in tandem and in any order. For example, a newly diagnosed diabetic can first engage in asynchronous learning by collecting and reviewing information individually by searching the Internet, reading pamphlets, or watching videos. Synchronous learning can occur when that individual attends a group class and receives information simultaneously with others.

CASE ANALYSIS 3

How could Julie create a handwashing curriculum using both asynchronous and synchronous learning?

Types of Visual Media

After considering what needs to be communicated and evaluating the audience needs, the food and nutrition professional selects the appropriate instructional media for the purpose. A single format or several options may be applicable. Box 14-2 outlines the possibilities. This section discusses the types of media to consider—from stationary formats to interactive use of real objects and multimedia presentations.

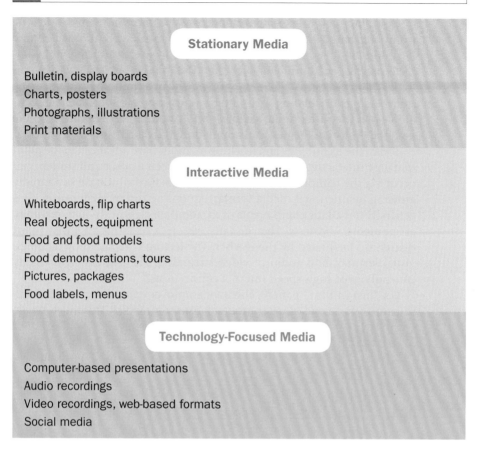

Box 14-2 ■ Examples of Visual Media

Stationary Media

Stationary media should be totally self-explanatory. They are often visual displays in a hallway, a classroom, or another public area. Visual media could also be a chart or a graph in a magazine, newspaper, or written handout. The audience is wide in scope and interest. Media are meant to attract attention and convey a simple message. The most effective stationary media also create immediate interest on first glance and promote the audience to spend more time with the media.[3,5]

Bulletin or Display Boards

Bulletin boards or display boards can spark interest in a topic. The concept should be simple, and the display should visually attract attention. The average adult spends 45 seconds looking at a display. Focus on one theme with three or fewer messages including the "take-home" message. Limit the number of words and use a type size of 18 to 24 points. Use creative headings, eye-catching graphics, and interesting photographs.[4] The bulletin and display boards are usually permanently affixed to a wall.

Charts and Posters

Information may be presented in charts or on posters that are self-made or purchased. They could be displayed on permanent wall locations such as framed cases or bulletin boards. A table, easel, or tripod could also be used to provide a moveable display. Consider laminating them so they can be rolled for storage or affixed to a foam mounting board to maintain quality. The United States Department of Agriculture's graphic design focusing on wasted food is an example (Figure 14-2).[13]

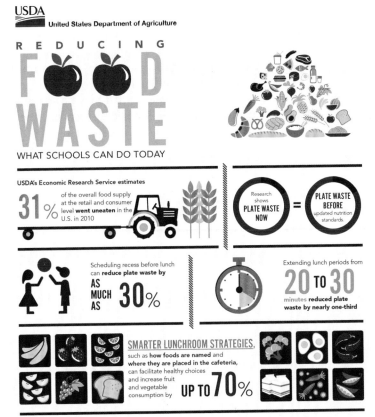

Figure 14-2 ▪ Infographics are effective media.

Numerical data can be visually presented in bar charts, pie-shaped charts, or line graphs. It is not necessary to read word for word from a visual. At most, you may tell why the visual is significant or paraphrase the content. Using interesting and thought-provoking comparisons of data to everyday examples can promote audience interest and increase the viewing time.[3,5] When used within a live presentation, remove it from view after discussing it to regain audience attention. Return to the visual as a way for the learner to rephase what they have learned.

Posters are also a medium for sharing research findings and other information at professional meetings. Poster content is divided into specific data segments that are combined on a single "page." Information should be free-standing and not require explanation. Data are often presented in clearly labeled charts accompanied by short explanatory text. Posters are typically generated using a computer software program, such as PowerPoint, and printed in a large-size format such as 36 in. by 48 in. Posters are then attached onto mounting boards at the meeting site for audience review. A digital file can also be e-mailed to a media service for printing at the meeting site. A recent trend is for web posting of the poster display prior to the meeting on the conference web site, which may be archived afterward for reference by the organization. Guidelines for poster computer generation are outlined in Figure 14-3. An example of a poster is illustrated in Figure 14-4.

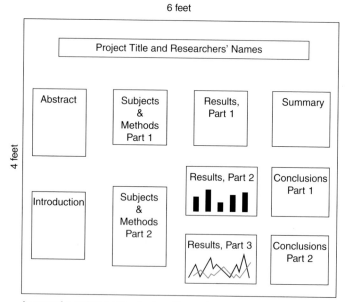

Layout of a typical poster display. Remember to express information with graphs, charts, or tables whenever possible. Place important information at eye level or higher on the poster.

Figure 14-3 ■ Guidelines for poster sessions.

APPLICATION OF HISPANIC CULTURE TO FOOD AND NUTRITION CURRICULUM PROJECTS PROMOTES STUDENT SELF-IDENTITY WHILE DISSEMINATING DIVERSITY TO A WIDER AUDIENCE

USDA Hispanic Serving Institution Grant Award 2011-38422-30864
PUENTES (Pathway of Undergraduate Education for Nutrition Training, Experience, and Success)

Judith Beto, PhD RD, Kathryn Montalbano MLS, Nancy Rivera BS, Krista Silverman BS, Katherine Schury BS, Ana Irizarry BS, Alexis Valenzuela BS from Nutritional Sciences, Dominican University, River Forest, IL 60305 USA

1. INTRODUCTION The broad objectives of PUENTES were: 1) to create an effective seamless coordinated undergraduate curriculum that could be replicated by others to provide an immediate solution to lack of sufficient numbers of Registered Dietitians (RD's) entering the workforce (125 new Hispanic RD's in 2009 compared to >2000 non-Hispanic RD) and 2) to increase local Hispanic student awareness of the RD career pathway through community outreach.

2. PURPOSE The purpose of this analysis was to evaluate the activities integrated within the PUENTES grant logic model to promote wider awareness of Hispanic culture both within and outside of the program.

3. METHODS Three primary activity areas were targeted: curriculum change (integrating cultural awareness within laboratory projects), community outreach (awareness of program, RD career options, and RD pathway), program accreditation (formal accreditation approval by ACEND (Accreditation Council on Education in Nutrition and Dietetics). Data was collected from September 2011 until May 2013.

4. OUTCOME MEASURES
The table shows outcome measures tracked for each of the three activity areas.

5. DATA ANALYSIS
Descriptive statistics were used to tabulate number of individuals attending each activity.

6. RESULTS A seamless BS-degree community college focused transfer program was implemented in Fall 2011, one semester ahead of plan. Number of PUENTES students = 22 (4 men, 18 women). Current status: 8 undergraduate, 8 post-BS (4 working interim year to save money, 4 enrolled in supervised practice), 6 completed program/studying for RD exam, 1 passed RD exam. Grant activities audience >2000; publication to 70,000 circulation.

TABLE: Outcome Measures for Selected Activity Areas

Activity Area	Activity Description with estimated "N" of audience	N
Curriculum Change	Experimental Foods – cultural food project laboratory emphasis with 4 food industry "showcases" inviting local professionals, present and future students	120
	Quantity Foods – cultural food menu focus with education handout; public patron audience; a total of 8 of 40 menus	400
Community Outreach	Two Diversity in Dietetics workshops for area health care professionals, students	300
	One peer-reviewed publication (J Acad Nutr Diet, June 2013**)	70000
	Booths at summer community health, food, and multicultural markets/local events to share Hispanic RD role models, career and nutrition resources (15 events)	900
	Community college career "tables" with PUENTES students and resources to "show" career path options (8 events)	500
Program Accreditation	Implemented Fall 2011; BS degree with additional 1200 hours supervised practice experience and eligibility to take RD exam	22

8. CONCLUSION The PUENTES program will provide by 2014 a minimum of 20 new Hispanic RDs to clinical practice in an innovative seamless accredited program that overcomes the known barriers to RD completion and practice.

**Publication
Strategies for addressing the internship shortage and lack of ethnic diversity in dietetics: White JH, Beto JA J Acad Nutr Diet 2013;113(6):771-775
doi:10.1016/j.jand.2013.012

Legend of grant activities:

A/B: Application of healthier empanadas recipe to experimental foods course laboratory project by PUENTES student : presented in food industry showcase setting to current and potential students and employers. C: Multicultural Market community booth in Maywood IL featuring fall dried bean soup recipe in a jar. D/E/F/G: Quantity food production course lab project incorporated 70-seat white table cloth public "restaurant" setting with PUENTES students planning traditional Hispanic meal; her family participated in training students in the course in authentic food preparation; picture of entrée plate.

Contact: Judith Beto, judybeto@dom.edu

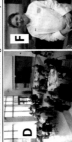
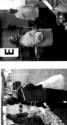

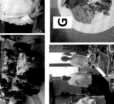
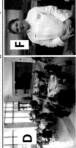

Figure 14-4 ■ An example of a poster display.

Photographs, Illustrations, and Flowcharts

Photographs can be generated using a digital or traditional camera or a professional photographer or illustrator. Photographs and illustrations may be available for free download or can be purchased from web sites or publication sources. For example, the ChooseMyPlate is available for free download to be used for education purposes, but other resources may have limitations on their use.[14] Be careful to obtain the correct media resolution to match final use. Generally, the higher the resolution, the clearer the picture quality, particularly when enlarged. Photographs may be used on bulletin boards and computer screens. If you are photographing people, such as employees and clients, a signed form releasing the use of the photos without limitation is required. Drawings and original computer graphics may need to be artist-generated, which can add to expense and time to produce. Flowcharts can also be computer-generated to demonstrate a process to a learner better than words alone. The use of logic models is becoming more prevalent to visually describe the process of a how a project will be conducted and evaluated. Clinical decision support tools are used to navigate through information databases.[15]

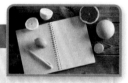

SELF-ASSESSMENT 1

Evaluate Figure 14-2 or Figure 14-4 for a specific audience using the art and design principles.

Print Handouts

Healthcare professionals tend to give patients and clients a great deal of verbal information. By the time they get home, most have probably forgotten at least half of the information. Trainers may do the same with new employees. Materials in print may be personalized using word processing and desktop publishing software.

Putting key points in writing so that clients, patients, employees, and other audiences can refer to them later solves this problem. In teaching about modified diets, for example, oral counseling is frequently supplemented with written materials. The printed handout lists the foods to eat often and those to limit. The format could offer recipe suggestions and suggest web sites to visit. Printed materials are effective in reinforcing individual counseling sessions and group classes.

Many printed handouts and brochures are now using quick response (QR) code symbols. These symbols can be scanned by mobile and smartphone devices that can access the Internet and are similar to universal product codes found on food packaging. The symbols direct the user to the current Internet site; thus, the information is always as current as possible and provides the learner a "link" to other resources. The use of QR symbols gives printed matters a longer life span with more flexible applications and are currently not copyright protected.[16]

When planning employee training, the presenter may consider giving an outline of the content, with space for note taking or a list of the main points to be remembered. PowerPoint and other slide-generation software provide options for printing outlines and slide handouts from created presentations. Listeners will be writing instead of listening, unless you distribute copies of the information on the slides.[2,7]

In teaching about normal nutrition, for example, the ChooseMyPlate and the Dietary Guidelines for Americans may be distributed. Government agencies and private organizations produce printed materials for a wide range of audiences, or you can make your own. If you are using materials produced by others, determine the right to reproduce the materials. If the material is copyright-free, just acknowledge the owner. If the material is copyrighted, obtain permission to reproduce the material. There may be a charge for this based on the number of items being used and the purpose of the use. Some materials may need to be purchased for distribution.

One-page instructional sheets written in short, simple words in active voice assist clients, even when more detailed materials are also being given. These one-page sheets can be posted on the refrigerator or hung at the office to remind clients of what to do and when to do it. Small give-away items such as pens, magnets, puzzles, and games may also be useful to remind the person of your message.

CASE ANALYSIS 4

What key components should Julie include on her handouts?

Interactive Media

Whiteboards and Flip Charts

Whiteboards and flip charts foster audience engagement when used in a participatory manner. Writing must be legible and clear. Writing should also be large and bold to be seen—at least 1 to 2 in. high or more for every 20 to 30 ft of audience space. Write key concepts before your audience arrives. This promotes face-to-face talking by limiting your writing with your back to the audience.[4]

Whiteboards, composed of erasable laminate surfaces, are mounted to walls or to moveable wheeled stands. Use appropriate water-based markers that can be erased when your presentation is over, without leaving a

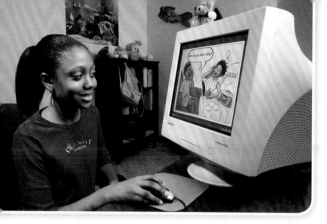

Visuals attract learners.

Source: US Department of Agriculture.

permanent image on the surface. Be prepared by bringing your own markers and eraser with you. You may need to use a board-cleaning fluid to remove marker buildup so your message can be clearly read. Whiteboards can also be planned to be used interactively by the audience. Learning teams can present information by writing their findings. Audience members can rotate among information written on the whiteboard and "vote" with supplied markers on concepts to determine opinions and consensus.

A flip chart with a display easel is composed of a tablet of large sheets of paper fastened together at the top. The sheets are "flipped" over to obtain a fresh sheet of paper. You can write or draw with crayon, felt pens, or markers. Select products that do not bleed through the paper. Presenters may want to ask someone to do the writing for them, particularly when audience comments and ideas are being generated. In this manner, the free-flowing of ideas (brainstorming or "brainwarming") can be recorded without distracting from the process.[17]

Flip charts can be used in multiple ways. Finished sheets can be torn off and attached to a wall to group or summarize ideas. When you need a record of audience participation, a flip chart is preferable to a whiteboard because each sheet can be saved after completion without recopying information. Alternately, one can prepare the sheets in advance and reveal them sequentially while standing facing the audience. It is advisable to leave a blank page when the audience focus should be on the presenter.

Real Objects

Nothing is more visual than showing real objects that a learner can touch and feel. A lesson on food labeling, for example, may include a variety of food packages so that the audience can participate hands-on with actual products in learning to read and understand the labels. To avoid audience distraction, introduce items when the visual impact is of greatest value and keep other items out of audience sight until required. Enhance involvement and decrease distraction by having one food package for each learner rather than passing a single item around.

A visit to a local supermarket or grocery store is another possibility to utilize real objects of foods and products. When an actual visit is not possible, a video tour or a virtual tour can be used.

Food demonstrations are also a common interactive learning opportunity. Preparing recipes to be tasted in group sessions when teaching about nutrition or modified diets increases familiarity with foods and cooking techniques. A person who has observed a professional create an actual recipe, was able to sample it, and has received the printed copy of the recipe is more likely to try it at home. In a series of classes, audience members may assist and provide recipes.

In training employees, it is preferable to train them using the real object.[7] Actual hands-on experience is preferable when learning how to use a piece of foodservice equipment such as a meat slicer, dish machine, or cash register. Touching a set of wooden blocks representing the size of ideal knife cuts helps a learner compare the proper size of his or her own diced carrot cubes. Breaking the teaching into small segments with a visual connection reinforced by implementing the skill is also preferable to facilitate learning.

Pictures, Packages, and Menus

Pictures or downloaded clip art may be displayed on posters or on computer screens. Sample packages and containers of recommended foods may also be provided as props. To teach food allergy awareness with a client, a file of actual food labels could promote learning interaction. Labels may be removed from packages and placed into a binder using clear page protectors. Labels could also be laminated or kept as photocopies. You may want to have different collections for different topics and audiences. For example, a file of food labels could be sorted by audience focus of carbohydrate or sodium content awareness.

Alternatively, clients could bring video pictures taken from their mobile phones of food labels or food items they consume. Mobile phone pictures have the advantage of documenting the date and time the food was consumed. The use of visual media like this helps create an interactive learning situation resembling a team effort.[12] Mobile technology programs linking Internet applications ("apps") are widely available to download for recording and storage of such information. Some programs can even be used to scan food labels and translate their nutrition information into diet exchanges or systems.

You can create a file of menus from local restaurant and fast-food chains to use to "practice" with your clients. Many menus can be found on the web sites of the restaurants themselves, which are often more current. Scanning the items into a computer will allow for presentation to a larger group.

Food Models and Measurements

Food models are representations of the real objects. Many professionals maintain an inventory of three-dimensional plastic food models. They are helpful in estimating client portion sizes, for example, during an assessment of food intake and in teaching portion sizes on controlled caloric

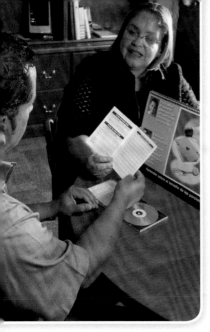

intakes. Besides the visual stimulation, putting the model in the person's hands makes a more active experience using another of the senses—touch. Life-sized food models may be purchased from commercial sources. You can also make your own food models using craft materials, such as illustrating different fluid volumes with resins in clear glassware.

You may need a variety of dishes in different sizes and shapes as well as disposable cups when demonstrating portion control. You should encourage using measuring cups at home to train the eye to serve correct portion sizes. Practicing weighing portions is helpful by comparing actual weight using a scale to reinforce perceived size. Actually dividing a box of cereal into the described portions is eye opening.

The counselor selects appropriate media.

Source: CDC/Amanda Knox.

Technology-Focused Media

Computer-Based Presentations

Most slides are computer-generated using word processing software. Typed-in words, pictures, clip art, and graphs are cut and pasted into the presentation. Active animation of text and graphics, insertion of video clips use a considerable amount of memory space but increase audience interest. It is best to use these illustrations to make a point not just because they are available.[18] In some cases, slides are available for purchase or from publishers promoting the use of their materials.

Presentations can be created with software templates. They can begin and end with a black slide or a title/logo slide to avoid the white glare of the screen without an image. If a very short part of the presentation does not include a slide, a black slide can be inserted or a key stroke can be used to create a computer screen change. It is important the information is concise and interesting rather than represent the full text of what the presenter will be saying. Reading the content of a slide is boring to the audience and decreases attention to the topic.[18]

To show the presentation to a large audience, the computer is connected to a projection device. A liquid crystal display (LCD) projector or other technology displays the images on a screen. Projectors vary in resolution, brightness, the ability to zoom picture size, weight, portability, and cost. The computer mouse or a laser pointer is used to illustrate points on the slides. It is important to use this method to intermittently point out information rather than consistently moving the pointer on the screen in a distracting manner. Laser pointers do not work on some projection systems due to the video resolution.

Download your presentation to a portable format in addition to storing on a computer-based file. Select the most appropriate devices from an array of options that are constantly evolving in technology and sophistication (i.e., memory sticks, flash drives, cloud storage). If for some reason your computer does not connect properly to the projector or monitor provided, you have the ability to move your presentation quickly to a computer that is compatible with the monitor provided.

Audio Recordings

Audio recordings, saved in a wide array of technology formats, can be pre-recorded to illustrate key educational points. Podcasts are effective ways to "hear" a message. Long recordings may be more appropriate for individual listening than for a group presentation. Short audios can be very effective in a large group presentation. Testimonials, several sentences from a key leader, or a commercial or radio segment can be used as a springboard for many messages. Create your audio presentation using an informal conversational tone of voice with slow, clear enunciation. Listen to the recording before using it to assess whether the sound quality is acceptable. Background noise on the recording can be very distracting.

Video Recordings and Web-Based Formats

The combination of sights and sounds from videos is pleasing to most people. Purchased or rented video media should be previewed to check for appropriateness. Visual materials are offered by many groups such as the Academy of Nutrition and Dietetics, American Heart Association, American Diabetes Association, National Dairy Council, Educational Foundation of the National Restaurant Association, commercial companies, government agencies, and private media companies.

An LCD projector with video signal capacities and monitor is generally necessary for audience viewing. Because audiences tend to view passively, they should be told what to look for before viewing. Preplanned activities or discussion questions should follow. A video may be viewed alone at the learner's own pace or viewed repeatedly to enhance learning. The presenter may use the "pause" feature to stop a video for discussion. Short video clips can highlight key points and help segment the talk.[18]

Capturing demonstrations and then placing on a web-based site can reinforce techniques and procedures in a step-by-step process. Whether you are illustrating how to easily remove the skin from chicken or how to interact with a client, the use of video can be a very effective tool for both learning new material and reinforcing skills.[2,9]

Many employee programs for orientation and training use video formats, sometimes with printed workbooks or learner's guides. If the employee views a video alone, discussions with the instructor should follow to explain the relationship of the video to the job. Videos can be placed on download formats or connected to a web-based site where demonstrations of learning can occur. The learner watches the video and periodically or at the end is asked questions about the content to assess learning.

Many employee education and orientation programs are moving a portion of their training to web-based training because it is convenient and available to all employees rather than those available on a particular day. Competencies can often be documented using employee response. Content can be offered in multiple languages or learning levels easily. The greatest advantage may be the ability to update content without creating new software. Customized unit-based training is also easier to facilitate via technology-based training. The employee or client can be directed to complete only the modules pertinent to the current role, providing on-demand or "just-in-time" training.[2,7] Videos should augment the learning. Teacher-facilitated discussion after the video should reinforce the concepts and promote active discussion. Short videos to take home after the presentation or counseling reinforce learning. This is especially useful for procedures such as preparing baby formula or conducting self-care.

Webinars and webcasts are produced, edited, narrated, and posted online. Similar techniques apply. Create short 3- to 8-minute presentations, keep them simple, and use key messages with graphics and demonstrations. Talk, don't read, when you create. For best quality, use the microphone and technology options that are available on most computers. Finally, be professional but do not worry about being perfect. If taping clients or employees, obtain a written release of use without limitations.

Social Media

Social media is a broad term used to describe the evolving area of the interactive technology using personal mobile devices that can access the Internet. Social media such as Facebook and LinkedIn are used to connect with others personally or professionally. "Tweeting" messages, writing "blogs," posting in chat rooms or "Listserv," and creating online forums are all used to disseminate information. The use of social media and the expected professional behavior expectations are still under research. A general rule is that anything posted cannot be retracted completely. It is important to evaluate these new media formats on a continuous basis as they evolve.[19-21]

Integrating Multiple Media Formats

Professionals should consider using more than one visual and/or type of media in a presentation. A common learning combination pairs a printed handout of the slides along with viewing the slides themselves. A more advanced option would be to add an audience-response system to this scenario.[22] This video feedback format allows the participants to share their opinions or answers to presenter questions using provided keypads or their mobile phones interactively when asked. Responses are tallied and displayed for the audience to view. A counseling session with a client may integrate actual foods and food labels to discuss a food diary.

A more advanced option would be to integrate the client's mobile phone technology and the Internet to further personalize the education session. Think of the message and select visual media that best fits the goals and teaching format. The focus is on the learners' needs.[19,23]

Numeracy and Literacy Considerations

The level of numeracy and literacy skill affects how learners remember and process information. Educational materials must be understandable to the people for whom they are intended. Printed materials in other languages may be needed for those with limited ability in English. Other materials need to be adapted to reading, writing, and math skills. Therefore, nutrition educators need to select or develop instructional materials that are easily comprehended.

Numeracy is defined as the ability to use numbers and math in ordinary life situations. The tasks involved may include correlations between measuring cup volume and portion size, relationships between time and intensity, or merely understanding what a number means on a glucose meter in relation to health risk. Numeracy commonly involves multistep processes. For example, diabetic clients must be able to use math to calculate the number of grams of carbohydrate they have eaten during a day by adding up the content of all foods consumed. In turn, they must apply this math to calculate sliding insulin doses. Numeracy is an essential component of correlating appropriate instructional materials with desired education outcomes.[24-26]

Literacy is the basic level of reading and writing that is required to understand basic information. Written materials can be assessed for the readability or grade level by measuring word and sentence length and difficulty. Several readability formulas are available, both as software programs and in print, to help assess the audience's readability, grade level, or both. The SMOG, FOG, Flesch, Raygor, and Fry tests are examples. The SMOG criteria are listed in Table 14-1. Because of the scientific and technical nature of health communications, vocabulary and wording of patient education materials may be incomprehensible to many adults. Readability formulas should be used to assess the approximate educational level a person must have to understand the material. Readability formulas, however, are only part of the process; developers should also "pilot-test," or try out materials on sample clients, or use more formal focus groups to find out if they will be understood by the target audience.[12] The overriding principle to remember is to be

1. Count 10 consecutive sentences near the beginning, in the middle, and near the end of the text. If the text has fewer than 30 sentences, use as many as are provided.
2. Count the number of words containing three or more syllables (polysyllabic) including repetitions of the same words.
   a. Hyphenated words are considered as one word.
   b. Numbers that are written out should be counted. If written in numerical form, they should be pronounced to determine if they are polysyllabic.
   c. Proper nouns, if polysyllabic, should be counted.
   d. Abbreviations should be read as though unabbreviated to determine if they are polysyllabic. However, abbreviations should be avoided unless commonly known.
3. Look up the approximate grade level on the SMOG conversion table:

Total Polysyllabic Word Count	Approximate Grade Level (+1.5 Grades)
0–2	4
3–6	5
7–12	6
13–20	7
21–30	8
31–42	9
43–55	10
56–72	11
73–90	12
91–110	13
111–132	14
133–156	15
157–182	16
183–210	17
211–240	18

Table 14-1 ■ SMOG Readability Formula

Source: From McLaughlin G. SMOG grading: a new readability formula. J Reading. 1969;12(8):639–646. Adapted with permission.

sensitive to the fact that many clients may have literacy and numeracy problems they may attempt to hide during the assessment process. Addressing literacy, especially health literacy, as a primary component of communication skills will dramatically increase the chances of successful counseling.[24–26]

Purchasing Prepared Media Materials

The question often arises about whether to prepare your own media materials or use existing materials. The most basic answer is to use the least expensive media to accomplish the goals with the best quality possible.[23] Factors such as the anticipated longevity of the material before it is outdated and the number of times you will use the material should influence the decision. The cost of purchased versus self-made media needs to be considered in terms of time, quality, and expertise. With so many presentations posted on the web, searching the Internet for presentations is valuable. If the materials fit the needs of the group, try to obtain permission to use the materials, referencing the original source. Many organizations and the government encourage individuals to use their materials without permission, but with proper acknowledgment.

The availability of technical expertise in design and production is essential, especially for audio and video production. The availability of prepared pamphlets or videos to meet the objectives is also important. In addition, the cost to reproduce the material is a consideration.

Regardless of who produces the instructional media, the materials should be evaluated on a continual basis. Box 14-3 offers some considerations when evaluating education materials. Eventually, you want to know what proves most effective in the shortest time frame in learning and retention, thus providing efficiency. Refer to Chapter 12 for more information on education evaluation.

General Evaluation Practices

Use a variety of printed education materials

Thoroughly preview education materials

Use a formal checklist to evaluate

Pilot-test modified or new education materials

Use education materials provided by a reputable source

Request feedback from clients

Conduct a client assessment before selecting materials

Consider the client's age, gender, and education level

Consider the client's ethnicity and cultural background

Consider the client's lifestyle and socioeconomic status

Box 14-3 ■ Evaluating Education Materials (*continued*)

Source: From Little D, Felten P, Berry C. Looking and Learning: Visual Literacy Across the Disciplines. *Philadelphia, PA: Jossey-Bass; 2015.*

Literacy Criteria

Readability and numeracy level
Length of sentences
Length of paragraphs
Number of syllables per word
Use of examples
Use of jargon, cliches, or idioms
Word appropriateness
Legibility, style, typeface
Size of print
Highlighting of specific information
Active or passive words
First, second, or third person
Typographical errors

Content Criteria

Addresses the needs of the client
Appropriateness to client
Applicability of information
Consistency of information
Objectivity of information
Implications of information
Motivational messages
Accuracy of information
Summarizes information
Credibility of information
Number of content errors
Date of publication
Flow of concepts, continuity
Scientific basis of information
Practicality of information
Focuses on behavioral change

Box 14-3 ■ Evaluating Education Materials (*continued*)

Format Criteria

Color scheme
Photographs, illustrations
Layout, balance
Use of white space
Use of highlighting techniques
Quality of copy
Captures attention
Interactive
Complexity of details
Illustrations that support messages
Web connection to current information
Quality of paper
Use of charts, graphs, and tables

Box 14-3 ■ *(continued)*

Summary

There is no doubt that use of instructional media enhances learning and retention from presentations while also having the potential to enhance the speaker's professional image. If you are not using at least five to eight visuals, you may be considerably less effective in your educational delivery.

The rapid evolvement of technology is having a profound impact on education and teaching. Clients want information right away, in small segments, and in easy-to-use formats. Food and nutrition professionals need to keep abreast of these changes as they utilize instructional media.

Review and Discussion Questions

1. What benefits does the use of visual media provide in presentations?
2. What should be considered in planning visuals?
3. Describe the concepts of literacy and numeracy. Why should the readability of printed materials be assessed?
4. Why is it important to evaluate visual media as one uses them?
5. When training employees, why is it preferable to train them using the real object, such as a meat slicer, dish machine, cash register, or other equipment?
6. What are some advantages of using computer-assisted formats for training and education?
7. What is the "rule of six?"
8. List at least 10 criteria for evaluating a presentation.
9. When would you use synchronous versus asynchronous learning? What is the value of each method?

Suggested Activities

1. Think about your earliest learning experiences. Can you remember any visual materials used by a teacher? Describe as much as you can remember and state your age at the time.
2. Prepare a chart or poster depicting one idea. Write a description of your objectives and intended audience. Write a critique of your visual explaining how you used art and design principles to enhance quality.
3. Prepare a video or webcast of a new employee procedure or a technique the employee needs to learn about. Some examples are procedure training (kitchen sanitation, food handling, or handwashing), preparation of a recipe for a modified diet, or a session on normal nutrition.

4. Create a computerized slide presentation, inserting at least one graphic.

5. Assign one student or a group of students to learn to use various types of visual media equipment. Each should write a task analysis (see Chapter 12) for the equipment and then train others in its use.

6. Select a commercially prepared visual media. Evaluate it in terms of its intended audience, objectives, effectiveness, art and design principles, and cost.

7. View a media-based educational program. Evaluate it using an evaluation form from the instructor.

8. Describe how one could use food labels or another form of visual media in teaching.

9. Select two educational pamphlets. Critique the content using a readability formula, if available. Critique the visuals as well. Determine whether the pamphlets can be reproduced and find out what the cost will be.

10. Using Box 14-2, make a list of limitations and advantages of each instructional media listed.

CHAPTER 15

Facilitating Group Learning

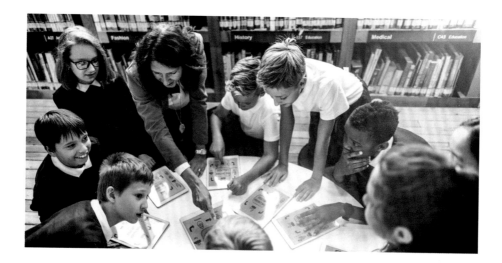

Objectives

- Explain the stages of group development.
- List the factors influencing group cohesiveness.
- Differentiate between formal and informal groups.
- Identify the characteristics of group and team dynamics.

- Describe the roles and responsibilities of a group leader or facilitator.
- Describe the roles and functions of both the facilitator and participants.
- Discuss the suggestions for promoting group change.
- Develop skill by leading a small group discussion.

Betty Smith, RD, CDE, is planning a series of meetings for a new support group for parents of children who have been recently diagnosed with type 1 diabetes mellitus. Her concern today is planning for optimum group participation in the first session, which will be 1 hour long. She also wants to be sure to meet the needs of the group so that they will return for future sessions.

The greater the loyalty of a group toward the group, the greater is the motivation among the members to achieve the goals of the group, and the greater the probability that the group will achieve the goals.

—Rensis Likert

Introduction

We all belong to groups. What groups do you belong to? A family group? Social group? Friends group? Religious group? Sports group? Service group? Work group? Professional group? Some groups meet together often; others less frequently. Face-to-face group meetings and committees are also common, including virtual online groups such as Facebook. We join groups to satisfy a need for belonging, for fun, to meet others for social contact, to unwind and reduce anxiety, to enhance a career, or because we have no choice at work.[1,2] Professionals are members and perhaps hold leadership positions in local, state, and national associations such as the Academy of Nutrition and Dietetics, the European Federation of the Associations of Dietitians, or special interest groups like the Council on Renal Nutrition of the National Kidney Foundation.

Providing nutrition services for individuals and groups and managing human resources are part of the scope of practice for nutrition professionals.[3,4] Dietitians and other healthcare professionals manage employee groups in addition to interacting with client groups, community groups, colleagues, and other healthcare professionals.

Consultation with or coordination of nutrition care with other providers or health professionals assists in managing and treating nutrition-related problems.[5] Some nutrition professionals are working on collaborative interdisciplinary or multidisciplinary healthcare teams dealing with nutrition support therapy, rehabilitation, nephrology care and dialysis, diabetes management, or other chronic disease management and attending patient care team meetings.[6-9] Specialists from several fields share knowledge, skills, and resources in working toward common goals to provide solutions to patient/client health problems. Solving the nation's obesity epidemic is an example of the need for interdisciplinary team approaches in public health, community groups, food companies, marketing, health professionals, and others. Practitioners group clients for small group counseling, such as for obesity, cardiovascular disease, or diabetes. Patient/client education sessions are often accomplished in a group setting.[7-9]

One of the primary goals of public health messages is to improve lifestyle habits of target audiences. People's ideas about health and behaviors are shaped by the communication of information by health professionals and by online health information technology. With the increasing complexity of health information and newer technology, nutrition practitioners are challenged to respond. The United States Department of Agriculture's SuperTracker Groups is an online free food, physical activity, and weight tracking tool available. This program allows nutrition professionals to create groups within schools, families, and other environments to share selected information and tracking reports to achieve common health goals.[10]

Managers are skilled in working with small employee groups. Activities such as conducting performance appraisals, counseling, disciplining staff, facilitating group or team meetings, team building, employee training, enhancing morale through the building of cohesiveness among staff, initiating change, and managing the resulting resistance all require well-honed communication skills.[8,11]

Small groups can be exciting and creative as well as boring and frustrating. One of the keys to effective working in a group, or leading one, is an understanding of group communication, facilitation, and dynamics. This chapter examines the stages of group development, characteristics of group and team dynamics, groupthink, group and team leadership, tasks of group leaders or facilitators, roles and functions of group members and facilitators, diversity in groups, and managing meetings.

CASE ANALYSIS 1

What suggestions do you have for the first session?

Groups and Teams Defined

What makes a group a group or a team a team and how does communication take place? A small group may be defined as a group consisting of "three to fifteen people who share a common purpose, who feel a sense of belonging to the group, and who exert influence on one another."[12] A group needs at least three people and if the group gets too large, it is better to divide it into subgroups so that everyone can participate and talk. In large groups, one or two more talkative members may dominate to the detriment of the others. Group size recommendations vary from an ideal number of 5 to 7 or no more than 20.[1,13]

Workplace employees are often organized into teams that have some of the characteristics of a sports team. Teams are made up of a small group of people, but teams are deliberately structured by management to achieve certain goals and to coordinate employee efforts to get work done. Expectations, responsibilities, and operating procedures are spelled out in advance.[11] Team leaders or facilitators require knowledge of group process skills and managing change.

Formal and Informal Groups

Groups may be either formal or informal. Formal groups are established by the organizational structure and by management. They are oriented to accomplishing work assignments, tasks, or goals. The members have established roles, responsibilities, and relationships.[1]

Informal groups develop because of the interests of the group members and often to fulfill social needs. They are not formally structured by the organization.[1,2] Yet, the group deeply affects members' behavior and performance. They may take breaks or lunch together, for example, and membership may cross departmental lines.

The informal group members communicate through the "grapevine," an important source of information for employees. This information is not controlled by management and is perceived as believable.[2] Managers need to be aware of the networks of communication that exist within employee groups as well as the formal communication within the organization.

CASE ANALYSIS   **2**

State a common educational goal applicable to this group.

Stages of Group Development

When groups or teams form, they go through a series of stages as they develop. These stages have been described in various ways. Commonly accepted is a four-stage interpretation, including Forming, Storming, Norming, and Performing.[1,14] Some add a fifth stage of Adjourning.[2] These stages are considered necessary and inevitable as the team grows over time, plans and accomplishes work, and finds solutions to problems.

Forming

The first stage, Forming, is a period of getting acquainted and overcoming uneasiness and uncertainty.[1,13] Because people desire to be liked, serious issues, controversies, and conflicts are avoided. The group focuses instead on getting organized for the goals and tasks ahead and getting started on the work. Unwritten group expectations, norms, and rules of behavior develop. Because members are more focused on themselves and avoiding conflicts, the facilitator may need to take a more directive approach at this stage.

Eventually members know one another and develop friendships, getting over their reluctance to talk. When you form a group made up of strangers, either clients or employees, the first session must allow time for people to become acquainted in order for them to communicate easily.[1]

Storming

In the second stage, called Storming, the polite phase is over and conflicts develop. Eventually different approaches and ideas develop as team members open up and disagree with or challenge other members over power, authority, responsibility, and other issues.[1,13] Although this stage can be contentious and uncomfortable, it is necessary for the full growth of the team.

In some groups, tolerance of differences develops and the differences are resolved; the team moves on. In other cases, especially when the background of members is very different, conflict continues and the real issues among group members are not addressed. At this stage, facilitators can encourage the sharing of views and opinions, but assume a more directive approach toward decision making and acceptable group behaviors.

The inevitable conflict must be replaced by effective discussion and interaction. A supportive climate needs to develop where members practice empathic listening and nonjudgmental responses.[1]

Norming

By the third stage, Norming, group members have become more accepting of the ideas of others and find ways to make the team members function together.[13] Members are more open and trusting when cooperation has developed.[1] Goals and plans are agreed upon and all members

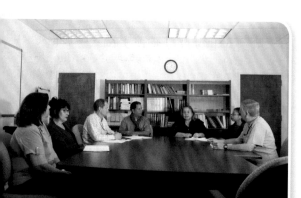

Groups should be seated in a circle so that all members can see each other.
Source: CDC.

take responsibility for the success of the team and its work. The facilitator's role is less important when the team or group can function on its own.

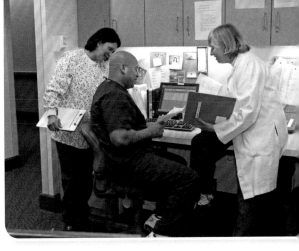

Employees consult as a team

Performing

The fourth stage, Performing, is not reached by all teams. High-performance teams work smoothly without conflict or the need for supervision. Members are highly motivated, competent, and able to make decisions.[2] They are interdependent and proud of their accomplishments when real work is accomplished in the cohesive group.[1,13] The facilitator may use a participative approach.

Teams may recycle to an earlier stage when changes occur. Employee turnover with newcomers joining the team, for example, or a change in supervisors may result in returning to the Storming stage as people need to become acquainted and learn to work together again.

Some add a fifth stage of Adjourning.[2] If the group's task is complete, the team may be dissolved. Because members' identities and prestige may be tied to the group, adjourning may create a difficult transition for employees.

CASE ANALYSIS 3

Give examples of how Betty might observe evidence of the stages of group development?

Characteristics of Group and Team Dynamics

A group or team without a task or purpose does not need to exist.[13] The task, purpose, or goal must be well defined and agreed upon by group members. The study of group dynamics includes the review of norms, roles, status, power, synergy, cohesiveness, and consensus.[12]

Norms

Norms are accepted standards of behavior or codes of conduct established in groups, whether one is a newcomer, a seasoned veteran, or the leader of the group.[1] Norms may be defined by an organization's culture, maintaining what is acceptable or unacceptable, appropriate or inappropriate behaviors in procedures, and shared values of the group.[1,2] These unwritten guidelines provide group identity, how members communicate and interact, and how tasks are approached, which leads to feelings of pride, inclusion, and superiority.[13] Norms may be tested when a member behaves in an inappropriate way. Unless the facilitator or a group member responds, norms will be tested again. When they are violated, there may be sanctions. How may you deal with a person in your friend group who is late too often, for example, when the norm is that people are on time?

Roles

While norms define the behavior of the group, roles apply to the behavior of an individual. Roles are behaviors that are learned.[13] Task roles tell who does what to complete a job or reach a goal, such as take minutes or seek information.[12] Social roles relate to enhancing the working relationships of group members. Members may take on more than one role in the group.[1,2] Some roles may be assigned, such as secretary/recorder or group leader, although more than one person can assume a group leadership role.[12]

Status

Status refers to a person's prestige, perceived importance, and influence on the group. A group with a high level of status may be referred to as the "in group" and most people want to be a part of it. Status influences group communication, both verbal and nonverbal, and the channels of interaction among people.[12]

Power

Power may be defined as "the ability to influence others' behavior" and to affect what group members do or how they behave. Power may come from being elected or appointed to a position, being the most knowledgeable person, or being a well-liked, popular individual. Although power and status are related, a person with power may not be able to influence everyone and power struggles may result.[12]

Synergy

All groups possess the potential to be a force for creative thinking or a force that preserves the status quo. Although not all groups achieve synergy, several people working together have the potential to produce more or better decisions or solutions than one person working alone.[1] The whole of the group is greater than the sum of its parts.

Cohesiveness

Developing cohesiveness in a team may contribute to producing qualitatively superior solutions and decision making. Cohesiveness is the "degree of attraction that members of a group feel toward one another and the group."[12] Cohesive group members listen to one another, like one another, have a high degree of loyalty to each other, have an increased self-esteem, and have a desire to stay in the group.[2,13] They talk in terms of "we" rather than "I" and refer to nongroup members as "they."[1] Although usually a good thing, groups can have too much cohesiveness, become autonomous, and all think alike.

Cohesiveness is not static and over time, a group may lose its cohesiveness. Because employee turnover is constant in many organizations, intense cohesiveness is rare. When a new member joins the group, interaction patterns and relationships may need to be developed again.[11] A summary of factors influencing group cohesiveness is found in Box 15-1.

1. All members perform worthwhile tasks, see the issues as important, and feel appreciated by the group.
2. Members clearly perceive the group's goals and consider them to be realistic.
3. Members recognize the group as an entity in its own right and refer to it as such, calling it "the group" or "our group."
4. The group develops a history and tradition. All cohesive groups (church, state, family, work, etc.) perform traditional rites and rituals, passing on to new members the "secrets" of the past and strengthening the existing ties among the group's veterans.
5. Group size is small rather than large.
6. Members possess knowledge or material needed by the group.
7. Member participation in the determination of the group's standards is full and direct.
8. The group is more homogeneous than heterogeneous.
9. Personal interaction among members is based on equality, with no one exercising much authority over anyone else. Members are not jealous of or competitive with one another.
10. Members share ideals and interests or a common satisfaction of the need for protection, security, and affection. The group has prestige.

Box 15-1 ■ Factors Increasing Group Cohesiveness

People in noncohesive groups feel unsure in expressing their opinions, argue less, and are more polite. When there are disagreements, they may feel less secure in contributing. If their own security is paramount, they do not challenge other group members.

CASE ANALYSIS 4

How should Betty introduce group members?

Consensus

Consensus occurs when all group members agree, support a decision, and commit to it.[12,13] It takes time before all members focus on a task and agree. Multidisciplinary healthcare teams, for example, have to come to consensus on patient treatment and other issues.[9] A consensus of expert opinions on knowledge and best practices is used to formulate evidence-based practice guidelines.[6]

Guidelines for Seeking Consensus

The training required to move a group from 25% to 75% efficiency in achieving consensus is based on a set of guidelines for group behavior. Professionals need to understand, however, that it may take several weeks of regularly reminding the group of the guidelines and interrupting each time the guidelines are not followed before the process becomes natural to the group. The following are guidelines for achieving consensus in groups[1,13]:

1. All group members have the responsibility and obligation to share opinions and ideas.
2. After group members have expressed opinions on a particular issue, they have the right to ask others to paraphrase these comments to their satisfaction.
3. After being paraphrased, they may not bring up their perspective again unless asked to do so by another group member. Insisting on one's own point of view or blocking discussion is not acceptable.
4. Differences of opinion should be viewed as natural, expected, and not criticized. Everyone has the responsibility to understand the ideas, arguments, and opinions of the other members and may ask questions for clarification.
5. After all perspectives are understood, the group needs to arrive at a solution or decision that can satisfy everyone. In accomplishing this task, the group may not immediately resort to the stress-reducing techniques of majority rule, trade-offs, averaging, coin-flipping, and bargaining.

Members need to be encouraged to seek out the perspectives of others so that everyone is involved in the decision-making process. Disagreements can help the group's decision because a wider range of information and opinions provides a greater chance that the group will develop superior solutions. Frequently, when the group members suspend their own judgment, new solutions emerge that no single individual would have been able to develop alone.

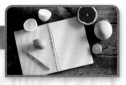

SELF-ASSESSMENT 1

The cafeteria work group has been a cohesive unit. Recently, Joyce Little, a popular 8-year employee, resigned. Tomorrow, Sarah Smith, a new employee, will be replacing her.

1. What effect will a change in employee have on the cohesiveness of the work group?
2. What can be done by the manager and current team members to recreate the cohesive unit?

Groupthink

Groupthink is a "mode of thinking members may engage in when they are deeply involved in a cohesive group."[13] When members reach consensus too quickly, are overly cohesive, or give in to avoid conflict, groupthink may occur.[2] The quality of a decision is reduced when the group stifles individual creativity, when the pros and cons are not examined, and when people do not challenge ideas.[12] Group pressures for conformity, or a goal of making a quick decision rather than finding the best solution, can lead to a faulty decision as members go along rather than give full consideration.[1] Members need to look for weaknesses in arguments.

Groupthink may also occur when members rely on compromise or majority rule rather than work toward consensus or when people with similar viewpoints, backgrounds, and opinions are grouped together.[13] Homogeneous groups with similar demographic, cognitive, and cultural backgrounds may make more errors in decision making and problem solving. Such groups may need to consult one or more outside experts. Have you ever thought of speaking up in a group, but decided against it? Being too uncritical and failing to raise questions about conclusions, solutions, or decisions can create a climate of groupthink.[17]

CASE ANALYSIS 5

How would the concept of "Groupthink" apply to this support group?

Group and Team Leadership

Leadership may be defined as "the ability to influence others through communication" and group process.[12] Some view leaders as those who delegate work and see that it is accomplished. The leader helps to focus the group's energy on its task until it is achieved. In fact, in many groups, members may influence each other and what is or is not accomplished. The leader influences the group and is influenced by the group as well.[1]

Despite all of the theories of leadership, there is no single explanation for every situation. In leaderless groups, one or more members may emerge to fulfill the leadership role. In your social group, who takes the leadership role and responsibility for making the plans and suggesting activities? Leadership depends on the members' willingness to follow in a given situation.[1] Most leaders have a vision for the group and are considered credible by the members.

Leaders may be appointed, elected, emergent, or shared. In the business world, the leader is appointed by management while elected leaders are selected through a formal, democratic process. Emergent leaders start out as a group member, but gradually provide services to the group. One or more members may emerge even with an existing, appointed leader. In your workplace, for example, is there a leader appointed by management, but also an employee who has a great influence on the group? Reticent and bossy people are not apt to emerge as leaders, but those who gain the respect and trust of members are.[1]

In shared leadership situations, the leader is a facilitator in a collaborative group effort, with members sharing power and responsibility. This is true in team management situations, for example. Facilitative leadership requires a cohesive group with well-defined tasks or goals.

Characteristics of an Effective Team

The contemporary leader recognizes that his or her role is not to dominate or unduly defer to the group or team. Different group members, because of their special knowledge or experience, may be in positions to act as resources for the group at various times.[1] The leader of a healthcare team, for example, needs to know the specific skills of the employees, so that appropriate people can be summoned to lead when appropriate. In such teams, there is generally little evidence of a struggle for power; the issue is not who controls, but how to get the job done.

The team leader motivates and reinforces members' behaviors that promote healthy team dynamics. A well-functioning team processes their progress and attempts to discern what may be interfering with the operation. The preferred method of resolution for the team is open discussion until a solution is found.

When all members of the team participate in the problem-solving and decision-making processes, team members feel responsible and commit to the successful implementation of the team's decisions and objectives. People who have an opportunity to voice their anxieties and questions, with their recommendations being incorporated whenever possible, are less likely to resist the changes and are more likely to assist in upholding them among others. The members of the group who later object are reminded that they had adequate opportunity to make suggestions, express their concerns, and that objecting now is inappropriate.

Although some group members may disagree with a change and revert to the old behavior, frequently group pressures and individuals' perceptions of their own dissonance cause them to abide by the group-accepted behavior. Suggestions for promoting group change are summarized in Box 15-2.

- If attitude change is desired, small open-ended, off-the-record discussion groups in which the person feels secure are most effective.
- When people need to change behaviors, participation in group discussions is 2 to 10 times more effective than a lecture that presents the reasons for and pleas for change.
- Active discussion by a small group to determine its goals, methods, and work or to solve other problems is more effective in changing group practices than separate instructions, supervisor's requests, or the imposition of new practices by an authority. Group involvement brings about better motivation, support for the change, and better implementation.
- Group change is easier to bring about and more permanent than change in the individual members of the group. The supposed greater permanence stems from the individual's assumed desire to live up to group norms. It follows that the stronger the group bonds, the more deeply based are the individual's attitudes. A public commitment to carry through the behavior decided on by group members creates an awareness of the expectations that members have for each other, thus creating forces on each member to comply.
- The best way for a manager to initiate change is to create an atmosphere that leads to a shared perception of the need for change. Then the members will call for the change themselves and enforce it. After all facts have been shared and all channels of communication have been opened, there is frequently a sudden but short-lived increase in hostility; however, without this complete sharing, there can be no real change, only mistrust and subtle hostility.
- High-status persons have more freedom from group control. The greater the prestige of individual group members, the greater the influence for change they can exert on the others.
- Change suggested by a peer is better than having it demanded by an authority figure.

Box 15-2 ■ Suggestions for Promoting Group Change

Source: Modified from Galanes G, Adams K, Brilhart J. Effective Group Discussion. *Dubuque, IA: McGraw-Hill; 2003.*

Managing Small Groups and Teams

People's attitudes, beliefs, and values are all rooted in the various groups to which they belong. The more genuinely attached people are to their groups and the more attractive these groups become in fulfilling the various needs of group members, the more likely these members will be in close and constant contact with their group. Under these conditions, group-anchored behaviors and beliefs are extremely resistant to change, with the group being able to exercise firm control over its members. The more attractive a group is to its members, the greater its influence over them. For the group itself to be used most effectively as an agent of change, it must first be cohesive with a strong sense of oneness.

CASE ANALYSIS 6

What are some things Betty can do to promote group change and participation?

Diversity in Small Groups and Teams

Diversity is a fact of life in our multicultural world made up of people of diverse cultures, values, beliefs, and customs that differ from our own. Diversity has an impact on many facets of verbal and nonverbal communication as well as on small group communication where it influences discussion and other issues. Since people do not have a common set of life experiences, communication in terms of shared meaning cannot be assumed and must be explored.

Today's management professional must possess competency in interpersonal skills, communication skills, and cultural diversity.[15] Putting diverse people together in a small group to work toward a common goal may lead to difficulties since perspectives and traditions are culturally defined. Research has shown that diverse groups that eat communal meals together may enhance group communication.[16] Homogeneous groups in which people have similar backgrounds may reach a more limited or defined consensus faster. Diverse groups, however, often bring a wider range of opinions that may strengthen the quality of solutions and decisions—and eventually the commitment to team goals.[1,13,15] We should not dismiss those who are quiet and slow to contribute because we need to hear and understand diverse perspectives from everyone to reach consensus resulting in creative solutions.

As a multicultural country, among both the workforce supervised and client groups served by healthcare professionals, no single approach will suffice. When managing groups, therefore, the professional's approach needs to be appropriate for the persons he or she is attempting to influence. When persons come from backgrounds in which they have not been encouraged to think or speak up, predictably in a work situation or a client group, they will lack the self-confidence to offer suggestions. If treated with patience, however, and given positive reinforcement each time they risk contributing an idea, they may gradually gain the confidence to become valuable group members.[15] Members of today's workforce, however, have grown up with a preference for egalitarian treatment—overt acknowledgment of each person's value, dignity, and worthiness of respect—and perform best in groups with a leader who acts as a facilitator, involving employees rather than prescribing to them.[11]

Group Facilitation Skills

To be successful as leaders, nutrition practitioners and managers must understand and utilize group facilitation skills. Facilitators are those who understand the value of group decision making and see their function as helping the group to get started, to establish a climate of work, to give support to others, to guide the group, and to keep the group on track so that its objectives are achieved. The group's activities and the facilitator's attitude toward the group are based on respect for what can be accomplished through group discussion and on the fostering of a group climate in which people feel comfortable and secure enough to contribute their ideas.[11,17]

Facilitator Preparation

Facilitators' responsibilities begin with the preparation of an appropriate meeting environment. They must make sure that the room is comfortable, with adequate ventilation, lighting, and with a consciously arranged seating pattern. Sitting in a circle, for example, allows group members to see one another's faces, which tends to increase interaction. When people are arranged at long rectangular tables, they tend to interact most with those in direct view and little with those on either side of them.

CASE ANALYSIS **7**

How should Betty set up the meeting room to encourage group interaction?

Nutrition professionals and managers need to assist in group problem solving by developing their roles as group facilitators. Effective facilitation requires training and discipline to stay in the role of guide, monitoring unobtrusively and adding interjections only as needed to maintain group process and functioning, while not actually becoming a participant. Described in the following paragraphs are specific skills that need to be practiced to develop group facilitation skills.[1,13]

Relieving Social Concerns

A tenet of group dynamics suggests that social concerns take precedence over task-related or work-related concerns. In other words, a person's first concern is with being accepted and acknowledged as worthy. If people feel anxiety about being with unknown others, they generally do not participate. One way in which a facilitator can attend to social concerns is to spend a few minutes at the beginning of each meeting allowing people to interact socially, providing "open time" to establish or reestablish positive regard for one another. Only after the members have had their social concerns met can they wholeheartedly participate in task concerns.

Tolerating Silence

After facilitators have made opening remarks, have made sure that everyone knows everyone else, have articulated the desire for everyone's participation, and have stated the reasons or purpose for the meeting, they might rephrase the topic in the form of a question and then invite someone to comment. Because members frequently hesitate to express opinions with which their superior or facilitator might disagree, they often wait to hear that person's opinion first.

At times, no one may want to initiate discussion. Silence is likely to occur most during the early stages of an ongoing group. After the group comes to understand that the facilitator truly does not intend to dominate, lead, or force opinions, members begin to use the meeting time to interact with one another. For those first few meetings, however, the facilitator should repeat the intention not to participate, should encourage others to participate, and then should just sit patiently.

Agenda

☐ Review / Approve Minutes
☐ District Reports
☐ Project Updates
  • Legislative Actions
  • Community Outreach
  • Labeling Changes
☐ New Business
☐ Adjournment

Meetings should have an agenda.

Guiding Unobtrusively and Encouraging Interaction

The facilitator guides indirectly, helping the members to relate better to one another and to complete the task. The facilitator can encourage interaction among the group members by looking away from speakers in the group as they attempt to harness his or her eyes.[14] Although this may seem rude, the speaker quickly gets the idea and looks to the other group members for feedback. The facilitator should resist the temptation to make a reply after others talk, but should instead wait for someone else to reply. If no one else comments, however, the facilitator can ask for reactions.

Reinforcing the Multisided Nature of Discussion

The facilitator can reinforce the nondogmatic, multisided nature of discussion by phrasing questions so that they are open-ended. Examples are "How do you feel about that?" "Who in your opinion . . .?" and "What would be some way to . . .?" Facilitators need to think before asking questions to avoid closed and leading questions, questions that can be answered by only one or two words, and questions that suggest a limited number of responses.

Controlling Overly Talkative Participants

A common problem that facilitators have is deciding what to say to a person who is overly talkative. There are many appropriate ways of handling this type of participant, keeping in mind that when facilitators interact with any single member of the group, all other participants experience the interaction vicariously.

Several techniques may be effective. The facilitator may interrupt the participant, commenting that the point has been understood, and begin immediately to paraphrase concisely so that the participant knows that he or she has been understood. Usually, this kind of participant stops talking after being paraphrased. Of course, this process may need to be repeated several times.

A second problem arises with participants who simply enjoy talking and perceive increased status from it. They do not stop talking after being paraphrased. They may need to be told that short concise statements are easier to follow, that they should limit the length and number of comments, or that the group is losing the point from their extensive commentary. The facilitator may need to talk with the person privately.

Encouraging Silent Members

For various reasons, including boredom, indifference, felt superiority, timidity, and insecurity, there are usually some members who refuse to participate. In some cultures, silence from subordinates or people younger than the group's leader is viewed as "respectful." The facilitator can arouse interest by asking for their opinions of what a colleague has said. If the silence stems from insecurity, the best approach is to reinforce positively each attempt at interjection. A smile, a nod, or a comment of appreciation for any expressed opinion is sufficient. If silent members have their heads down and blank facial expressions, it would be a mistake to force them into the discussion.

Halting Side Conversation

Generally, the facilitator should not embarrass members who are engaged in private conversations by drawing attention to them. If the side conversation becomes distracting to others, those engaged in the conversation might be called by name and asked an easy question. For example, one might say, "John, I would be interested in your perspective on this issue."

Discouraging Wisecracks

If someone in the group disrupts with too much humor, the facilitator needs to determine at what point the humor stops being a tension reliever and starts to interfere with the group's progress. When the humor is bringing the focus onto the joker, facilitators need to interrupt, preferably smiling, with a comment such as "Now let's get back to business."

Helping the Group Stay on Topic

When the group seems unable to stick to the agenda and wanders, a device underused by facilitators is a flip chart to jot down points that have been agreed on as a way to chart the group's progress. The facilitator can prod the group on by simply summarizing and writing down the points.

Avoiding Acknowledgment of the Facilitator's Preferences

Facilitators hinder the group when they praise the ideas they like and belittle those they dislike. It is important to avoid making comments that may be taken as disapproval, condescension, or sarcasm. Because facilitators are in a position to reward or punish attendees, group members quickly learn when supervisors want to be followed and not disagreed with, and that is how they will respond.

SELF-ASSESSMENT 2

Jane Jones, RD, is meeting with a group of pregnant women to discuss the nutritional needs during pregnancy. All are having a second or third child. As a result, she has chosen group discussion as the method of presentation.

1. How should she prepare the environment for group discussion?
2. What is her role as facilitator of the group?

Facilitator and Participant Functions and Roles

In addition to the specific skills required of facilitators, there are numerous group skills that both participants and facilitators should possess. There is a mistaken notion that it is the facilitator's responsibility alone to see that the group's tasks are accomplished and that a healthy group spirit is maintained. In reality, these responsibilities belong to anyone who has the training and insight to diagnose the group's weaknesses and has the skills to correct them.

Because most people are used to being "led" in groups, the facilitator may need to reinforce verbally the functions that all participants are expected to perform. Box 15-3 describes some of these skills and roles that both facilitators and participants have a mutual obligation to develop in themselves.[1,12-14] Some are task roles that enhance discussion in reaching

Task Roles	
Initiator	Proposes new ideas, goals, procedures; offers suggestions; gets group moving
Information/opinion seeker	Asks questions; seeks information, facts, opinions
Information/opinion giver	Offers judgments, beliefs, facts, opinions; raises issues
Elaborator	Expands on suggestions or ideas
Clarifier	Clarifies what was said; adds examples, illustrations, explanations
Coordinator	Puts together relationships among facts, ideas, suggestions, activities
Summarizer	Reviews points of discussion; restates ideas; offers conclusion
Evaluator	Expresses judgments on the value of ideas or suggestions; applies criteria for evaluation; helps group assess quality
Orienter	Clarifies group's purpose or goal; defines the position of the group; summarizes or suggests the direction of the discussion
Supporter/encourager	Praises, agrees, indicates warmth and solidarity; verbally supports members

Box 15-3 ■ Group Task and Social Roles (*continued*)

Social Roles	
Harmonizer	Mediates differences among members; reconciles disagreement; brings collaboration from conflict
Tension reliever	Reduces the formality or status differences; offers humor
Gatekeeper	Ensures all have an equal chance to be heard; protects those who prefer to be silent

Box 15-3 ■ (continued)

a goal; others are social roles that relate to the relationships and cohesion of the group members. There are also roles that are not helpful to group progress.

The supporter plays a valuable role, for example, because without verbal support from others, good ideas and suggestions are often disregarded. If no one supports a minority opinion, it is quickly dismissed. Generally, if only one person supports the idea, the group will seriously consider the merits of the proposal and a minority opinion can gain majority support. Verbal support remarks are "I agree," "Well said," or "I wish I had said that."

Gatekeepers tend to say things such as "You look like you have strong feelings" or "I can tell by your face that you disapprove." Such comments are generally all the prodding the silent participant needs to enter the discussion.

All members—participants as well as facilitators—are responsible, and they need to be alert to perform as many of the functions as they see a need for. Some people may be natural harmonizers or orienters, while others are summarizers. While members of the group are talking, other group members need to be reflecting on the dynamics of the group and on the needs at the moment. This process leads to an understanding of which functions need to be performed to help the group accomplish its task.

Some group members assume negative roles that are not helpful and inhibit the group. These include being an aggressor, dominator, withdrawer, recognition seeker, objector/blocker, joker, and special interest or self-interest pleader.[12,14]

CASE ANALYSIS 8

What would you suggest that Betty can do to implement "group facilitation skills"?

Paradox of Group Dynamics

There is a paradox inherent in groups. Groups possess the potential to stimulate creative thinking and to promote a decision or solution that is superior to what any individual could accomplish alone. On the other hand, groups possess the potential to stifle creative thinking and thus promote an outcome inferior to what an individual working alone might accomplish. Ordinarily, no one person is solely responsible for what happens in any given session. However, whether a group becomes a force to promote creative thinking and problem solving or a force that inhibits these functions depends primarily on the skills of its leader and, to a lesser degree, on the skills of the participants. Knowing how to facilitate positive behavior in groups and how to inhibit the negative behavior is an asset to nutrition practitioners and managers.

Problem Solving and Decision Making

Decision making and problem solving require the generation of alternatives and making choices among them.[1] When a group is unable to agree on a solution, several other methods—each with its advantages and disadvantages—may be used. One method is for the leader to make the decision. The advantage is that the decision is arrived at quickly; the disadvantage is that those who dislike it may not support it. Members who feel that they have "lost" may attempt to subvert the decision or solution later.

A second possibility is for some members to accommodate others by no longer insisting on their preferred solution. This method immediately relieves the group of conflict, but those who accommodated may later resent having done so and may not feel obliged to uphold the solution. Third and perhaps the most common method is compromise, each side giving in a little until both can agree. The problem with compromise is that often what is given up is sought back eventually. Compromise solutions tend to be short-lived. Other conflict-reducing techniques such as majority rule, trade-offs, and coin-flipping also tend to be short-lived.

Brainstorming

Brainstorming is a group method for stimulating creativity in problem solving by developing a large number of original ideas that one might not think of alone. Freewheeling is encouraged since quantity, rather than quality, is desired in order to obtain a large number of creative ideas and solutions. Suggestions are written on a flip chart or white board. All ideas are acceptable, even if unusual, and none are criticized or evaluated. Combining or improving on another's idea is encouraged as one idea may stimulate others. After a period of time, decisions are made on which one or ones are usable and the ideas are prioritized.[1,2,13]

Nominal Group Process

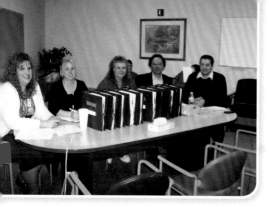

Groups can often provide solutions more effective than those of an individual.

Source: Photo used with permission from Allegiance Behavioral Health, Plainview, TX.

Nominal group process may be thought of as a type of silent brainstorming at first.[12] This method requires group members to work alone for a short period of time, generating their ideas without group interruption. In the second step, each member reads one idea in round-robin fashion without discussion until all ideas are recorded on a flip chart. In the third step, members work as a group and ideas are discussed and clarified without evaluation. In the final step, members vote independently to prioritize the list.[1,13] This method has an advantage for those who have difficulty organizing their thoughts during the fast moving discussion of brainstorming and for those who do not share ideas or solutions readily.

Focus Groups

Focus groups are another creative technique. They are a qualitative approach for eliciting the perceptions of a defined group of 5 to 15 people. Participants are selected according to their knowledge of the subject. In an hour or longer session, a facilitator can assist in finding answers to problems, issues, topics, and solutions. To obtain specific information, the topic or issue is introduced by the facilitator who has compiled a list of open-ended questions to pose to the group for their exploration. With signed consent forms, the discussion may be recorded so that it may be replayed or transcribed for analysis.[1]

Meetings as a Function of Group Dynamics

For most of us, meetings are an inescapable fact of life. They require the collaboration of members and the use of effective communication skills, such as listening and interpreting verbal and nonverbal behaviors. Most meetings are designed to share information, to discuss information, or to take action as a group.[18,19] Yet, attending meetings can be a negative experience. Common complaints are that the meeting did not start on time, people did not stay on the subject or were unprepared and did not contribute, or the meeting went on too long and nothing was accomplished.

The remedy for these complaints lies in many of the group communication skills that have been discussed and starts with a clear written agenda. The leader or facilitator is responsible for setting the goals for the meeting, keeping to the meeting time constraints, guiding the group participants to stay focused on the agenda, and ending with a clear plan of action for participants.

The leader uses group facilitation skills to empower members to contribute, to manage any conflict, and promote group cohesiveness or change as appropriate.[15,18,19]

When meetings involve persons who do not know one another, the facilitator should allow time for group members to introduce themselves or send biographical information in advance. An individual's tone of voice, dress, diction, and manner provide valuable clues to his or her character. Often, negative inferences disappear after the other's voice is heard and some information regarding the person's background is offered.

Group members may need to receive the agenda and advance information if they are expected to discuss an unfamiliar topic. Most meetings require some form of documentation: someone to take and distribute minutes of the meeting, audio or video recording of the meeting for later transcription and dissemination, or informal meeting summary points on a dry-erase board or projected digital tablet screen. This documentation will also help define the plan of action for the participants to build upon for subsequent meetings.

The facilitator's most important role is to keep the meeting focused on the agenda, but all group members should consider this responsibility their own as well.[18,19] Members should note whether or not everyone is participating, call on quiet members, and try to limit people who talk too long. Examples of supportive statements are "Ann, we haven't heard from you yet. What are your thoughts?" or "Thanks for sharing, John, but we need to hear from others also." To someone off topic, "I'm not sure how your comments fit our discussion." One should avoid comments that create a defensive reaction, such as "You are way off topic."

Summary

As professionals, we all belong to groups and attend meetings. We also manage, facilitate, and lead groups. This chapter discusses the several stages of group development, group and team dynamics and their characteristics, the roles and functions of the leader or facilitator as well as the roles and functions of both the facilitator and the group member. Increasing group cohesiveness, promoting change in groups, and managing meetings are included. Readers can start applying the information now in their own groups, whether social, work, professional, or other groups.

Review and Discussion Questions

1. What are the responsibilities of a group facilitator?
2. What are the responsibilities of a group or team member?
3. Discuss the stages of group development.
4. What are the characteristics of group dynamics?
5. Discuss the differences between the formal and the informal work group.
6. What are the ways to increase group cohesiveness?
7. Discuss several of the participant functions and how they generally either aid in promoting the group's effectiveness or assist in accomplishing the group's task.

Suggested Activities

1. In groups of three, discuss the best small group experiences you have ever had. What occurred that qualifies them as superior? Describe specific behaviors of both the group's leader or facilitator and the participants that seem to have made a difference. Time should be allotted for each group to share its insights with the others.
2. In groups of three, plan to meet in two different settings over the next 2 days, with different seating, room size, lighting, and the like. Report your observations on the effects of the environment to the entire class. Notice whether different groups had similar reactions and were influenced by the same factors. A simpler variation on this activity would be to hold a discussion for 10 minutes with the group arranged in a circle and then to continue the discussion with the group sitting in a straight row.
3. Make a list of two small groups in which you have been active and describe the functions you performed in each. Compare your perceptions of yourself as a contributing group member with the perceptions that

your friends or classmates had of you. Do you notice that you performed different functions in different groups? Do some functions overlap from group to group? Are your classmates in agreement with you regarding your functions within their group?

4. Thinking back to some recent experiences in group discussions, complete each of the following statements:

    A. "My strengths as a group participant are . . ."

    B. "My strengths as a group facilitator are . . ."

    C. "What is keeping me from being more effective both as a participant and as a facilitator is . . ."

    D. "My plans for improvement are . . ."

5. Write a question or description of a food or nutrition problem or issue, preferably from your own personal or professional experience, for which you do not have a solution. Present it to a small group and facilitate their discussion. Possible questions might include "What populations need to take vitamin supplements?" "What are the best food choices when eating at a fast-food outlet?" "What recommendations should one give to someone who desires to reduce calories or exercise more?"

6. Group together four to five people who have a common problem such as wanting (1) to lose weight, (2) to start eating breakfast, (3) to control excess consumption of snacks, (4) to select nutritious meals, (5) to increase the fiber content of their diets, or (6) to exercise more often. State the problem and have the group attempt to solve it.

References

Chapter 1: Expanding Scope of Nutrition Practice

1. Worsfold L, Grant BL, Barnhill GD. The essential practice competencies for the Commission on Dietetic Registration's Credential Nutrition and Dietetics Practitioners. *J Acad Nutr Diet*. 2015;115:978–984.
2. European Federation of Associations of Dietitians. http://www.efad.eu /everyone/1468/5/0/32. Accessed December 15, 2015.
3. Dietitians of Canada. http://dietitians.ca. Accessed September 28, 2016.
4. Dietitians Association of Australia. http://daa.asn.au. Accessed September 28, 2016.
5. International Confederation of Dietetic Associations. http://www .internationaldietetics.org/About-ICDA.aspx. Accessed December 15, 2015.
6. Marcason W. Dietitian, dietician, or nutritionist? *J Acad Nutr Diet*. 2015;115:484.
7. Wilson B. *First Bite: How We Learn to Eat*. New York, NY: Basic Books; 2015.
8. Healthy People 2020. http://www.healthypeople.gov. Accessed December 15, 2015.
9. NHANES. http://cdc.gov/nchs/nhanes. Accessed September 28, 2016.
10. United States Department of Agriculture. ChooseMyPlate. http://ChooseMyPlate.gov. Accessed November 1, 2015.
11. Tagtow A, Nguyen J, Jonson-Bailey D, et al. Food waste reduction efforts at the USDA. *J Acad Nutr Diet*. 2015:115;1914–1919.
12. Chang S, Gavey E. Supertracker groups: connecting registered dietitian nutritionists with clients. *J Acad Nutr Diet.* 2015:115:1755–1757.
13. Dietary Guideline Dietary Guidelines for Americans. http://health.gov /dietaryguidelines. Accessed November 1, 2015.
14. Eating Well with Canada's Food Guide. http://healthycanadians.gc.ca /eating-nutrition/healthy-eating-saine-alimentation/food-guide-aliment /index-eng.php. Accessed November 15, 2015.
15. World Health Organization. Global targets 2025. http://who.int/en. Accessed November 15, 2015.
16. International Food Information Council Foundation. Tenth Food & Health Survey: consumer attitudes toward food safety, nutrition & health. http://www.ific.org. Accessed January 24, 2016.
17. Pew Report 2015. http://pewresearch.org/2015. Accessed September 28, 2016.

18. Academy Quality Management Committee, Scope of Practice Subcommittee of Quality Management Committee. Academy of Nutrition and Dietetics: Revised 2012 standards of practice in nutrition care and standards of professional performance for registered dietitians. *J Acad Nutr Diet.* 2015;113:S29–S45.

19. Academy Quality Management Committee, Scope of Practice Subcommittee of Quality Management Committee. Academy of Nutrition and Dietetics: Revised 2012 standards of practice in nutrition care and standards of professional performance for dietetic technicians, registered. *J Acad Nutr Diet.* 2015;113:S56–S71.

20. Academy of Nutrition and Dietetics, Nutrition Care Process. http://www.eatrightpro.org/resources/practice/nutrition-care-process. Accessed November 1, 2015.

21. Commission on Dietetic Registration. RDN credential. http://cdrnet.org/certifications. Accessed September 28, 2016.

22. Kent PS, McCarthy MP, Burrowes JD, et al. Academy of Nutrition and Dietetics and National Kidney Foundation: Revised 2014 standards of practice and standards of professional performance for registered dietitian nutritionists (competent, proficient, and expert) in nephrology nutrition. *J Acad Nutr Diet.* 2014;114:1448–1457.e45.

23. Academy of Nutrition and Dietetics. Standards of practice. http://www.eatrightpro.org/resources/practice/quality-management/standards-of-practice. Accessed January 15, 2016.

24. Academy of Nutrition and Dietetics. Nutrition terminology reference manual (eNCPT): dietetic language for nutrition care. http://ncpt.webauthor.com. Accessed September 28, 2016.

25. Academy of Nutrition and Dietetics. Evidence-based analysis library. http://www.andeal.org. Accessed September 28, 2016.

26. Thompson KL, Davidson P, Swan WI, et al. Nutrition care process chains: the "missing link" between research and evidence-based practice. *J Acad Nutr Diet.* 2015;115:1491–1497.

27. Subjective Global Assessment. http://subjectiveglobalassessment.com. Accessed January 15, 2016.

28. Kelly MP. Nutrition physical assessment in chronic kidney disease. In: Byham-Gray LD, Burrowes JD, Chertow GM. *Nutrition in Kidney Disease.* New York, NY: Humana Press, Springer Science; 2014:69–89.

29. Peregrin T. Enhanced bedside manner heals patient-practitioner communication. *J Acad Nutr Diet.* 2014;114:529–532.

30. Mueller C, Rogers D, Brody RA, et al. Report from the advanced-level clinical practice audit task force of the Commission on Dietetic Registration: results of the 2013 advanced-level clinical practice audit. *J Acad Nutr Diet.* 2015;115:624–634.

31. Kohn JB. Stories to tell: conducting a nutrition assessment with the use of narrative medicine. *J Acad Nutr Diet.* 2016;116:10–14.

32. Boyce B. Emerging paradigms in dietetics practice and healthcare: patient-centered medical homes and accountable care organizations. *J Acad Nutr Diet.* 2015;115:1765–1770.

33. Volgiano C, Steiber A, Brown K. Linking agriculture, nutrition, and health: the role of the registered dietitian nutritionist. *J Acad Nutr Diet*. 2015;115:1710–1714.
34. Volgiano C, Brown K, Miller AM, et al. Plentiful, nutrient-dense food for the world: a guide for registered dietitian nutritionists. *J Acad Nutr Diet*. 2015;115:2014–2018.

Chapter 2: Communication

1. Gates GE, Amaya L. Registered dietitian nutritionists and nutrition and dietetics technicians, registered, are ethically obligated to maintain personal competence in practice. *J Acad Nutr Diet*. 2015;115:811–815.
2. Worsfold L, Grant BL, Barnhill GD. The essential practice competencies for the Commission on Dietetic Registration's Credentialed Nutrition and Dietetics Practitioners. *J Acad Nutr Diet*. 2015;115:978–984.
3. Commission on Dietetic Registration. Code of ethics. http://www.eatrightpro.org/resources/career/code-of-ethics. Accessed September 28, 2016.
4. Beebe SA, Beebe SJ, Ivy DK. *Communication: Principles for a Lifetime*. 6th ed. Upper Saddle River, NJ: Pearson; 2015.
5. Boyce B. HIPAA compliance from a private practice purview. *J Acad Nutr Diet*. 2014;114:1341–1346.
6. Healthy People 2020. Health communication and health information technology. www.healthypeople.gov. Accessed November 1, 2015.
7. http://www.healthypeople.gov/2020/topics-objectives/topic/health-communication-and-health-information-technology. Accessed September 28, 2016.
8. Literacy and Health Outcomes. http://archive.ahrq.gov/clinic/epcsums/litsum.htm. Accessed November 1, 2015.
9. Robbins SP, Judge TA. *Essentials of Organizational Behavior*. 16th ed. Englewood Cliffs, NJ: Prentice Hall; 2014.
10. Duggan A, Street L. Interpersonal communication in health and illness. In: Glanz K, Rimer BK, Viswanath R, eds. *Health Behavior: Theory, Research, and Practice*. 5th ed. San Francisco, CA: Jossey-Bass; 2015:243–268.
11. Stewart CJ, Cash WB. *Interviewing: Principles and Practices*. 14th ed. New York, NY: McGraw Hill; 2014.
12. www.mindtools.com. Accessed November 5, 2015.
13. Frey WH. *Diversity Explosion: How New Racial Demographics Are Remaking America*. Washington, DC: Brookings Institute; 2015.
14. Luquis RR. Culturally appropriate communication. In: Perez MA, Luquis RR, eds. *Cultural Competence in Health Education and Health Promotion*. 2nd ed. San Francisco, CA: Jossey-Bass; 2014:193–216.
15. Diaz-Cueller AL, Evans SF. Diversity and health education. In: Perez MA, Luquis RR, eds. *Cultural Competence in Health Education and Health Promotion*. 2nd ed. San Francisco, CA: Jossey-Bass; 2014:23–58.

Chapter 3: Interviewing

1. Jortberg B, Myers E, Giglotti L, et al. Academy of Nutrition and Dietetics: standards of practice and standards of professional performance for registered dietitian nutritionists (competent, proficient, and expert) in adult weight management. *J Acad Nutr Diet*. 2015;115:609–623.

2. Writing Group of the Nutrition Care Process, Standardized Language Committee. Nutrition care process and model part 1: The 2008 update. *J Am Diet Assoc*. 2008;108:1113–1117.

3. Stewart CJ, Cash WE. *Interviewing Principles and Practices*. 14th ed. New York, NY: McGraw-Hill; 2014.

4. Dessler G. *Fundamentals of Human Resource Management*. 2nd ed. Upper Saddle River, NJ: Prentice-Hall; 2012.

5. Morris SS, Snell SA, Bohlander GW. *Managing Human Resources*. 17th ed. Mason, OH: South-Western; 2015.

6. Thompson FE, Suber AF. Dietary assessment methodology. In: Ferrizzo M, Coulston AM, Boushey CJ, eds. *Nutrition in the Prevention and Treatment of Disease*. 3rd ed. San Diego, CA: Elsevier; 2013:5–46.

7. Lee R, Nieman D. *Nutritional Assessment*. 6th ed. Boston, MA: McGraw Hill; 2013.

8. Johnson RK, Yon BA, Hankin JH. Dietary assessment and validation. In: Monsen ER, Van Horn L, eds. *Research Successful Approaches*. 3rd ed. Chicago, IL: American Dietetic Association; 2008:187–204.

9. Stumbo PJ. New technology in dietary assessment: a review of digital methods in improving food record accuracy. *Proc Nutr Soc*. 2013;72:70–76.

10. Kirkpatrick SI, Subar AF, Douglass D, et al. Performance of the automated self-administered 24-hour recall relative to a measure of true intakes and to an interviewer-administered 24-h recall. *Am J Clin Nutr*. 2014;100:233–240.

11. Subar A, Kirkpatrick SL, Mittl B, et al. The automated self-administered 24-hour dietary recall (ADA24): a resource for researchers, clinicians, and educators from the National Cancer Institute. *J Acad Nutr Diet*. 2012;112:1134–1136.

12. Diep CS, Hingle M, Chen TA, et al. The automated self-administered 24-hour dietary recall for children, 2012 version, for youth aged 9 to 11 years: a validation study. *J Acad Nutr Diet*. 2015;115:1591–1598.

13. http://dietassessmentprimer.cancer.gov. Dietary Assessment Primer: National Cancer Institute (NCI); Accessed November 1, 2015.

14. Ptomey LT, Willis EA, Honas JJ, et al. Validity of energy intake estimated by digital photography plus recall in overweight and obese young adults. *J Acad Nutr Diet*. 2015;115:1392–1399.

15. Gemming L, Utter J, Mhurchu CN. Image-assisted dietary assessment: a systematic review of the evidence. *J Acad Nutr Diet*. 2015;115:64–67.

16. Kristal AR, Kolar AS, Fisher JL, et al. Evaluation of web-based, self-administered, graphical food frequency questionnaire. *J Acad Nutr Diet*. 2014;114:613–621.

17. Hutchesson MJ, Rollo ME, Callister R, et al. Self-monitoring of dietary intake by young women: online food records completed on computer or smartphone are as accurate as paper-based food records but more acceptable. *J Acad Nutr Diet*. 2015;115:87–94.

18. Gemming L, Rush E, Maddison R, et al. Wearable cameras can reduce dietary under-reporting: doubly labelled water validation of a camera-assisted 24 h recall. *Br J Nutr*. 2014;28:1–8.
19. Gemming L, Doherty A, Utter J, et al. The use of a wearable camera to capture and categorize the environmental and social context of self-identified eating episodes. *Appetite*. 2015;19:118–125.
20. Martin CK, Nicklas T, Gunturk B, et al. Measuring food intake with digital photography. *J Hum Nutr Diet*. 2014;27:72–81.
21. Mochari H, Gao Q, Mosca L. Validation of the MEDFICTS dietary assessment questionnaire in a diverse population. *J Am Diet Assoc*. 2008;108:817–822.
22. Friedeburg AMW, MacIntyre E, Rheeder P. Reliability and validity of a modified MEDFICTS dietary fat screener in South African school children are determined by use and outcome measures. *J Acad Nutr Diet*. 2014;114:870–880.
23. Ollberding NJ, Gilsanz V, Lappe JM, et al. Reproducibility and intermethod reliability of a calcium food frequency questionnaire for use in hispanic, non-hispanic black, and non-hispanic white youth. *J Acad Nutr Diet*. 2015;115:519–527.
24. Yang YJ, Martin BR, Boushey CJ. Development and evaluation of brief calcium assessment tool for adolescents. *J Am Diet Assoc*. 2010;110:111–115.
25. Sublette ME, Segal-Isaacson CJ, Cooper TB, et al. Validation of a food frequency questionnaire to assess intake of n-3 polyunsaturated fatty acids in subjects with and without major depressive disorder. *J Am Diet Assoc*. 2011;111:117–123.
26. Beebe SA, Beebe SJ, Ivy DK. *Communication: Principles for a Lifetime*. 6th ed. Upper Saddle River, NJ: Pearson; 2015.
27. Peregrin T. Competency-based hiring: the key to recruiting and retaining successful employees. *J Acad Nutr Diet*. 2014;114:1330–1339.
28. AbuSabha R. Interviewing clients and patients: improving the skill of asking open-ended questions. *J Acad Nutr Diet*. 2013;113:624–633.

Chapter 4: Communication and Cultural Competence

1. Academy Quality Management Committee, Scope of Practice Subcommittee of Quality Management Committee. Academy of Nutrition and Dietetics: Revised 2012 standards of practice in nutrition care and of professional performance for registered dietitians. *J Acad Nutr Diet*. 2015;113:S29–S45.
2. Academy Quality Management Committee, Scope of Practice Subcommittee of Quality Management Committee. Academy of Nutrition and Dietetics: Revised 2012 standards of practice in nutrition care and standards of professional performance for dietetic technicians, registered. *J Acad Nutr Diet*. 2015;113:S56–S71.
3. The Joint Commission. Crosswalk of Joint Commission Ambulatory Program and the National CLAS (Culturally and Linguistically Appropriate) Standards. http://www.jointcommission.org/crosswalk_of_joint_commission_ambulatory_program_and_the_national_clas_standards. Accessed September 28, 2016.
4. U.S. Census Bureau, 2009-2013 American Community Survey. http://www.census.gov/acs. Accessed September 28, 2016.

5. U.S. Department of Health and Human Services, Office of Disease Prevention and Health Promotion, Healthy People 2020, Washington, DC. http://www.healthypeople.gov/2020/topicsobjectives2020/default.aspx. Accessed January 10, 2016.

6. Alizadeth S, Chavan M. Cultural competence dimensions and outcomes: a systematic review of the literature. *Health Soc Care Community*. 2015. doi:10.1111/hsc.12293.

7. Academy of Nutrition and Dietetics. Practice tips: cultural competence resources. http://www.eatrightpro.org/10877.pdf. Accessed January 10, 2016.

8. Academy of Nutrition and Dietetics. *Cultural Competency for Nutrition Professionals*. Chicago, IL: Academy of Nutrition and Dietetics; 2015.

9. Goody CM, Drago L, eds. *Cultural Food Practices*. Chicago, IL: American Dietetic Association; 2010.

10. United States Department of Health and Human Services, Office of Minority Health and Health Disparities, Center for Linguistic and Cultural Competence in Healthcare. http://hhs.org/omh. Accessed January 10, 2016.

11. Lynch EW, Hanson MU. *Developing Cross-Cultural Competence: A Guide for Working with Children and Their Families*. 4th ed. Baltimore, MD: Brookes Publishing; 2011.

12. Bilyk H. Role of registered dietitian nutritionists in the research and promotion of native and cultural foods. *J Acad Nutr Diet*. 2015;115(S1):531–533.

13. Frank GC. Simplifying education to improve health food purchases by Latina women. *Adelante LAHIDAN*, Newsletter of the Member Interest Group Latinos and Hispanics in Dietetics and Nutrition of the Academy of Nutrition and Dietetics. 2016;9:4–8.

14. Ayala GX, Baquero B, Klinger S. A systematic review of the relationship between acculturation and diet among Latinos in the United States: implications for future research. *J Am Diet Assoc*. 2008;108:1330–1344.

15. Barak MM. *Managing Diversity: Toward a Globally Inclusive Workplace*. 3rd ed. Los Angeles, CA: Sage Publications; 2013.

16. Pew Report 2015. http://pewresearch.org/2015. Accessed September 28, 2016.

17. Luquis RR. Culturally appropriate communication. In: Perez MA, Luquis RR, ed. *Cultural Competence in Health Education and Health Promotion*. 2nd ed. San Francisco, CA: Jossey-Bass; 2014:193–216.

18. U.S. Bureau of Labor Division of Information and Marketing Services. Projected growth of labor for participation of seniors, 2006-2016. http://www.bls.gov/opub/ted/2008/jul/wk4/art04.htm. Accessed September 28, 2016.

19. Robbins SP, Judge TA. *Essentials of Organizational Behavior*. 16th ed. Englewood Cliffs, NJ: Prentice Hall; 2014.

20. Cliffe S. Companies don't go global, people do. *Harv Bus Rev*. 2015;86:83–85.

21. Dauvrin M, Lorant V. Leadership and cultural competence in healthcare professionals. A social network analysis. *Nurs Res*. 2015;64:200–210.

22. Campinha-Bacote J. Coming to know cultural competence: an evolutionary process. *Int J Hum Caring*. 2011;15(3):42–48.

23. Mackay B, Harding T, Jurlina L, et al. Utilizing the hand model to promote culturally safe environment for international nursing students. *Nur Prac NZ*. 2011;27:13–24.

24. Cassel KD, Boushey CJ. Leveraging cultural knowledge to improve diet and health among affiliated Pacific Islanders populations. J Acad Nutr Diet. 2015;115:885–888.

25. Eckhardt CL, Lutz T, Karania N, et al. Knowledge, attitudes, and beliefs can influence infant feeding practices in American Indian mothers. *J Acad Nutr Diet.* 2014;114:1587–1593.

26. Everett-Murphy K, De Villiers A, Ketterer E, et al. Using formative research to develop a nutrition education resource aimed at assisting low-income households in South Africa adopt a healthier diet. *Health Educ Res.* 2015;6:882–896.

27. Wilson B. *First Bite: How We Learn to Eat.* New York, NY: Basic Books: 2015.

28. Steiber A, Hegazi R, Herrera M, et al. Spotlight on global malnutrition: a continuing challenge in the 21st century. *J Acad Nutr Diet.* 2015;115:1335–1341.

29. Kaholokula JK, Mau MK, Efird JT, et al. A family and community focused lifestyle program prevents weight regain in Pacific Islanders: a pilot randomized controlled trial. *Health Educ Behav.* 2011;5:1–10.

30. Fleischhacker S. Emerging opportunities for registered dietitian nutritionists to help raise a healthier generation of Native American youth. *J Acad Nutr Diet.* 2015;115:219–225.

31. Mechanick JI, Marchetti AE, Apovian C, et al. Diabetes-specific nutrition algorithm: a transcultural program to optimize diabetes and pre-diabetes care. *Curr Diab Rep.* 2012;180–194.

32. Duggan A, Street L. Interpersonal communication in health and illness. In: Glamz K, Rimer BK, Viswanath R, eds. *Health Behavior: Theory, Research, and Practice.* 5th ed. San Francisco, CA: Jossey-Bass; 2015:243–268.

33. Patterson RE, Laughlin GA, LaCroix AZ, et al. Intermittent fasting and human metabolic health. *J Acad Nutr Diet.* 2015;115:1203–1212.

34. Pinzon-Perez HP, Perez MA. *Complementary, Alternative, and Integrative Health: A Multicultural Perspective.* San Francisco, CA: Jossey-Bass; 2016.

35. Kittler PG, Sucher KP, Nelms J. *Food and Culture.* 6th ed. Belmont, CA: Wadsworth; 2011.

36. USDA. Myplate Spanish. http://www.choosemyplate.gov /multilanguage-spanish. Accessed March 23, 2016.

37. USDA. My Plate, Other languages. http://www.choosemyplate.gov/other-languages. Accessed March 23, 2016.

Chapter 5: Stages and Processes of Health Behavior Change

1. Salazar LF, Crosby RA, DiClemente RJ. Health behavior in the context of the "new" public health. In: DiClemente RJ, Salazar LF, Crosby RA, eds. *Health Behavior Theory for Public Health: Principles, Foundations, and Applications.* Burlington, MA: Jones & Bartlett Learning; 2013:2–26.

2. Nutrition counseling: behavior change theories. http://www.andeal.org/topic.cfm?menu=3151&cat=1397. Accessed September 28, 2016.

3. Prochaska JO, Norcross JC. *Systems of Psychotherapy: A Transtheoretical Analysis.* 7th ed. Stanford, CT: Cengage Learning; 2013.

4. Prochaska JO, Redding CA, Evers KE. The transtheoretical model and stages of change. In: Glanz K, Rimer BK, Viswanath K, eds. *Health Behavior: Theory, Research, and Practice.* 5th ed. San Francisco, CA: Jossey-Bass; 2015:125–148.

5. Rhee KE, McEachern B, Jelalian E. Parent readiness to change differs for overweight child dietary and physical activity behaviors. *J Acad Nutr Diet.* 2014;114:1601–1610.
6. Maslellos N, Gunn LH, Felix LM, et al. Transtheoretical model stages of change for dietary and exercise modification in weight loss management for overweight and obese adults. *Cochrane Database Syst Rev.* 2014;2:CD008066.
7. DiClemente RJ, Redding CA, Crosby RA, et al. Stage models for health promotion. In: DiClemente RJ, Salazar LF, Crosby RA, et al. *Health Behavior Theory for Public Health: Principles, Foundations, and Applications.* Burlington, MA: Jones & Bartlett Learning; 2013:105–128.
8. Manuvinakurike R, Velicer WF, Bickmore TW. Automated indexing of Internet stories for health behavior change: weight loss attitude pilot study. *J Med Internet Res.* 2014;16:e285.
9. Cunningham E. How can I support my clients in setting realistic weight loss goals. *J Acad Nutr Diet.* 2014:114;176.
10. Haas L, Maryniuk M, Beck J, et al. National standards for diabetes self-management education and support. *Diab Care.* 2014;37:S144–S153.
11. Miller CK, Bauman J. Goal setting: an integral component of effective diabetes care. *Curr Diab Rep.* 2014;14:509.
12. Miller CK, Headings A, Peyrot M, et al. Goal difficulty and goal commitment affect adoption of a lower glycemic index diet in adults with type 2 diabetes. *Patient Educ Couns.* 2012;86:84–90.
13. Rahani E, Stoody RE, Rhiane C. Updating the dietary guidelines for Americans: status and looking ahead. *J Acad Nutr Diet.* 2015;115:180.
14. Dietary Guidelines for Americans 2015. www.health.gov/dietaryguidelines. Accessed January 28, 2016.
15. Ries AV, Blackman LT, Page RA, et al. Goal setting for health behavior change: evidence from an obesity intervention for rural low-income women. *Rural Remote Health.* 2014;14:2682.
16. Martin LR, Haskard-Zolnierek KB, DiMatteo MR. *Health Behavior Change and Treatment Adherence: Evidence-Based Guidelines for Improving Healthcare.* New York, NY: Oxford University Press; 2010.
17. Appelhans BM, Whited MC, Schneider KL, et al. Time to abandon the notion of personal choice in dietary counseling for obesity? *J Am Diet Assoc.* 2011;111:1130–1136.
18. Morris M. *Goal Setting: 10 Easy Steps to Keep Motivated & Master Your Personal Goals.* San Francisco, CA: Globalized Healing; 2014.
19. Wiggins D. *How to Set Goals.* 2014. http://www.amazon.in/How-Set-Goals-Personal-Achievement-ebook/dp/B00BOVMRYG. Accessed October 13, 2016.
20. Nutrition counseling: behavioral change strategies. http://www.andeal.org/topic.cfm?cat=3946. Accessed September 28, 2016.
21. Scientific Report of the 2015 Dietary Advisory Committee. Part D. Chapter 3. Individual diet and PA behavior change. pp. 13–14. www.nel.gov/topic.cfm?eat=3342. Accessed January 25, 2016.
22. Nutrition care process. www.andeal.org.ncp. Accessed January 8, 2016.
23. Hutchesson MJ, Rollo ME, Callister M, et al. Self-monitoring of dietary intake by young women: online food records completed on computer or smartphone are

as accurate as paper-based food records but more acceptable. *J Acad Nutr Diet.* 2015;115:87–94.

24. Kristal AR, Kolar AS, Fisher JL, et al. Evaluation of web-based, self-administered, graphical food frequency questionnaire. *J Acad Nutr Diet.* 2014;114: 613–621.

25. Boyce B. HIPAA Compliance from a Private Practice Purview. *J Acad Nutr Diet.* 2014;114:1341–1346.

26. US Department of Health and Human Services. Health information privacy. www.hhs.gov/ocr/privacy/hipaa/understanding/consumers. Accessed January 28, 2016.

27. Rollo ME, Hutchesson MJ, Burrows TL, et al. Video consultations and virtual nutrition care for weight management. *J Acad Nutr Diet.* 2015;115:1213–1225.

28. HIPAA: Health Insurance Portability and Accountability Act. http://www.hhs.gov /hipaa/for-professionals/FAQ. Accessed September 28, 2016.

29. Office for Civil Rights. Health information privacy rights. www.hhs.gov/ocr. Accessed January 28, 2016.

Chapter 6: Person-Centered Counseling

1. Clark NM, Janevic MR. Individual theories. In: Riekert KA, Ockene JK, Pbert L, eds. *The Handbook of Health Behavior Change.* New York, NY: Springer; 2014:3–26.

2. The Editors. Theory, research, and practice in health behavior. In: Glanz K, Rimer BK, Viswanath K, eds. *Health Behavior: Theory, Research, and Practice.* 5th ed. San Francisco, CA: Jossey-Bass; 2015:23–41.

3. Rogers CR. *On Becoming a Person.* Boston, MA: Houghton Mifflin; 1961.

4. Rogers CR. *Client-Centered Therapy. It's Current Practice, Implications and Theory.* London: Constable & Robinson; 2003.

5. Prochaska JO, Norcross JC. *Systems of Psychotherapy: A Transtheoretical Analysis.* 8th ed. Stanford, CT: Cengage Learning; 2014.

6. Rollnick S, Miller WR, Butler CC. *Motivational Interviewing in Health Care: Helping Patients Change Behaviors.* New York, NY: Guilford Press: 2008.

7. Miller WR, Rollnick S. *Motivational Interviewing: Helping People Change.* 3rd ed. New York, NY: Guilford Press; 2013.

8. Berger BA, Villaume WA. *Motivational Interviewing for Health Care Professionals: A Sensible Approach.* Washington, DC: *American Pharmacists Association*; 2013.

9. Hollis JL, Williams LT, Collins CE, et al. Does motivational interviewing align with international scope of practice, professional competency standards, and best practice guidelines in dietetics practice? *J Acad Nutr Diet.* 2014;114:676–687.

10. Steinberg MP, Miller WR. *Motivational Interviewing in Diabetes Care.* New York, NY: Guilford Press; 2015.

11. Clifford D, Curtis L. *Motivational Interviewing in Nutrition and Fitness.* New York, NY: Guilford Press; 2015.

12. Resnicow K, McMaster F. Motivational interviewing: moving from why to how with autonomy support. *Int J Behav Nutr Phys Act.* 2012;9:19.

13. Haas L, Maryniuk M, Beck J, et al. National standards for diabetes self-management education and support. *Diabetes Care.* 2014;37:S144–S153.

14. Smart H, Clifford D, Moris MN. Nutrition students gain skills from motivational interviewing curriculum. *J Acad Nutr Diet.* 2014;114:1712–1722.

15. Hall K, Gibbie T, Lubman DI. Motivational interviewing techniques–facilitating behavior change in the general practice setting. *Aust Fam Physician.* 2012;41:660–667.

16. Martin LR, Haskard-Zolnierek KB, DiMatteo MR. *Health Behavior Change and Treatment Adherence: Evidence-Based Guidelines for Improving Healthcare.* New York, NY: Oxford University Press; 2010.

17. Rollnick S, Butler CC, Kinnersley P, et al. Motivational interviewing. *BMJ.* 2010;340:c1900.

18. Spahn JM, Reeves RS, Keim KS, et al. State of the evidence regarding behavior change theories and strategies in nutrition counseling to facilitate health and food behavior change. *J Am Diet Assoc.* 2010;110:879–891.

19. Resnicow K, McMaster F, Bocian A, et al. Motivational interviewing and dietary counseling for obesity in primary care: an RCT. *Pediatrics.* 2015;135:649–657.

20. Lundahl B, Moleni T, Burke BL, et al. Motivational interviewing in medical care settings: a systematic review and meta-analysis of randomized controlled trials. *Patient Educ Couns.* 2013;93:157–168.

21. Borelli B, Tooley EM, Scott-Sheldon LA. Motivational interviewing for parent-child health interventions: a systematic review and meta-analysis. *Pediatr Dent.* 2015;37:254–265.

22. Crosby RA, Salazar LF, DiClemente RJ. Value expectancy theories. In: DiClemente RJ, Salazar LF, Crosby RA, eds. *Health Behavior Theory for Public Health: Principles, Foundations, and Applications.* Burlington, MA: Jones & Bartlett; 2013:65–80.

23. Skinner CS, Tiro J, Champion VL. The health belief model. In: Glanz K, Rimer BK, Viswanath K, eds. *Health Behavior: Theory, Research, and Practice*, 5th ed. San Francisco, CA: Jossey-Bass; 2015:75–94.

24. Salazar LF, Crosby RA, Noar SM, et al. Models based on threat and fear appeals. In: DiClemente RJ, Salazar LF, Crosby RA, eds. *Health Behavior Theory for Public Health: Principles, Foundations, and Applications.* Burlington, MA: Jones & Bartlett; 2013:83–95.

25. Freeland-Graves JH, Nitzke S, Academy of Nutrition and Dietetics. Position of the Academy of Nutrition and Dietetics: total diet approach to healthy eating. *J Acad Nutr Diet.* 2013;113:307–317.

26. Morris, SS, Snell SA, Bohlander GW. *Managing Human Resources.* 17th ed. Mason, OH: South-Western; 2015.

27. Beebe SA, Beebe SJ, Ivy DK. *Communication: Principles for a Lifetime.* 6th ed. New York, NY: Pearson; 2015.

Chapter 7: Counseling for Behavior Modification

1. Peltier B. *The Psychology of Executive Coaching: Theory and Application.* 2nd ed. New York, NY: Taylor & Francis Group LLC; 2010.

2. Sarafino EP. *Applied Behavior Analysis: Principles and Procedures for Modifying Behavior.* Hoboken, NJ: Wiley; 2012.

3. Academy of Nutrition and Dietetics. Nutrition terminology reference manual eN-CPT: dietetics language for nutrition care. http://ncpt.webauthor.com. Accessed November 3, 2015.

4. McLean PS, Wing RR, Davidson T, et al. NIH working group report: innovative research to improve maintenance weight loss. *Obesity.* 2015;23:7–15.

5. Farmer RF, Chapman AL, American Psychological Association. *Behavioral Interventions in Cognitive Behavior Therapy: Practical Guidance for Putting Theory into Action.* 2nd ed. Washington, DC: American Psychological Association; 2016.

6. Nairne JS. *Psychology.* 6th ed. Belmont, CA: Thomson/Wadsworth; 2012.

7. Bandura A. *Self-Efficacy: The Exercise of Control.* New York, NY: WH Freeman; 1997.

8. Cromley T, Neumark-Sztainer D, Story M, et al. Parent and family associations with weight-related behaviors and cognitions among overweight adolescents. *J Adolesc Health.* 2010;47(3):263–269.

9. van der Kruk JJ, Kortekaas F, Lucas C, et al. Obesity: a systematic review on parental involvement in long-term European childhood weight control interventions with a nutritional focus. *Obes Rev.* 2013;14:745–760. doi:10.1111/obr.12046.

10. Eckel RH, Jakicic JM, Ard JD, et al. 2013 AHA/ACC guideline on lifestyle management to reduce cardiovascular risk: a report of the American College of Cardiology/American Heart Association Task Force on practice guidelines. *Circulation.* 2014;129:S76–S99.

11. Wadden T, Butryn M, Hong P, et al. Behavioral treatment of obesity in patients encountered in primary care settings. *JAMA.* 2013;312(17):1779–1791.

12. Lin JS, O'Connor E, Whitlock EP, et al. Behavioral counseling to promote physical activity and a healthful diet to prevent cardiovascular disease in adults: a systematic review for the U.S. Preventive Services Task Force. *Ann Intern Med.* 2010;153:736–750.

13. Di Noia J, Prochaska J. Mediating variables in a transtheoretical model dietary intervention program. *Health Educ Behav.* 2010;37(5):753–762.

14. Phelan S, Wing RR, Raynor HA, et al. Holiday weight management by successful weight losers and normal weight individuals. *J Consult Clin Psychol.* 2008;76(3):442–448.

15. Spahn JM, Reeves RS, Keim KS, et al. State of the evidence regarding behavior change theories and strategies in nutrition counseling to facilitate health and food behavior change. *J Am Diet Assoc.* 2010;110(6):879–891.

16. American Health Information Management Association. The 10 security domains updated. *J AHIMA.* 2012;83(5):48–52.

17. Burke LE, Wang J, Sevick MA. Self-monitoring in weight loss: a systematic review of the literature. *J Am Diet Assoc.* 2011;111:92–102.

18. Skinner BF. *Science and Human Behavior.* New York, NY: Macmillan; 1953.

19. Academy of Nutrition and Dietetics. Interventions for the treatment of obesity and overweight in adults. *J Acad Nutr Diet.* 2016;116:129-147.

20. Niemeier HM, Phelan S, Fava JL, et al. Internal disinhibition predicts weight regain following weight loss and weight loss maintenance. *Obesity.* 2007;15:2485–2494.

21. Peterson N, Middleton K, Nackers L, et al. Dietary self-monitoring and long-term success with weight management. *Obesity.* 2014;22(9):1962–1967.

22. National Weight Control Registry. http://www.nwcr.ws. Accessed November 3, 2015.

23. Donnelly JE, Blair SN, Jakicic JM, et al. American College of Sports Medicine position stand. Appropriate intervention strategies for weight loss and prevention of weight regain for adults. *Med Sci Sports Exerc*. 2009;41:459–482.

24. Andrade AM, Coutinho SR, Silva MN, et al. The effect of physical activity on weight loss is mediated by eating self-regulation. *Patient Educ Couns*. 2010;79(3):320–326.

25. Pearson E. Review: Goal setting as a health behavior change strategy in overweight and obese adults: a systematic literature review examining intervention components. *Patient Educ Couns*. 2012;87:32–42.

26. Jensen MD, Ryan DH, Apovian CM, et al. 2013 AHA/ACC/TOS guideline for the management of overweight and obesity in adults a report of the American College of Cardiology/American Heart Association Task Force on Practice Guidelines and The Obesity Society. *J Am Coll Cardiol*. 2013;63:2985–3025.

27. Purnell J, Gernes R, Stein R, et al. A systematic review of financial incentives for dietary behavior change. *J Acad Nutr Diet*. 2014;114(7):1023–1035.

28. Gregg E, Chen H, Bertoni A, et al. Association of an intensive lifestyle intervention with remission of type 2 diabetes. *JAMA*. 2012;308(23):2489–2496.

29. American Association of Diabetes Educators. Seven self care behaviors. http://www.diabeteseducator.org/ProfessionalResources/AADE7/. Accessed November 4, 2015.

30. Monroe C, Thompson D, Bassett D, et al. Usability of mobile phones in physical activity–related research: a systematic review. *Am J Health Educ*. 2015;464:196–206.

31. National Diabetes Education Program. http://ndep.nih.gov. Accessed November 4, 2015.

32. Lloyd-Jones DM, Hong Y, Labarthe D, et al. Defining and setting national goals for cardiovascular health promotion and disease reduction: the American Heart Association's strategic impact goal through 2020 and beyond. *Circulation*. 2010;121:586–613.

33. Artinian NT, Fletcher GF, Mozaffarian D, et al. Interventions to promote physical activity and dietary lifestyle changes for cardiovascular disease risk factor reduction in adults: a scientific statement from the American Heart Association. *Circulation*. 2010;122:406–441.

34. Arena R, Guazzi M, Shurney D, et al. Special article: Healthy lifestyle interventions to combat non-communicable disease—a novel nonhierarchical connectivity model for key stakeholders: a policy statement from the American Heart Association, European Society of Cardiology, European Association for Cardiovascular Prevention and Rehabilitation, and American College of Preventive Medicine. *Mayo Clin Proc*. 2015;90:1082–1103.

Chapter 8: Counseling for Cognitive Change

1. Beck JS. *Cognitive Therapy: Basics and Beyond*. 2nd ed. New York: Guilford Press; 2011.

2. Writing Group of the Nutrition Care Process/Standardized Language Committee. Nutrition care process and model part 1: the 2008 update. *J Am Diet Assoc*. 2008;108:1113–1117.

3. Burke LE, Froehlich RA, Zhena Y, et al. Current theoretical bases for nutrition intervention and their uses. In: Coulston AM, Boushey CJ, Ferrazzi M, eds. *Nutrition in the Prevention and Treatment of Disease*. 3rd ed. Boston, MA: Elsevier; 2013:141–155.

4. McKay M, Davis M, Fanning P. *Thoughts & Feelings: Taking Control of Your Moods & Your Life*. 4th ed. Oakland, CA: New Harbinger Pub; 2011.

5. Fairburn CG, Bailey-Straebler S, Basden S, et al. A transdiagnostic comparison of enhanced cognitive behavior therapy and interpersonal psychotherapy in the treatment of eating disorders. *Behav Res Ther*. 2015;70:64–71.

6. Position of the American Dietetic Association. Nutrition intervention in the treatment of eating disorders. *J Am Diet Assoc*. 2011;111:1236–1241.

7. Turner H, Marshall E, Stopa L, et al. Cognitive-behavioural therapy for outpatients with eating disorders: effectiveness for a transdiagnostic group in a routine clinical setting. *Behav Res Ther*. 2015;68:70–75.

8. Dobson KS, Dozois DJA. Historical and philosophical basis of the cognitive-behavioral therapies. In: Dobson KS, ed. *Handbook of Cognitive-Behavioral Therapies*. 3rd ed. New York, NY: Guilford Press; 2010:3–38.

9. The Editors. The scope of health behavior. In: Glanz K, Rimer BK, Viswanath K, eds. *Health Behavior: Theory, Research, and Practice*. 5th ed. San Francisco, CA: Jossey-Bass; 2015:3–22.

10. Adult weight management: executive summary of recommendations. www .andeal.org/topic.cfm?menu=52760. Accessed December 1, 2015.

11. Bandura A. Exercise of personal and collective efficacy in changing societies. In: Bandura A, ed. *Self-Efficacy in Changing Societies*. New York, NY: Cambridge University Press; 1995:1–45.

12. Yu Z, Sealey-Potts C, Rodriguez J. Dietary self-monitoring in weight management: current evidence on efficacy and adherence. *J Acad Nutr Diet*. 2015;115:1931–1938.

13. Burke LE, Wang J, Sevick MA. Self-monitoring in weight loss: a systematic review of the literature. *J Am Diet Assoc*. 2011;111:92–102.

14. Hoy MK, Winters BL, Chlebowski RT, et al. Implementing a low-fat eating plan in the Women's Intervention Nutrition Study. *J Am Diet Assoc*. 2009;109:688–696.

15. Prochaska JO, Redding CA, Evers KE. The transtheoretical model and stages of change. In: Glanz K, Rimer BK, Viswanath K, eds. *Health Behavior: Theory, Research, and Practice*. 5th ed. San Francisco, CA: Jossey-Bass; 2015:125–148.

16. Bandura A. Health promotion by social cognitive means. *Health Educ Behav*. 2004;31:143–164.

17. Anderson-ES, Winett RA, Wojcik JR. Social cognitive determinants of nutrition and physical activity among web-health users enrolling in an online intervention: the influence of social support, self-efficacy, outcome expectations, and self regulation. *J Med Internet Res*. 2011;17:13.

18. Clark NM, Janevic MR. Individual theories. In: Riekert KA, Ockene JK, Pbert L, eds. *The Handbook of Health Behavior Change*. 4th ed. New York, NY: Springer Pub; 2014:3–26.

19. Bandura A. *Social Foundations of Thought and Action: A Social Cognitive Theory*. Englewood Cliffs, NJ: Prentice-Hall; 1986.

20. Bandura A. *Self-Efficacy: The Exercise of Control*. New York, NY: WH Freeman; 1997.
21. Kelder SH, Hoetscher D, Perry CL, et al. How individuals, environments, and health behaviors interact. In: Glanz K, Rimer BK, Viswanath K, eds. *Health Behavior: Theory, Research, and Practice*. 5th ed. San Francisco, CA: Jossey-Bass; 2015:159–181.
22. Heiss VJ, Petosa FL. Social cognitive theory correlates of moderate-intensity exercise among adults with type 2 diabetes. *Psychol Health Med*. 2015;10:1–10.
23. Olander EK, Fletcher H, Williams S, et al. What are the most effective techniques in changing obese individuals' physical activity self-efficacy and behavior: a systematic review and meta-analysis. *Int J Behav Nutr Phys Act*. 2013;10:29.
24. Stacey FG, James EL, Chapman K, et al. A systematic review and meta-analysis of social cognitive theory-based physical activity and/or nutrition behavior change interventions for cancer survivors. *J Cancer Surviv*. 2015;9:305–338.
25. Marlatt GA, Witkiewitz K. Relapse prevention for alcohol and drug problems. In: Marlatt GA, Donovan DM, eds. *Relapse Prevention: Maintenance Strategies in the Treatment of Addictive Behaviors*. 2nd ed. New York, NY: Guilford Press; 2005:1–44.
26. Donovan DM. Assessment of addictive behaviors for relapse prevention. In: Donovan DM, Marlatt GA, eds. *Assessment of Addictive Behaviors*. 2nd ed. New York, NY: Guilford Press; 2005:1–48.
27. Teixeira PJ, Carraca EV, Marques MM, et al. Successful behavior change in obesity interventions in adults: a systematic review of self-regulation mediators. *BMC Med*. 2015;13:84.
28. Hendershot CS, Witkiewitz K, George WH, et al. Relapse prevention for addictive behaviors. *Sust Abuse Treat Prev Policy*. 2011;6:17.
29. Collins RL. Relapse prevention for eating disorders and obesity. In: Marlatt GA, Donovan DM, eds. *Relapse Prevention: Maintenance Strategies in the Treatment of Addictive Behaviors*. 2nd ed. New York: Guilford Press; 2005:249–269.
30. Prochaska JO, Norcross JC. *Systems of Psychotherapy: A Transtheoretical Analysis*. 8th ed. Stamford, CT: Cengage Learning; 2014.
31. Witkiewitz K, Marlatt GA. Overview of relapse prevention. In: Witkiewitz K, Marlatt GA, eds. *Therapist's Guide to Evidence-Based Relapse Prevention*. Boston, MA: Elsevier; 2007:3–18.
32. Witkiewitz K, Marlatt GA. High-risk situations: relapse as a dynamic process. In: Witkiewitz K, Marlatt GA, eds. *Therapist's Guide to Evidence-Based Relapse Prevention*. Boston, MA: Elsevier; 2007:19–35.
33. Kristeller JL, Wolever RQ. Mindfulness-based eating awareness training for binge eating disorder: the conceptual foundation. *Eat Disord*. 2011;19:49–61.
34. Wansink B. Under the influence: how external cues make us overeat. *Nutrition Action Health Letter*. 2011;38:3–7.
35. Burke LE, Turk MW. Obesity. In: Richert KA, Ockene JK, Pbest L, eds. *The Handbook of Health Behavior Change*. New York, NY: Springer Publishing;2014:363–378.

Chapter 9: Counseling Through the Lifespan

1. Healthy People 2020. http://www.healthypeople.gov/2020/topics-objectives. Accessed January 3, 2016.
2. ChooseMyPlate. http://www.choosemyplate.gov/MyPlate. Accessed January 3, 2016.
3. Graham DJ, Jeffery RW. Location, location, location: eye-tracking evidence that consumers preferentially view prominently positioned nutrition information. *J Acad Nutr Diet*. 2011;111:1704–1711.
4. Jortberg B, Meyers E, Gigliotti L, et al. Academy of Nutrition and Dietetics: Standards of Practice and Standards for Professional Performance for Registered Dietititan Nutritionists (Competent, Proficient, and Expert) in adult weight management. *J Acad Nutr Diet*. 2015;115:609–618.
5. Procter SB, Campbell CG. Position of the Academy of Nutrition and Dietetics: nutrition and lifestyle for a healthy pregnancy outcome. *J Acad Nutr Diet*. 2015;115:1099–1103.
6. Berry D, Verbiest S, Hall EG, et al. A postpartum community-based weight management intervention designed for low-income women: feasibility and initial efficacy testing. *J Natl Black Nurses Assoc*. 2015;26:29–39.
7. Raiten DJ, Steiber AL, Carlson SE, et al. Working group reports: evaluation of the evidence to support practice guidelines for nutritional care of preterm infants-the Pre-B Project. *Am J Clin Nutr*. 2016;103:648S–678S.
8. Lesson R, Kavanagh K. Position of the Academy of Nutrition and Dietetics: promoting and supporting breastfeeding. *J Acad Nutr Diet*. 2015;115:444–449.
9. Schwartz R, Ellings A, Baisden A, et al. Washington "steps up": a 10-step quality improvement initiative to optimize breastfeeding support in community health centers. *J Hum Lact*. 2015;31:651–659.
10. The American Academy of Pediatrics. Feeding and nutrition. http://healthychildren .org/English/ages-stages/baby/feeding-nutrition/Pages/default.aspx. Accessed September 28, 2016.
11. Hayes D. Getting started on eating right. October 1, 2014. http://www.eatright .org/resource/food/nutrition/dietary-guidelines-and-myplate/getting-started-on-eating-right. Accessed September 28, 2016.
12. Maalouf J, Cogswell ME, Yuan K, et al. Top sources of dietary sodium from birth to age 24 mo, United States, 2003-2010. *Am J Clin Nutr*. 2015;101:1021–1028.
13. Ogata BN, Hayes D. Position of the Academy of Nutrition and Dietetics: nutrition guidances for healthy children ages 2 to 11 years. *J Acad Nutr Diet*. 2014;114:1257–1276.
14. Izumi BT, Eckhardt CL, Hallman JA, et al. Harvest for Healthy Kids pilot study: associations between exposure to a farm-to-preschool intervention and willingness to try and liking of target fruits and vegetables among low-income children in Head Start. *J Acad Nutr Diet*. 2015;115:2003–2013.
15. Wilson B. *First Bite: How We Learn to Eat*. New York, NY: Basic Books; 2015.
16. Amuta AO, Jacobs W, Idoko EE, et al. Influence of home food environment on children's fruit and vegetable consumption: a study of rural low-income families. *Health Promot Pract*. 2015;16:689–698.

17. Hingle MD, Castonquay IS, Ambuel DA, et al. Alignment of children's food advertising with proposed federal guidelines. *Am J Prev Med*. 2015;48:707–713.
18. Sharman SJ, Skouteris H, Powell MB, et al. Factors related to the accuracy of self-reported dietary intake of children aged 6 to 12 years elicited with interviews: a systematic review. *J Acad Nutr Diet*. 2016;116:76–114.
19. Spears-Lanoix EC, McKyer EL, Evans A, et al. Using family-focused garden, nutrition, and physical activity programs to reduce childhood obesity: the Texas! Go! Eat! Grow! pilot study. *Child Obes*. 2015;11:707–714.
20. Briggs M, Fleischhacker S, Mueller CG. Position of the American Dietetic Association, School Nutrition Association, and Society for Nutrition Education: comprehensive school nutrition services. *J Am Diet Assoc*. 2010;110:1738–1749.
21. Brown CL, Halvorson EE, Cohen GM, et al. Addressing childhood obesity: opportunities for prevention. *Pediatr Clin North Am*. 2015;62:1241–1261.
22. Council on Community Pediatrics, Committee on Nutrition, American Academy of Pediatrics. Promoting food security for all children. *Pediatrics*. 2015;136:e1431–e1438.
23. Berge JM, MacLehose RF, Meyer C, et al. He said, she said: examining parental concordance on home environment factors and adolescent health behaviors and weight status. *J Acad Nutr Diet*. 2016;116:45–60.
24. Hoffman JA, Rosenfeld L, Schmidt N, et al. Implementation of competitive food and beverage standards in a sample of Massachusetts schools: the NOURISH study (Nutrition Opportunities to Understand Reforms Involving Student Health). *J Acad Nutr Diet*. 2015;115:1299–1307.
25. Sattler M, Hopkins L, Anderson Steeves E, et al. Characteristics of youth food preparation by low-income, African American homes: associations with healthy eating index scores. *Ecol Food Nutr*. 2015;54:380–396.
26. Society for Adolescent Health and Medicine, Golden NH, Katzman DK, et al. Position Paper of the Society for Adolescent Health and Medicine: medical management of restrictive eating disorders in adolescents and young adults. *J Adolesc Health*. 2015;56:121–125.
27. Food and Nutrition Information Center, United States Department of Agriculture. Fitness and sports nutrition. http://fnic.nal.usda.gov/lifecycle-nutrition/fitness-and-sports-nutrition. Accessed September 28, 2016.
28. Ptorney LT, Willis EA, Honas JJ, et al. Validity of energy intake estimated by digital photography plus recall in overweight and obese young adults. *J Acad Nutr Diet*. 2015;115:1392–1399.
29. Wakabayashi H, Matsushima M. Dysphagia assessed by the 10-item eating assessment toll is associated with nutritional status and activities of daily living in elderly individuals requiring long-term care. *J Nutr Health Aging*. 2016;20:22–27.
30. U.S. Department of Health and Human Services, United States Department of Agriculture. 2015-2020 Dietary guidelines. Executive summary. http://health.gov/dietaryguidelines/2015/guidelines/?platform-hootsuite. Accessed January 22, 2016.
31. Weaver CM, Alexander DD, Boushey CJ, et al. Calcium plus vitamin D supplementation and risk of fractures: an updated meta-analysis from the National Osteoporosis Foundation. *Osteoporos Int*. 2016;27:367–376.

32. Bernstein M, Munoz N. Position of the Academy of Nutrition and Dietetics: food and nutrition in older adults: promoting health and wellness. *J Acad Nutr Diet*. 2014;112:1255–1277.
33. Forbes SC, Holroyd-Leduc JM, Poulin MJ, et al. Effect of nutrients, dietary supplements and vitamins on cognition: a systematic review and meta-analysis of randomized controlled trials. *Can Geriatr J*. 2015;18:231–245.
34. American Dietetic Association. Position paper of the American Dietetic Association: nutrition intervention in the treatment of eating disorders. *J Am Diet Assoc*. 2011;111:1236–1241.
35. Baek MH, Heo YR. Evaluation of the efficacy of nutritional screening tools to predict malnutrition in the elderly at a geriatric care hospital. *Nutr Res Pract*. 2015;9:637–643.
36. Franz MJ, Boucher JL, Rutten-Ramos S, et al. Lifestyle weight-loss interventions outcomes in overweight and obese adults with type 2 diabetes: a systematic review and meta-analysis of randomized clinical trials. *J Acad Nutr Diet*. 2015;115:1447–1463.
37. The MacColl Center. The chronic care model. http://improvingchroniccare.org/index.php?p=The-Chronic-Care-Model&xs2. Accessed September 28, 2016.
38. Kohn JB, Schofield M. Is medical nutrition therapy considered a form of preventive care and is it reimbursable? *J Acad Nutr Diet*. 2015;115:1904.
39. Yu Z, Sealey-Potts C, Rodriguez J. Dietary self-monitoring in weight management: current evidence on efficacy and adherence. *J Acad Nutr Diet*. 2015;115:1931–1938.
40. Beto JA, Schury KA, Bansal VK. Strategies to promote adherence to nutritional advice in patients with chronic kidney disease: a narrative review and commentary. *Int J Nephro Renovascular Dis*. 2016;9:1–13.
41. Powers MA, Bardsley J, Cypress M, et al. Diabetes self-management education and support in type 2 diabetes: a joint position statement of the American Diabetes Association, the American Association of Diabetes Educations, and the Academy of Nutrition and Dietetics. *J Acad Nutr Diet*. 2015;115:1323–1334.
42. Kent PS, McCarthy MP, Burrowes JD, et al. Academy of Nutrition and Dietetics and National Kidney Foundation: Revised 2014 standards of practice and standards for professional performance for registered dietitian nutritionists (competent, proficient, and expert) in nephrology nutrition. *J Acad Nutr Diet*. 2014;114:1448–1457e45.
43. Women's Health Initiative. http://www.nhlbi.nih.gov/whi. Accessed September 28, 2016.

Chapter 10: Principles and Theories of Learning

1. Wilson B. *First Bite: How We Learn to Eat*. New York, NY: Basic Books; 2015.
2. Woolfolk AE. *Educational Psychology*. 11th ed. Boston, MA: Pearson/Allyn & Bacon; 2010.
3. Health Canada. Eating well with Canada's food guide. http://healthycanadians.gc.ca/eating-nutrition/healthy-eating-saine-alimentation/food-guide-aliment/index-eng.php. Accessed November 15, 2015.

4. United States Department of Agriculture. MyPlate. http://choosemyplate .gov. Accessed November 15, 2015.

5. Glanz K, Viswanath K, eds. *Health Behavior and Health Education: Theory, Research, and Practice*. 5th ed. San Francisco, CA: Jossey-Bass; 2015.

6. Caine RN, Caine G. *Natural Learning for a Connected World. Education, Technology, and the Human Brain*. New York, NY: Teachers' College Press; 2011.

7. Taylor K, Marienau C. *Facilitating Learning with the Adult Brain in Mind*. San Francisco, CA: Jossey-Bass; 2016.

8. Scott D. *New Perspectives on Curriculum, Leaning and Assessment*. New York, NY: Springer; 2016.

9. Kliveri M. Bridging competence and skills gap in food safety with continuing professional development. *Perspect Public Health*. 2014;134:194–195.

10. Dunn J. How I did it... The CEO of Bolthouse farms on making carrots cool. *Harv Bus Rev*. 2015;93:43–46.

11. Wittner J, Renkl A. How effective are instructional explanations in example-based learning? A meta-analytic review. *Educ Psychol Rev*. 2010;22:393–409.

12. Pleschova G, McAlpine L. Helping teachers to focus on learning and reflect on their teaching: what role does teaching context play? *Stud Educ Eval*. 2016;48:1–9.

13. Knowles MS, Holton EF, Swanson RA. *The Adult Learner: The Definitive Classic in Adult Education and Human Resource Development*. 10th ed. Houston, TX: Gulf Publishing; 2005.

14. Lucas RW. *Energize Your Training: Creative Techniques to Engage Learners*. Alexandria, VA: ASTD Press; 2010.

15. Schunk DH. *Learning Theories: An Educational Perspective*. 7th ed. Old Tappan, NJ: Pearson; 2016.

16. Paolini A. Enhancing teaching effectiveness and student learning outcomes. *J Effective Teaching*. 2015;1:20–33.

17. Halem CJ, Searle NS, Gunderman R, et al. The educational attributes and responsibilities of effective medical educators. *Acad Med*. 2011;86:474–480.

18. Costa A, Kallick B. *Learning and Leading with Habits of Mind: 16 Essential Characteristics for Success*. Alexandria, VA: Association for Supervision and Curriculum Development; 2008.

19. Glanz K, Rimer BK, Viswanath K, eds. *Health Behavior and Health Education: Theory, Research, and Practice*. 5th ed. San Francisco, CA: Jossey-Bass; 2015.

20. Sawyer K, ed. *The Cambridge Handbook of the Learning Sciences*. 2nd ed. New York, NY: Cambridge University Press; 2014.

21. Quintana C, Zhang M, Kracjcik J. A framework for supporting metacognitive aspects of online inquiry through software-based scaffolding. *Educ Psychologist*. 2010;40:235-244.

Chapter 11: Planning Learning

1. Worsford L, Grant BL, Barnhill GD. The essential practice competencies for the Commission on Dietetic Registration's Credentialed Nutrition and Dietetics Practitioner. *J Acad Nutr Diet*. 2015;115:978–984.

2. International Confederation of Dietetics Associations. International definition of dietitians, 2010. http://www.internationaldietetics.org/International-Standards /International-Definition-of-Dietitian.aspx. Accessed September 28, 2016.

3. The Joint Commission. *Comprehensive Accreditation Manual for Hospitals (CAMH)*. Oak Brook, IL: The Joint Commission; 2015. http://www.jointcommission.org/ accreditation/accreditation_main.aspx. Accessed September 28, 2016.

4. Dali'Oglio I, Nicolo R, Di Ciommo V, et al. A systematic review of hospital food-service patient satisfaction studies. *J Acad Nutr Diet*. 2015:115:567–584.

5. Gibson S, Dart J, Bone C, et al. Dietetic student preparedness and performance on clinical placements: perspectives of clinical educators. *J Allied Health*. 2015;44:101–107.

6. Roy R, Kelly B, Rangan A, et al. Food environment intervention to improve the dietary behavior of young adults in a tertiary education setting: a systematic literature review. *J Acad Nutr Diet*. 2015;115:1647–1681.

7. Wallace R, Lo J, Devine A. Tailored nutrition education in the elderly can lead to sustained dietary behavior change. *J Nutr Health Aging*. 2016;20:8–15.

8. Olsho LE, Klerman JA, Ritchie L, et al. Increasing child fruit and vegetable intake: findings from the US Department of Agriculture Fresh Fruit and Vegetable Program. *J Acad Nutr Diet*. 2015;115:1283–1290.

9. Weaver RD, Hemmelgarn BR, Rabi DM, et al. Association between participation in a brief diabetes education programme and glycaemic control in adults with newly diagnosed diabetes. *Diabet Med*. 2014;31:1610–1614.

10. Kliveri M. Bridging competence and skills gap in food safety with continuing professional development. *Perspect Public Health*. 2014;134:194–195.

11. Scott D. *New Perspectives on Curriculum, Learning and Assessment*. New York, NY: Springer; 2016.

12. Caine RN, Caine G. *Natural Learning for a Connected World. Education, Technology, and the Human Brain*. New York, NY: Teachers' College Press; 2011.

13. Wittwer J, Renkl A. How effective are instructional explanations in example-based learning? A meta-analytic review. *Educ Psychol Rev*. 2010;22:393–409.

14. Monroe JT. Mindful eating: principles and practice. *Am J Lifestyle Med*. 2015;9:217–220.

15. Sleddens EF, Kroeze W, Kohl LF, et al. Correlates of dietary behavior in adults: an umbrella review. *Nutr Rev*. 2015;73:477–499.

16. Harris JE, Gleason PM, Sheean PM, et al. An introduction to qualitative research for food and nutrition professionals. *J Am Diet Assoc*. 2009;109:80–90.

17. Magids S, Zorfas A, Leemon D. The new science of customer emotions: a better way to drive profit and profitability. *Harv Bus Rev*. 2015;97:68–74.

18. Graham DJ, Heidrick C, Hodgin K. Nutrition label viewing during food-selection task: Front-of-package labels vs nutrition facts labels. *J Acad Nutr Diet*. 2015;115:1636–1646.

19. Murphy KE, De Villiers A, Ketterer E, et al. Using formative research to develop a nutrition education resource aimed at assisting low-income households in South Africa adopt a healthier diet. *Health Educ Res*. 2015;30:882–896.

20. Mager RF. *Preparing Instructional Objectives: A Critical Tool in the Development of Effective Instruction*. 3rd ed. Atlanta, GA: CEP Press; 1997.

21. Bloom BS. *Taxonomy of Educational Objectives. Handbook I: Cognitive Domain*. New York, NY: Longman; 1956. (Copyright renewed 1984 by Bloom BS, Krathwohl D.)

22. Anderson LW, Sosniak LA, eds. *Bloom's Taxonomy: A Forty-Year Retrospective*. Chicago, IL: University of Chicago; 1994.

23. Anderson LW, Krathwohl D, eds. *A Taxonomy for Learning, Teaching, and Assessing: A Revision of Bloom's Taxonomy of Educational Objectives*. New York, NY: Longman; 2001.

24. Krathwohl D, Bloom BS, Masia B. *Taxonomy of Educational Objectives. Handbook II: Affective Domain*. New York, NY: David McKay; 1964.

25. Simpson E. *The Classification of Educational Objectives in the Psychomotor Domain*. Washington, DC: Gryphon House; 1972.

26. Harrow A. *A Taxonomy of the Psychomotor Domain*. New York, NY: David McKay; 1972.

27. Robbins SP, Judge TA. *Essentials of Organizational Behavior*. 16th ed. Englewood Cliffs, NJ: Prentice Hall; 2014.

Chapter 12: Implementing and Evaluating Learning

1. Lucas RW. *Energize Your Training: Creative Techniques to Engage Learners*. Alexandria, VA: ASTD Press; 2010.

2. Rosciano A. The effectiveness of mind mapping as an active learning strategy among associate degree nursing students. *Teach Learn Nurs*. 2015;10:93–99.

3. Wittwer J, Renkl A. How effective are instructional explanations in example-based learning? A meta-analytic review. *Educ Psychol Rev*. 2010;22:393–409.

4. Scott D. *New Perspectives on Curriculum, Leaning and Assessment*. New York, NY: Springer; 2016.

5. Rosas LC, Thlyagarajan S, Goldstein BA, et al. The effectiveness of two community-based weight loss strategies among obese, low-income US Latinos. *J Acad Nutr Diet*. 2015;115:537–550.

6. Ptorney LT, Willis EA, Honas JJ, et al. Validity of energy intake estimated by digital photography plus recall in overweight and obese young adults. *J Acad Nutr Diet*. 2015;115:1392–1399.

7. Caine RN, Caine G. *Natural Learning for a Connected World. Education, Technology, and the Human Brain*. New York, NY: Teachers' College Press; 2011.

8. Beck AM, Christensen AG, Hansen BS, et al. Multidisciplinary nutrition support for undernutrition in nursing home and home care: a cluster randomized controlled trial. *Nutrition*. 2016;32:199–205. doi:10.106//j.nut.2015.08.009.

9. Henry BW, Smith TJ. Evaluation of the FOCUS (feedback on counseling using simulation) instrument for assessment of client-centered nutrition counseling. *J Nutr Educ Behav*. 2010;42:57–62.

10. Monroe JT, Lofgren IE, Sartini BL, et al. The Green Eating Project: web-based intervention to promote environmentally conscious eating behaviours in US university students. *Public Health Nutr*. 2015:18;2368–2378.

11. Baim S. Digital storytelling: conveying the essence of a face-to-face lecture in an on-line learning environment. *J Effective Teaching*. 2015;15:47–58.

12. Holthaus V, Sergais G, Rohrig I, et al The impact of interprofessional simulation on dietetic student perception of communication, decision-making, roles, and self-efficacy. *Top Clin Nutr*. 2015;30:127–142.

13. Diaz-Cueller AL, Evans SF. Diversity and health education. In: Perez MA, Luquis RR, eds. *Cultural Competence in Health Education and Health Promotion*. 2nd ed. San Francisco, CA: Jossey-Bass; 2014:23–58.

14. Resnicow K, McMaster F, Bocian A, et al. Motivational interviewing and dietary counseling for obesity in primary care. *Pediatrics*. 2015;135:649–657.

15. Castro Y, Fernandez ME, Strong LL, et al. Adaptation of counseling intervention to address multiple cancer risk factors among overweight/obese Latino smokers. *Health Educ Behav*. 2015;42:65–72.

16. Edmondson AC. The kinds of teams health care needs. *Harv Bus Rev*. December 16, 2015. http://hbr.org/2015/12/the-kinds-of-teams-health-care-needs. Accessed December 12, 2015.

17. Grote D. *How to be Good at Performance Appraisals: Simple, Effective, Done Right*. Boston, MA: Harvard Business Review; 2011.

18. Mager RF, Beach KM. *Developing Vocational Instruction*. Belmont, CA: Fearon Publishers; 1967.

19. Molinsky A. Employee training needs more than a script. *Harv Bus Rev*. April 24, 2014. http://hbr.org/2014/04/employee-training-needs-more-than-a-script. Accessed November 13, 2015.

20. Mager RF. *Analyzing Performance Problems, or, You Really Oughta Wanna*. Belmont, CA: Pitman Management and Training; 1984.

21. Gravelis A, Simpson S. *Planning and Enabling Learning in the Lifelong Learning Sector*. Exeter, UK: Learning Matters; 2010.

22. Derrick JW, Bellini SG, Spelman J. Using the hospital nutrition environment scan to evaluate health initiative in hospital cafeterias. *J Acad Nutr Diet*. 2015;115:1855–1860.

23. National Network of Libraries of Medicine. Define how a program will work – the logic model. http://nnlm.gov/outreach/community/logicmodel.html. Accessed September 28, 2016.

24. Knowles MS. *The Adult Learner: A Neglected Species*. 4th ed. Houston, TX: Gulf Publishing; 1990.

25. Marzano RL, Yanoski DC, Paynter DE. *Proficiency Scales for the New Science Standards. A Framework for Science Instruction and Assessment*. Bloomington, IN: Marzano Research; 2015.

26. Pleschova G, McAlpine L. Helping teachers to focus on learning and reflect on their teaching: what role does teaching context play? *Stud Educ Eval*. 2016;48:1–9.

27. Mager RF. *C.R.I.: Criterion-Referenced Instruction: Analysis, Design, and Implementation*. Los Altos Hills, CA: Mager Associates; 1976.

28. Kim II, Hannafin M. Developing situated knowledge about teaching with technology via web-enhanced case-based activity. *Computers Educ*. 2011;57:1378–1388.

29. Arntfield S, Parlett B, Meston CN, et al. A model of engagement in reflection writing-based portfolios: interactions between points of vulnerability and acts of adaptability. *Med Teach*. 2015;4:1–10.

30. Cordier R, McAuliffe T, Wilson NJ, et al. The appropriateness and feasibility of an online e-Portfolio for assessment of undergraduate allied health students. *Aust Occup Ther J.* 2016;63:154–163. doi:10.1111/1440-1630.12226.
31. The Joint Commission. *Comprehensive Accreditation Manual for Hospitals (CAMH).* Oak Brook, IL: The Joint Commission; 2015. http://www.jointcommission.org/accreditation/accreditation_main.aspx. Accessed September 28, 2016.
32. Rolio ME, Hutchesson MJ, Burrows TL, et al. Video consultations and virtual nutrition care for weight management. *J Acad Nutr Diet.* 2015;115:1213–1225.
33. Academy of Nutrition and Dietetics. *International Dietetics and Nutrition Terminology (IDNT): Standardized Language for the Nutrition Care Process.* Chicago, IL: Academy of Nutrition and Dietetics; 2016. http://ncpt.webauthor.com. Accessed September 28, 2016.

Chapter 13: Delivering Oral Presentations

1. Academy Quality Management Committee, Scope of Practice Subcommittee of Quality Management Committee. Academy of Nutrition and Dietetics: Revised 2012 standards of practice in nutrition care and standards of professional performance for registered dietitians. *J Acad Nutr Diet.* 2015;113:S29–S45.
2. Academy Quality Management Committee, Scope of Practice Subcommittee of Quality Management Committee. Academy of Nutrition and Dietetics: Revised 2012 standards of practice in nutrition care and standards of professional performance for dietetic technicians, registered. *J Acad Nutr Diet.* 2015;113:S56–71.
3. International Confederation of Dietetics Associations. International definition of dietitians, 2010. http://www.internationaldietetics.org/International-Standards/International-Definition-of-Dietitian.aspx. Accessed September 28, 2016.
4. Dietitians Association of Australia. National competency standards for entry-level dietitians. http://www.daa.asn.au/universities-recognition/national-competency-standards. Accessed November 15, 2015.
5. Dietitians of Canada. Mission, vision, and values. http://www.dietitians.ca/About-Us/MissionVisionValues.aspx. Accessed November 15, 2015.
6. DeVito JA. *Essential Elements of Public Speaking.* 5th ed. Boston, MA: Allyn & Bacon; 2015.
7. Beebe SA, Beebe SJ, Ivy DK. *Public Speaking: An Audience-Centered Approach.* 9th ed. Boston, MA: Allyn & Bacon; 2015.
8. Coopman SJ, Lull L. *Public Speaking: The Evolving Art.* 2nd ed. Boston, MA: Wadsworth Cengage Learning; 2012.
9. Verderber RF, Sellnow DD, Verderber KS. *The Challenge of Effective Speaking in a Digital Age.* 16th ed. Boston, MA: Wadsworth Cengage Learning; 2015.
10. Gallo C. *Talk Like TED: The 9 Public-Speaking Secrets of the World's Top Minds.* New York, NY: St. Martin's Press; 2014.
11. Duarte N. HBR *Guide to Persuasive Presentations.* Boston, MA: Harvard Business Review; 2015.
12. Hewlett SA. *Executive Presence: The Missing Link between Merit and Success.* New York, NY: Harper Collins; 2014.
13. Cuddy A. *Presence: Bringing Your Boldest Self to Your Biggest Challenges.* New York, NY: Little, Brown, and Company; 2015.

14. Cant RP. Communication competence within dietetics: dietitians' and clients' views about unspoken dialogue—the impact of personal presentation. *J Hum Nutr Diet*. 2009;22:504–510.
15. Maxey C, O'Connor KE. *Speak Up! A Woman's Guide to Presenting Like a Pro*. New York, NY: St. Martins' Griffin; 2008.
16. Petrilli CM, Mack M, Petrilli JJ, et al. Understanding the role of physician attire on patient perceptions: a systematic review of the literature—targeting attire to improve likelihood of rapport (TAILOR) investigators. *BMJ Open*. 2015;5:e006578. doi:10.1136/bmjopen-2014-006578.
17. Mauruani A, Leger J, Giraudeau B, et al. Effect of physician dress style on patient confidence. *J Eur Acad Dermatol Venereol*. 2013;27:333–337.
18. Palacios-Gonzalwz C, Lawrence DR, Substance over style: is there something wrong with abandoning the white coat? *J Med Ethics*. 2015;41:433–436.

Chapter 14: Using Instructional Media

1. Beebe SA, Beebe SJ, Ivy DJ. *Communications: Principles for a Lifetime*. 6th ed. Upper Saddle river, NJ: Pearson; 2015.
2. O'Neil J, Marsick VJ. *Understanding Adult Action Learning*. New York, NY: American Management Association; 2007.
3. Tufte E. *The Visual Display of Quantitative Information*. 2nd ed. Cheshire, CT: Graphics Press; 2001.
4. Smaldino SE, Lowther DL, Russell JD. *Instructional Media and Technologies for Learning*. 10th ed. Englewood Cliffs, NJ: Allyn and Bacon; 2012.
5. Tufte E. *Enivisioning Information*. Cheshire, CT: Graphics Press; 2004.
6. Furio J. Being objective. *San Francisco Mag*. 2012;59:42–43.
7. Arthur D. *Recruiting, Interviewing, Selecting and Orienting New Employees*. 5th ed. New York, NY: American Management Association; 2012.
8. Potter J. *Introduction to Media Literature*. Thousand Oaks, CA: Sage Publications; 2015.
9. Mytton G, Diem P, Van Dam PH. *Media Audience Research: A Guide for Professionals*. Thousand Oaks, CA: Sage Publications; 2016.
10. http://www.ChooseMyPlate.gov/multiple-language. Accessed February 1, 2016.
11. Benavides S, Polen HH, Goncz CE, et al. A systematic evaluation of paediatric medicines information content in clinical decision support tools on smartphones and mobile devices. *Inform Prim Care*. 2011;19:39–46.
12. Kan TW, Teng CH, Chen MY. QR code-based augmented reality applications. In: Borko F, ed. *Handbook of Augmented Reality*. New York, NY: Springer; 2011:339–354.
13. McCaffrey T, Pearson J. Find innovation where you least expect it. *Harv Bus Rev*. 2015;93:82–89.
14. Gallo C. *Talk Like TED: The 9 Public-Speaking Secrets of the World's Top Minds*. New York, NY: St. Martin's Press; 2014.
15. Stein K. Remote nutrition counseling: considerations in a new channel for client communication. *J Acad Nutr Diet*. 2015;115:1561–1576.
16. Myerholtz L, Schirmer J, Carling M. Sailing smooth across the cultural divide: constructing effective behavioral science presentations for medical audiences. *Int J Psychiatry Med*. 2015;50:115–127.

17. IMS Institute for Healthcare Informatics. Engaging patients through social media: is the healthcare industry ready for empowered and digitally demanding patients? January 2014. http://www.imshealth.com. Accessed June 5, 2015.
18. Rollo ME, Hutchesson MJ, Burrows TL, et al. Video consultations and virtual nutrition care for weight management. *J Acad Nutr Diet*. 2015;115:1213–1225.
19. James K, Albreacht JA, Litchfield R, et al. Social marketing campaigns: comparison of social and traditional media. *J Am Diet Assoc*. 2011;111(suppl):abstract.
20. Center for Medicare Services. Toolkit for making written material clear and effective. www.cms.gov/Outreach-and-Education/Outreach/WrittenMaterialsToolkit/index.html?redirect=/writtenmaterialstoolkit. Accessed September 28, 2016.
21. Ethomed. Patient education. http://ethnomed.org/patient-education. Accessed February 1, 2016.
22. U. S. Census Bureau. American Community Survey data. http://www.census.gov/newsroom/press-releases/2015/cb15-185.html. Accessed February 1, 2016.
23. Little D, Felten P, Berry C. *Looking and Learning: Visual Literacy across the Disciplines*. Philadelphia, PA: Jossey-Bass; 2015.
24. Hutchesson MJ, Rollo ME, Callister R, et al. Self-monitoring of dietary intake by young women: online food records completed on computer or smartphone are as accurate as paper-based food records but more acceptable. *J Acad Nutr Diet*. 2015;115:87–94.
25. Flynn L, Jalali A, Moreau KA. Learning theory and its application to the use of social media in medical education. *Postgrad Med J*. 2015;91:556–560.
26. http://www.usda/gov. Accessed February 1, 2016.

Chapter 15: Facilitating Group Learning

1. Harris TE, Sherblom JC. *Small Group and Team Communication*. 5th ed. Boston, MA: Pearson; 2010.
2. Robbins SP, Judge TA. *Essentials of Organizational Behavior*. 12th ed. Upper Saddle River, NJ: Prentice Hall; 2013.
3. Academy Quality Management Committee, Scope of Practice Subcommittee of Quality Management Committee. Academy of Nutrition and Dietetics: Revised 2012 standards of practice in nutrition care and standards of professional performance for registered dietitians. *J Acad Nutr Diet*. 2015;113:S29–S45.
4. Academy Quality Management Committee, Scope of Practice Subcommittee of Quality Management Committee. Academy of Nutrition and Dietetics: Revised 2012 standards of practice in nutrition care and standards of professional performance for dietetic technicians, registered. *J Acad Nutr Diet*. 2015;113:S56–S71.
5. Academy of Nutrition and Dietetics. *International Dietetics and Nutrition Terminology (IDNT): Standardized Language for the Nutrition Care Process*. Chicago, IL: Academy of Nutrition and Dietetics; 2016. http://ncpt.webauthor.com. Accessed September 28, 2016.
6. Fanzo JC, Graziose MM, Kraemer K, et al. Educating and training a workforce for nutrition in a post-2015 world. *Adv Nutr*. 2015;6:639–647.

7. Jortberg B, Myers E, Gigliotti L, et al. Academy of Nutrition and Dietetics: Standards of practice and standards of professional performance for registered dietitian nutritionists (competent, proficient, and expert) in adult weight management. *J Acad Nutr Diet*. 2015;115:609–618.

8. Berthelsen RM, Barkley WC, Oliver PM, et al. Academy of Nutrition and Dietetics: Standards of practice and standards of professional performance for registered dietitian nutritionists in management of food and nutrition systems. *J Acad Nutr Diet*. 2014;114:1104–1112.

9. Eliot KA, Kolasa KM. The value in interprofessional, collaborative-ready nutrition and dietetics practitioners. *J Acad Nutr Diet*. 2015;115:1578–1588.

10. Chang S, Gavey E. SuperTracker groups: connecting registered dietitian nutritionists with clients. *J Acad Nutr Diet*. 2015;115:1755–1763.

11. Torrington D, Hall L, Taylor S, et al. *Human Resource Management*. 9th ed. Philadelphia, PA: Transatlantic Publications; 2014.

12. Beebe SA, Beebe SJ, Ivy DK. *Communication Principles for a Lifetime*. 6th ed. Boston, MA: Allyn & Bacon; 2015.

13. Myers SA, Anderson CM. *The Fundamentals of Small Group Communication*. Los Angeles, CA: Sage; 2008.

14. Jacobs EE, Masson RL, Harvill RL, et al. *Group Counseling: Strategies and Skills*. 7th ed. Belmont, CA: Brooks/Cole; 2012.

15. Neeley T. Global teams that work: a framework for bridging social distance. *Harv Bus Rev*. 2015;93:75–81.

16. Kniffin IM, Wansink B, Devine CM, et al. Eating together at the firehouse: how workplace commensality relates to the performance of firefighters. *Hum Perform*. 2015;4:281–306.

17. Fertman CI. *Workplace Health Promotion Programs: Planning, Implementation, and Evaluation*. San Francisco, CA: Jossey-Bass; 2015.

18. Saunders EG. Do you really need to hold that meeting? *Harv Bus Rev*. March 20, 2015. http://hbr.org/2015/03/do-you-really-need-to-hold-that-meeting. Accessed November 15, 2015.

19. HBR Press Toolkit. *HBR Tools: Better Meetings. Digital Monograph TLBMS1-ZIP-ENG*. Boston, MA: Harvard Business Review; 2015.

INDEX

Note: The letters f and t following locators refer to figures and tables respectively.

Behavior modification (*continued*)
  definition, 166
  eating behavior changes, 172–183
    "ABC" framework, example, 173
    antecedents, 173–178
    behavior, 178
    consequences, 178–183
  modes
    classical conditioning, 168–169
    modeling, 171–172
    operant conditioning, 169–171
  nutrition counseling, 167
  role of counselor, 167
  self-management, 184
  self-monitoring, 183–184
  social support, 185
  therapy, 190
  types, 168
Body mass index (BMI), 15, 19
Brainstorming, 403
Brief Calcium Assessment Tool (BCAT), 53
Bulimia nervosa, 194, 201
Bulletin boards, 366–367

C
Caloric needs, 239t
Campinha-Bacote model, 91
Carbohydrate counting, 18, 129, 279, 284, 285, 316, 377
Cardiovascular diseases (CVDs), 167, 188, 236, 239, 276, 323, 386
Catharsis, 118
CBT. *See* Cognitive-behavioral therapy (CBT)
Characterization level, 291t, 293
Charts, stationary media, 367
Checklist, oral presentations, 347
Children
  life span counseling of, 222–230
  preschool-aged, 223–226
  school-aged, 226–230
ChooseMyPlate, 229, 236, 256, 260, 276, 370, 371
Chronic care model, 240
Chronic diet-related diseases, 239–241
  education strategies, 240
    electronic medical record, use, 240
    self-management concept, barriers, 240
  metabolic syndrome, 239
  specialty care strategies, 240–241
    nutrition intervention recommendations, 241t
  treatment models, 239
    chronic care model, 240

Classical conditioning, 168–169
  animal study/research (Pavlov)
    conditioned response/stimulus, 169
    unconditioned response/stimulus, 169
  responses to, types, 169
Client autonomy, honoring, 143
Client-centered approach. *See* Nondirective counseling
Client change talk, 149–150
Closed *vs.* open question, 65–66, 67t
Coaching, teaching method, 308
Code of Ethics, 12, 25
Cognition(s), 195–197
  behavior modification, phases
    making changes, 203
    recognizing, 199–201
  definition, 194, 195
  perceptions, influence on behaviors, 196
  positive/negative/neutral, types, 196
  restructuring/self-assessment, 197
  self-talk, examples, 196
  stream of consciousness in, 195
Cognition-rational/linguistic learning theory, 258
Cognitive appraisal, 209
Cognitive-behavioral therapy (CBT), 194–195
  assumptions, 195
  bulimia nervosa, treatment for, 194
  fundamental proposals, 194
  problem-oriented, approach, 195
Cognitive behavior modification
  exploring problem, 201–202
    negative cognitions, testing of, 202
    open-end questions, outcomes (Socratic method), 202
  making changes, 203
    power of positive thinking, 203
  recognizing problem, 199–201
    self-monitoring records, assessment, 199t–200t, 200
Cognitive behavior theory, 193
  behavioral approach, 193
  cognitive approach, 193
Cognitive change, counseling for
  cognitions, 195–197
  cognitive-behavioral therapy, 194–195
  cognitive distortions, 197–198
  cognitive restructuring techniques, 198
  dietary habits, impact, 195
  models and theories of change, 217
  relapse prevention, 209–217
  self-efficacy and, 203–209
  validated theories, 194

11-27-17